Current Topics in Microbiology and Immunology

93

Editors

W. Henle, Philadelphia · P.H. Hofschneider, Martinsried
H. Koprowski, Philadelphia · F. Melchers, Basle · R. Rott,
Gießen · H.G. Schweiger, Ladenburg/Heidelberg
P.K. Vogt, Los Angeles

Initiation Signals in Viral Gene Expression

Edited by Aaron J. Shatkin

With 30 Figures

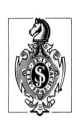

Springer-Verlag
Berlin Heidelberg New York 1981

Aaron J. Shatkin, Ph.D. Head,
Laboratory of Molecular Virology
Roche Institute of Molecular Biology
Nutley, New Jersey 07110
U.S.A.

QRI
E6
vol.93

ISBN 3-540-10804-1 Springer-Verlag Berlin Heidelberg New York
ISBN 0-387-10804-1 Springer-Verlag New York Heidelberg Berlin

Typesetting: Fotosatz Service Weihrauch, Würzburg
Printing and binding: Universitätsdruckerei H. Stürtz AG, Würzburg
2121/3321-543210

Table of Contents

A.J. Shatkin: Introduction – Elucidating Mechanisms of Eukaryotic Genetic Expression by Studying Animal Viruses   1

R. Tjian: Regulation of Viral Transcription and DNA Replication by the SV40 Large T Antigen   5

T. Shenk: Transcriptional Control Regions: Nucleotide Sequence Requirements for Initiation by RNA Polymerase II and III 25

S.J. Flint: Splicing and the Regulation of Viral Gene Expression 47

M. Kozak: Mechanism of mRNA Recognition by Eukaryotic Ribosomes During Initiation of Protein Synthesis . 81

R.M. Krug: Priming of Influenza Viral RNA Transcription by Capped Heterologous RNAs 125

J. Perrault: Origin and Replication of Defective Interfering Particles 151

Subject Index 209

Indexed in Current Contents

Introduction
Elucidating Mechanisms of Eukaryotic Genetic Expression by Studying Animal Viruses

AARON J. SHATKIN*

Eukaryotic genetic expression is carefully regulated. Normal cell growth and division, tissue differentiation, and organism development all depend on a strictly ordered progression of specific events. Perturbation of the control of these processes, for example by exposure to harmful chemicals or infection with viruses leads to aberrant forms of metabolism, often resulting in malignancies and cell death. One of the most challenging problems in biology is to define at the molecular level the mechanisms that govern gene function in higher organisms, including ultimately man. This goal serves to unify the diverse efforts of many investigators, whether studying the precise patterns of embryogenesis, the loss of control that occurs during neoplastic growth or the redirection of biosynthetic pathways in virus-infected cells.

Recently there has been remarkable and exciting progress toward understanding the molecular biology of eukaryotic expression. Much of this rapidly increasing new information has come from studies of animal virus systems. Just as investigations of the relatively simple, rapidly assayed, and easily manipulated bacteriophages lead to basic discoveries about prokaryotic cells, analyses of animal viruses and their interactions with host cells have provided fundamental information about how eukaryotic nucleic acids are organized for regulated replication, transcription, and translation. For example, the small genome of SV_{40}, like cellular DNA in chromatin, is associated with histones to form nucleosomal arrays (*Griffin* 1975). In SV_{40}-infected cells these viral "minichromosomes" are replicated and transcribed by cellular enzymes, thus providing an excellent experimental system that has been effectively exploited as detailed in the review by *Tjian*.

Other studies on SV_{40} (*Lavi* and *Groner* 1977; *Aloni* et al. 1977) and on adenovirus transcription earlier (*Chow* et al. 1977; *Klessig* 1977; *Berget* et al. 1977) provided the first evidence for splicing of mRNA precursors. With this striking finding came a new appreciation of eukaryotic genes as structures consisting of highly specific functional subdivisions, not simply blocks of contiguous nucleotides. This organization is most readily apparent at the level of pre-mRNA cutting and ligation, processes that result in retention of some RNA sequences (exons) in gene transcripts and removal of others (introns). As described in the paper by *Flint,* reconstitution of stretches of pre-RNA by splicing in different ways can enormously increase coding potential without genome alteration.

Discovery of this fundamental mechanism of expression depended partly on another recently described characteristic feature of eukaryotes, the "cap" structure, $m^7G(5')ppp(5')N$ (Figure 1). It is present on the 5'-termini of most viral and cellular messengers and their precursors (*Shatkin* 1976). The structure, synthesis, and functional consequences of capping have been reviewed in detail recently (*Filipowicz* 1978; *Banerjee*

---

*Roche Institute of Molecular Biology, Nutley, New Jersey 07110, USA

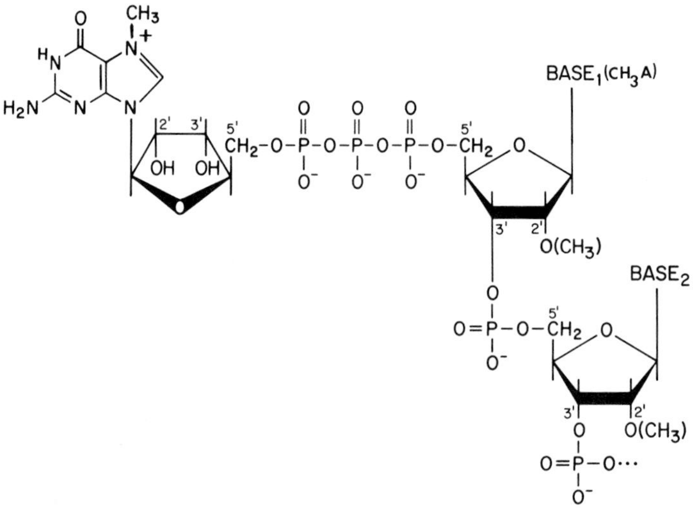

Fig. 1

1980). The steps involved in cellular mRNA capping (*Venkatesan* and *Moss* 1980) are probably the same as those deciphered by studying the enzymatic activities associated with human reovirus type 3 (*Furuichi* et al. 1976). These steps and the enzymes that catalyze them include:

(1) $p\overset{*}{p}pX + pppY \rightarrow p\overset{*}{p}pXpY + PP_i$ RNA polymerase

(2) $p\overset{*}{p}pXpY \rightarrow \overset{*}{p}pXpY + P_i$ Nucleotide phospho-hydrolase

(3) $pppG + \overset{*}{p}pXpY \rightarrow Gp\overset{*}{p}pXpY + PP_i$ Guanylyl transferase

(4) $Gp\overset{*}{p}pXpY + S\text{-adenosylmethionine} \rightarrow m^7Gp\overset{*}{p}pX^mpY$ Methyl transferases

From this scheme it is evident that the cap is added early in transcription, probably during initiation or very soon after nascent chains are started. The cap on nuclear transcripts is retained during conversion of pre-mRNA to mature mRNA. Like the poly(A) detected on the 3'-termini of vaccinia virus mRNA (*Kates*, 1970) and subsequently on most eukaryotic messengers, the cap provides a unique marker for mRNA 5'-termini. With the possibility of defining precisely the 5'-ends of mRNAs came a renewed interest in studying mechanisms of initiation of eukaryotic transcription. The resulting recent findings are reviewed in the chapter by *Shenk*.

Caps also were found to promote the formation of protein synthesis initiation complexes (*Both* et al. 1975), and a cap binding protein that stimulates capped mRNA translation was purified from initiation factor preparations by affinity chromatography on m^7 GDP-Sepharose (*Sonenberg* et al. 1979, 1980). The importance of the 5' end of mRNA as the site of ribosome attachment is an essential element of the scanning model recently proposed to explain how ribosomes recognize a single initiation site in mRNA (*Kozak* 1978). New evidence concerning monocistronic function of eukaryotic mRNAs is described and the scanning model of protein synthesis initiation is evaluated in the paper by *Kozak*.

Another particularly intriguing finding related to caps is the priming of influenza transcription by capped heterologous mRNAs. Although purified influenza virus contains RNA polymerase associated with its RNA genome, virus replication is dependent on cellular DNA-dependent RNA polymerase II activity (*Lamb* and *Choppin* 1977). Furthermore, influenza mRNAs isolated from infected cells are capped (*Krug* et al. 1976), although capping activity is not associated with the virion transcriptase (*Plotch* et al. 1978). These paradoxes were resolved by the finding that influenza transcriptase is primed, and the cap and approximately 10–15 adjacent nucleotides of the primer mRNA are incorporated into the viral transcripts as preformed 5'-ends. Chimeric influenza messages consisting of viral coding sequences and cellular 5'-termini have also been isolated from infected cells (*Dhar* et al. 1980). While primer-dependence may not be a general property of transcriptases, recent studies of the mRNA synthesizing systems present in two other RNA viruses, human reovirus (*Yamakawa* et al. 1981) and insect cytoplasmic polyhedrosis virus (*Furuichi* 1981), indicate that short 5'-terminal oligonucleotides are made in great molar excess relative to full-length mRNAs. It remains to be determined if these are prematurely terminated, abortive transcripts or if they represent initiator oligonucleotides that function as primers for mRNA synthesis. RNA priming and the mechanism of initiation of influenza mRNA formation is described in the chapter by *Krug;* both the early background work and more recent experiments are summarized.

The last paper in the collection is a comprehensive review of nucleotide sequences involved in the formation and replication of defective interfering particles of animal viruses. Defective particles are generated by members of almost all virus groups. Exactly how they arise is of considerable intrinsic interest. In addition, there is a strong possibility that defective interfering particles are important elements in virus disease, especially in persistent infections. The long-term interactions that may occur between virus- and host-directed pathways of expression are considered by *Perrault.*

It seems likely that future investigations of animal virus systems by such powerful new techniques as recombinant DNA technology and monoclonal antibody production will provide additional insights into eukaryotic gene expression. Hopefully, the following review articles will help stimulate some of these studies.

References

Aloni Y, Dhar R, Laub O, Horowitz M, Khoury G (1977) Novel mechanism for RNA maturation: the leader sequences of simian virus 40 mRNA are not transcribed adjacent to the coding sequences. Proc Natl Acad Sci USA 74:3686–3690

Banerjee AK (1980) 5'-Terminal cap structure in eucaryotic messenger ribonucleic acids. Microbiol Reviews 44:175–205

Berget SM, Moore C, Sharp PA (1977) Spliced segments at the 5' terminus of adenovirus 2 late mRNA. Proc Natl Acad Sci USA 74:3171–3175

Both GW, Furuichi Y, Muthukrishnan S, Shatkin AJ (1975) Ribosome binding to reovirus mRNA in protein synthesis requires 5'-terminal 7-methylguanosine. Cell 6:185–195

Chow LT, Gelinas RE, Broker TR, Roberts RJ (1977) An amazing sequence arrangement at the 5' ends of adenovirus 2 messenger RNA. Cell 12:1–8

Dhar R, Chanock RM, Lai C-J (1980) Non-viral oligonucleotides at the 5' terminus of cytoplasmic influenza viral mRNA deduced from cloned complete genomic sequences. Cell 21:495–500

Filipowicz W (1978) Function of the 5'-terminal ^{7}mG cap in eukaryotic mRNA. FEBS Lett 96:1–11

Furuichi Y (1981) Allosteric stimulatory effect of S-adenosylmethionine on the RNA polymerase in cytoplasmic polyhedrosis virus. J Biol Chem 256:483–493

Furuichi Y, Muthukrishnan S, Tomasz J, Shatkin AJ (1976) Mechanism of formation of reovirus mRNA 5'-terminal blocked and methylated sequence, ^{7}mGpppGmC. J Biol Chem 251:5043–5053

Griffith JD (1975) Chromatin structure: deduced from a minichromosome. Science 187:1202–1203

Kates J (1970) Transcription of the vaccinia virus genome and the occurrence of polyriboadenylic acid sequences in messenger RNA. Cold Spring Harbor Symp Quant Biol 35:743–752

Klessig DF (1977) Two adenovirus mRNAs have a common 5' terminal leader sequence encoded at least 10 kb upstream from their main coding regions. Cell 12:9–21

Kozak M (1978) How do eucaryotic ribosomes select initiation regions in messenger RNA? Cell 15:1109–1123

Krug RM, Morgan MA, Shatkin AJ (1976) Influenza viral mRNA contains internal N^6-methyladenosine and 5'-terminal 7-methylguanosine in cap structures. J Virol 20:45–53

Lamb RA, Choppin PW (1977) Synthesis of influenza virus polypeptides in cells resistant to α-amanitin: evidence for the involvement of cellular RNA polymerase II in virus replication. J Virol 23:816–819

Lavi S, Groner Y (1977) 5'-Terminal sequences and coding region of late simian virus 40 mRNAs are derived from noncontiguous segments of the viral genome. Proc Natl Acad Sci USA 74:5323–5327

Plotch SJ, Tomasz J, Krug RM (1978) Absence of detectable capping and methylating enzymes in influenza virions. J Virol 28:75–83

Shatkin AJ (1976) Capping of eucaryotic mRNAs. Cell 9:645–653

Sonenberg N, Rupprecht KM, Hecht SM, Shatkin AJ (1979) Eukaryotic mRNA cap binding protein: purification by affinity chromatography on Sepharose-coupled m^{7}GDP. Proc Natl Acad Sci USA 76:4345–4349

Sonenberg N, Trachsel H, Hecht S, Shatkin AJ (1980) Differential stimulation of capped mRNA translation in vitro by cap binding protein. Nature 285:331–333

Venkatesan S, Moss B (1980) Donor and acceptor specificities of HeLa cell mRNA guanylyltransferase. J Biol Chem 255:2835–2842

Yamakawa M, Furuichi Y, Nakashima K, LaFiandra AJ, Shatkin AJ (1981) Excess synthesis of viral mRNA 5'-terminal oligonucleotides by reovirus transcriptase. J Biol Chem 256:6507–6514

Regulation of Viral Transcription and DNA Replication by the SV40 Large T Antigen

Robert Tjian*

1 Introduction 5
2 Primary Structure of the SV40 Large T Antigen 7
3 Purification of T Antigen. 7
4 DNA Binding Properties 9
5 Regulation of Early Viral Transcription 13
6 T Antigen Binding and Viral Replication 17
7 Induction of Cellular DNA Synthesis and Gene Expression 18
8 Enzymatic Properties of T Antigen 18
9 Summary 20
References 20

1 Introduction

Simian Virus 40 (SV40) provides a particularly useful model for studying gene regulation at the molecular level because it is one of the simplest and most thoroughly characterized (*Tooze* 1980) viral systems known to undergo a well-defined developmental cycle in mammalian cells. The entire nucleotide sequence of the 5243 base pair genome of SV40 has been determined (*Reddy* et al. 1978; *Fiers* et al. 1978) and important regions such as the origin of replication, transcriptional promoters, structural gene boundaries, splice junctions, and positions of mutations have been located. The small double-stranded circular genome of SV40 encodes only five or six genes and consequently relies in large part on the host cell machinery to carry out complex regulated processes such as transcription and replication. During lytic infection of monkey cells, SV40 undergoes a temporal program of gene expression that is controlled in part by viral coded proteins (*Tegtmeyer* 1972; *Cowan* et al. 1973; *Tegtmeyer* et al. 1975; *Reed* et al. 1976). Immediately after infection, the SV40 A and F genes, encoding the large T (*Black* et al. 1963; *Tegtmeyer* 1975) and small t (*Prives* et al. 1978; *Crawford* et al. 1978; *Sleigh* et al. 1978) antigens respectively, are expressed. Transcription of these early viral genes by the host RNA polymerase II originates from a region of the genome located at approximately 0.67–0.70 fractional units on the conventional genome map (Fig. 1) (*Sambrook* et al. 1973; *Khoury* et al. 1973; *Jackson* and *Sugden* 1972; *Khoury* et al. 1975). During this early phase of the lytic cycle, SV40 DNA replication does not occur (*Tegtmeyer* 1972) and expression of the structural

*Department of Biochemistry, University of California, Berkeley, California 94720, USA

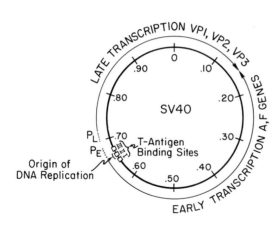

Fig. 1. Map of the SV40 genome depicting the origin of replication, T-antigen binding sites, approximate starts of early and late transcription and coding regions for viral genes

capsid proteins is detectable only at very low levels (*Cowan* et al. 1973; *Alwine* et al. 1977). However, after the intracellular concentration of large T antigen reaches a certain threshold (*Graessmann* et al. 1978), viral DNA replication is initiated. This A-gene-dependent synthesis of SV40 DNA originates from a unique position on the genome (*Danna* and *Nathans* 1972; *Fareed* et al. 1972) at 0.67 map units and proceeds bidirectionally (*Jaenisch* et al. 1971; *Kelly* and *Nathans* 1977). The discontinuous strand synthesis during SV40 DNA replication (*Fareed* and *Salzman* 1972) is thought to be catalyzed by the host DNA polymerase and is primed by short RNA sequences located at intervals along the DNA template (*Su* and *DePamphilis* 1976). After the onset of viral DNA replication, transcription of the early genes is reduced while late gene RNA synthesis becomes activated to a high level. Analysis of temperature sensitive mutants in the A gene revealed that, at the restrictive temperature, early viral mRNAs and proteins are overproduced (*Cowan* et al. 1973; *Tegtmeyer* 1975; *Reed* et al. 1976; *Alwine* et al. 1977). Thus, it appears that the product of the SV40 A gene, large T antigen, plays a pivotal role in viral gene expression by initiating DNA synthesis and autoregulating early transcription. There is also a wealth of evidence that implicates large T antigen in functions involving the initiation and maintenance of virally induced transformation of nonpermissive cells (*Kimura* and *Dulbecco* 1972; *Tegtmeyer* 1975; *Brugge* and *Butel* 1975; *Martin* and *Chou* 1975; *Osborn* and *Weber* 1975b; *Steinberg* et al. 1978). By contrast, mutations in gene F have only a small and poorly defined effect on viral gene expression during lytic infection of permissive cells (*Sleigh* et al. 1978; *Topp* pers. comm.). There is, however, some evidence that implicates small t antigen in functions involving the initiation of virally induced cellular transformation in certain established cell lines but not in primary cultures or rapidly dividing cells (*Sleigh* et al. 1978; *Bouck* et al. 1978; *Martin* et al. 1979; *Martin* 1981).

A comprehensive general review of papovaviruses has recently been published in the second edition of Tooze's *Molecular Biology of Tumor Viruses*. I will therefore not attempt to cover both the lytic and transformation functions of SV40 tumor antigens. Instead, the purpose of this review will be to analyze critically the various lines of investigation pertaining specifically to the molecular mechanisms by which the large T antigen of SV40 regulates viral transcription and replication. In particular, I will focus on the experimental strategies that have been employed to study the biochemical properties of purified SV40 T antigen.

2 Primary Structure of the SV40 Large T Antigen

The SV40 A gene product is a nuclear protein with an apparent molecular weight of 96,000 as determined by sodium dodecyl sulfate gel electrophoresis (*Tegtmeyer* 1975). However, the primary structure of the T antigen polypeptide deduced from the DNA sequence indicates that its actual molecular weight should be closer to 82,000 (*Fiers* et al. 1978; *Paucha* et al. 1978). Chromatography of a denatured T antigen related protein isolated from an SV40 transformed-cell line confirms that its molecular weight is approximately 80,000 (*Griffin* et al. 1978). The discrepancy between the electrophoretic mobility of T antigen and its actual molecular weight may be due in part to postanslational modifications of the T antigen polypeptide. For instance, the amino terminus of T antigen is known to be acetylated in vivo and there is evidence for phosphorylated residues (*Rundell* et al. 1977; *McCormick* et al. 1980; *Mann* and *Hunter* 1980; *Walter* and *Flory* 1979). However, these documented modifications of T antigen do not appear sufficient to account for its aberrant mobility in sodium dodecyl sulfate gels, suggesting that additional modifications altering the primary structure of the polypeptide may have gone undetected.

3 Purification of T Antigen

The isolation of biochemically useful quantities of active SV40 large T antigen presented a formidable problem because most SV40 infected or transformed cells produce relatively low amounts of the viral protein. For instance, large T antigen represents only 0.01–0.03% of the total soluble protein in lytically infected monkey cells. Consequently, a significant amount of effort has gone towards finding or isolating a convenient source from which the SV40 A gene product can be purified.

Early investigators chose to purify T antigen from SV40 transformed cells such as the human cell line, SV80, because these cells were easy to obtain in large quantities and they produced relatively high amounts of viral early proteins (*Livingston* et al. 1974; *Osborn* and *Weber* 1974). It had been assumed that the 96,000 dalton protein purified from transformed cells would be identical in structure and function to authentic SV40 T antigen produced in lytically infected monkey cells. However, a recent study indicates that the commonly used SV80 cells actually produce a T protein that is defective in at least its viral DNA replication functions (*Gish* and *Botchan*, personal communication). Analysis of SV40 sequences rescued from SV80 cells also revealed a lesion in the carboxyl portion of the protein. In retrospect, the finding that SV80 cells contain a mutant A gene is not surprising. Human cells, which are normally semipermissive for SV40 DNA replication, should contain free viral DNA at a low frequency when transformed by SV40. The fact that SV80 cells are stably transformed but do not contain any free viral DNA implies that excision and replication of viral DNA is somehow blocked. Inhibition of viral DNA synthesis can occur as a result of mutations in the cellular replication machinery or, alternatively, a defect could have arisen either in the viral origin of replication or in the A gene. In the case of SV80 cells, viral DNA can be efficiently rescued and replicated by providing exogenous wildtype T antigen (*Gish* and *Botchan*, personal communication). This finding indicates that a mutation has occurred that affects the replication functions of T antigen. Thus, the SV80 protein may not be appropriate for studies involving the lytic functions of the A gene product. However, the SV40 A gene product is apparently a multifunctional protein with several distinct activities, some involved in lytic functions and others in transformation and induction of cellular gene expression. If so, partially defective products such as SV80 protein could still be useful for investigating properties of the A gene product that are not directly involved with DNA binding and regulation of lytic processes. Moreover, the SV80 protein also provides a source of a mutant protein that can be used to study specific A gene defects affecting viral DNA replication and transcription (see below).

As an alternative source of protein, cells infected with adenovirus-SV40 hybrid viruses have been used for purification of the SV40 T antigen (*Lewis* et al. 1969; *Black* and *White* 1967; *Lewis* and *Rowe* 1970; *Hassell* et al. 1978; *Tjian* 1978b). One naturally occurring virus designated Ad2$^+$D2 directs the synthesis of a T antigen related protein in quantities 50 times greater than cells either lytically infected or transformed by SV40 (*Tjian* 1978a). Moreover, it is easier to isolate viral protein from cells infected with this hybrid virus because Ad2 inhibits host protein synthesis late in infection and extracts of HeLa cells grown in suspension contain less proteolytic activity than either CV1 or SV80 cells. The D2 protein isolated from cells infected with Ad2$^+$D2 is a 107,000 dalton hybrid protein comprised of approximately 10% of an Ad2 protein at its amino terminus and about 90% of the SV40 gene A protein carboxy terminus (*Hassell* et al. 1978). Because the D2 protein lacks the amino terminal portion of the SV40 T antigen molecule, it is possible that its biochemical properties would not accurately reflect those of authentic T antigen. To overcome this problem, and at the same time retain the advantages of overproduction in the adenovirus system, a number of novel adenovirus-SV40 recombinants were recently constructed in vitro (*Thummel* et al. 1981b). These hybrid viruses were designed to overproduce the SV40 A gene product under the control of adenovirus promoters. HeLa cells infected with a novel hybrid virus (AdSVR6) synthesize high levels of a 96,000 dalton T antigen that is structurally indistinguishable from the authentic lytic product made in SV40-infected monkey cells. These hybrid viruses have provided a convenient source for the purification of SV40 T antigen.

A typical procedure for purifying T antigen involves isolating nuclei at pH 6.9 in a low salt buffer, extracting the nuclei with a high ionic strength buffer at pH 8.1 (*Tjian* 1978a), ammonium sulfate fractionation followed by three to four chromatographic columns (*Livingston* et al. 1974; *Tjian* 1978a; *Tjian* et al. 1979). In general, some combination of gel filtration, DEAE sephadex, phosphocellulose and heparin or DNA agarose has given the best results. During purification, proteolysis of the T protein is sometimes observed, especially in the case of CV1 or SV80 cells. However, once T antigen has been purified to near homogeneity, it can be stored at −70 °C in 10–20% glycerol without loss of biological activity for up to 2 years. The yields of T antigen purified to greater than 90% homogeneity from various sources of cells are shown in Table 1.

Table 1. Levels of T antigen production and yields of purified protein from different cells

Source of T antigen	Total protein (%)	T antigen in 10 g of cells (µg)	T antigen actually purified from 10 g of cells (µg)	Yield (%)
SV40 in-fected CV1 cells	0.01–0.04	50– 200	5–10	5
SV80 cells	0.03–0.06	150– 300	30–50	10
Ad-SVR6 in-fected Hela cells	0.2 –0.3	1000–1500	150	10
Ad2+D2 in-fected Hela cells	1.0 –1.5	5000–8000	700	15–20

The amount of T antigen related proteins produced by different sources was calculated by quanti-tating anti-T immunoprecipitates from extracts of labeled as well as unlabeled cells. The values in yields of purified T antigen were determined from an average of many preparations isolated to near homogeneity by published procedures

4 DNA Binding Properties

It was suspected that the SV40 T antigen might be a DNA binding protein even before there was any direct biochemical evidence to support this idea. Its nuclear location in the cell (*Black* et al. 1963) as well as its involvement in viral DNA synthesis (*Tegtmeyer* 1972) and transcription (*Tegtmeyer* 1975; *Reed* et al. 1976) led workers in the field to hypothesize that the SV40 A gene encoded a regulatory protein that interacts directly with DNA to in-fluence gene expression. The remainder of this review will largely be devoted towards documenting the experiments that have confirmed these early predictions.

The general affinity of T antigen for double-stranded DNA was first demonstrated by DNA cellulose chromatography (*Carrol* et al. 1974). Shortly thereafter, the possibility that wild type T antigen from lytically infected cells may bind selectively to the origin region of the SV40 genome was demonstrated by electron microscopy of antibody-T antigen complexes isolated from infected cell lysates (*Reed* et al. 1975). Using a filter binding assay, it was subsequently shown that partially purified SV80 T protein binds with equal affinity to SV40 DNA and a number of phage DNAs (*Jessel* et al. 1975). Moreover, binding of SV40 DNA restriction fragments by the SV80 protein suggested preferential binding to several different regions on the viral genome (*Jessel* et al. 1976). These initial filter binding studies were difficult to interpret because they involved impure preparations of SV80 protein. Moreover, the binding of isolated restriction frag-ments often correlated with the size of the DNA fragment rather than sequence.

In order to increase the sensitivity and specificity of the filter binding assay, pure D2 protein was used to protect specific sequences of uniformly labelled SV40 DNA from di-gestion by pancreatic DNAse I (*Tjian* 1978a). These DNAse protection experiments established that specific binding of D2 protein occurred at three closely spaced sites on

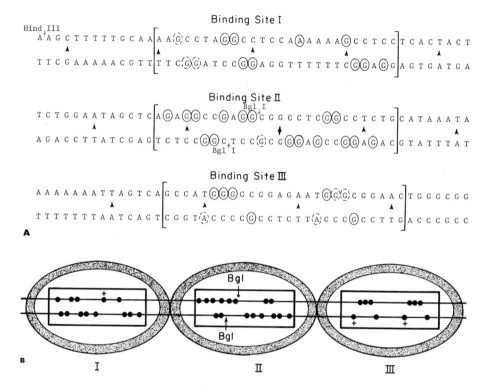

Fig. 2. A,B. SV40 T antigen binding sites. *A* Sequence of nucleotides containing the triple binding sites. *B* A schematic representation of binding sites determined by DNAse protection and dimethyl sulfate protection. The nucleotide sequence in the region overlapping the SV40 origin of DNA replication was reproduced from Fiers, et al. 1978 and Reddy, et al. 1978. The numbered nucleotides are according to the BBB system (*Tooze* 1980). Arrows indicate cleavage sites of restriction enzyme Bgl I. The three tandem binding sites as defined by dimethylsulfate protection experiments are shown in brackets (A) and boxes (B). The ellipses (B) depict the region of DNA sequence protected by T antigen from DNAse digestion. Guanine residues specifically shielded from methylation by T antigen are encircled by solid and broken lines (A) and solid dots (B). Adenine residues enhanced for methylation by T antigen are encircled by broken lines (A) and solid dots with (+) (B). Double arrowhead equals position of first nucleotide and single arrowhead indicates ten-nucleotide spacing

SV40 DNA that extended over a region of 120–140 bp containing the origin of viral DNA replication. Binding of the D2 protein to its three recognition sites occurs in a sequential manner with the strongest affinity at site I and progressively lower affinity to sites II and III (Fig. 2). In addition, dimethylsulfate methylation studies revealed that the D2 protein (*Tjian* 1978b) makes symmetrical contacts with the binding sequences almost exclusively in the major groove of the DNA duplex (Fig. 2).

Papovaviruses such as polyoma and BK contain origin DNA sequences that exhibit a high degree of homology to the SV40 origin (*Soeda* et al. 1979; *Friedmann* et al. 1979; *Fiers* et al. 1978; *Reddy* et al. 1978; *Seif* et al. 1979; *Yang* and *Wu* 1978). Therefore, the ability of the SV40 T antigen to bind origin DNA sequence from these other papovaviruses has also been tested. DNAse protection experiments reveal that the D2 protein binds preferentially to multiple binding sites in the region of BK and polyoma virus DNA that are analogous to the SV40 origin sequences (*Tjian* 1980). Although the specificity and general features of the interactions at these binding sites are similar, there are some significant differences that probably reflect minor alterations in the nucleotide sequence of the three viruses. For example, SV40 sites I, II, and III bind in a sequential manner while polyoma virus sites I and II bind with equal efficiency and site III binds less well. By contrast, site I of BKV binds most efficiently and sites II and III bind with similar affinities. Presently, it is not clear how these protein-DNA interactions relate to the ability of the SV40 T antigen to carry out replication functions at the different papovavirus origin sequences.

A quantitative filter binding assay recently revealed that purified SV80 protein binds to the specific SV40 origin DNA sequences approximately 20 times less efficiently than D2 protein (*Myers* et al. 1981b). However, the nonspecific DNA binding capabilities of the SV80 protein and D2 protein were very similar. This weakened binding of SV80 protein for origin sequences may help to explain the inability of earlier studies to demonstrate specific DNA binding. Several studies have confirmed that binding of SV80 protein, although weak, occurs predominantly at the origin sequence (*Shalloway* et al. 1980; *Myers*, personal communication). A recent study using an exonuclease III assay reported a fourth T antigen binding site located adjacent to site III (*Shalloway* et al. 1980). However, the SV80 protein was used in these experiments and extremely high concentrations of this defective binding protein were required (500 : 1 molar ratio of protein to DNA) in order to detect binding sites that are protected from exonuclease digestion. Consequently, the assays were performed under conditions that are known to allow nonspecific binding of T antigen to many sites on the SV40 DNA. Moreover, this additional site has not been detected by DNAse footprinting or DMS protection using either SV80 protein or D2 protein under conditions that promote only specific DNA binding (*Tjian* 1978b; *Myers* et al. 1981a).

It is possible that neither the mutant SV80 protein nor the truncated D2 protein bind DNA with the same specificity as wild-type SV40 T antigen. To settle this issue, intact wild-type SV40 T antigen was purified from the newly constructed hybrid viruses (*Thummel* et al. 1981b) and shown by filter binding, DNAse protection, and DMS methylation studies to bind SV40 DNA origin sequences with a specificity identical to that of D2 protein (*Myers* et al. 1981a). Thus, it appears that the DNA binding properties of SV80 protein are aberrant and do not accurately reflect either the strength or the specificity of DNA binding by wild-type SV40 T antigen. Moreover, it is clear that the amino-terminal portion of T antigen is not required for specific DNA binding because both D2 and intact T antigen bind to the triple recognition sites in the same manner.

The size of SV40 DNA fragments protected by T antigen (30–35 bp) from DNAse digestion and the symmetrical contacts made between protein and DNA suggested that the active binding promoter is likely to be either a dimer or tetramer (*Tjian* 1978b; *Myers* et al. 1981a). Moreover, a number of studies reported oligomeric forms of native T antigen by gel filtration and velocity sedimentation (*Osborn* and *Weber* 1974; *Tegtmeyer* pers. comm., *Tjian*, unpublished). Direct electron microscopic examination of purified D2 protein in free form reveals monomers, tetramers, and dodecamers (*Myers* et al. 1981c). However, the predominant species bound to SV40 DNA appears to be a tetramer (Fig. 3).

Quantitative studies of T-antigen binding suggested that interactions at the three sites is not only sequential but may also be cooperative (*Myers* et al. 1981a). This idea was tested

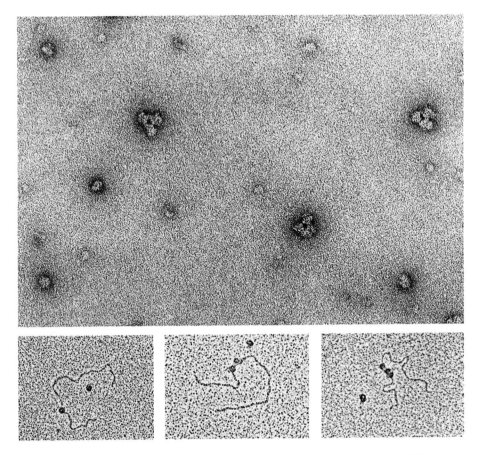

Fig. 3. Electron micrographs of purified D2 protein. *Top Panel:* A preparation of D2 protein negatively stained with uranyl formate. Small particles (monomers), medium size particles (tetramers), and large triangular shaped structures (dodecamers) are seen. *Lower Panels:* Micrographs showing D2 protein bound to the SV40 origin of DNA replication. The origin sequence is approximately 32% from one end of the DNA fragment. Either one, two or three particles of tetramer size are seen bound specifically to the origin region of SV40 DNA. The D2 concentration was 1 µg/ml and protein DNA complexes were visualized after rotary-shadowing

by measuring the quantitative differences between the efficiency of T antigen to bind cloned DNA sequences lacking specific portions of binding site I, II, and III. Removal of sites II and III has no detectable influence on the binding of T antigen to site I, the strongest binding site ($K_d = 6 \times 10^{-10}$ M) (*Myers*, personal communication). By contrast, DNAse protection experiments revealed that T antigen binds site II much less efficiently in the absence of binding to site I. Similarly, binding to site III appears to be influenced by binding to site I and II. Thus, there is direct evidence that a cooperative binding interaction occurs between T antigen at sites I and II and possibly between site II and III. It is interesting to note that potential protein-protein interactions between tetramers of T antigen at the binding sites may be similar to those observed during formation of T-antigen dodecamer structures seen in the electron microscope (*Myers* et al. 1981c).

A number of recent studies have attempted to correlate the DNA binding properties of T antigen with various physical states of the A gene product. For instance, it was found in one study that newly synthesized T-antigen molecules exhibit a greater affinity for SV40 origin sequences than "aged" molecules (*Oren* et al. 1980). Other reports suggested that T-antigen molecules phosphorylated to different extents bind DNA with altered affinities. However, there is presently no clear indication of the biochemical or structural difference between new and old T-antigen molecules nor is there a definitive correlation between the phosphorylated state of the protein and its DNA binding properties. In short, there is no conclusive evidence to indicate the physiological importance of the various T-antigen forms that have been detected in SV40 infected and transformed cells.

Recently, there have been several attempts to determine the binding of T antigen to chromatin rather than naked DNA in vitro. Two such studies report that, in fact, the predominant binding site on chromatin is a region at the origin of viral replication, thus confirming the findings obtained with purified DNA (*Reiser* et al. 1980; *Segawa* et al. 1980). It is worthwhile to note that a region of DNA containing the SV40 origin of replication and transcriptional promoters has been found to be relatively free of nucleosomes when isolated from infected cells (*Varshavsky* et al. 1979). However, the relationship between T-antigen binding and the nucleosome structure of SV40 minichromosomes remains undefined.

5 Regulation of Early Viral Transcription

Having established the specific DNA binding properties of T antigen, it became important to determine how the binding of T antigen to its recognition sites can control viral gene expression. Why does T antigen bind in a cooperative manner to three specific binding sites? What is the spatial arrangement of binding sites to the viral origin of replication and transcriptional promoters? What are the molecular mechanisms by which T antigen is able to initiate viral DNA synthesis and repress early transcription? Although these questions have not all been answered, a number of recent studies have provided some insights into the function of T antigen during the lytic cycle.

Analysis of temperature-sensitive mutants in the A gene of SV40 indicated that both T antigen and its mRNA are overproduced under nonpermissive conditions (*Tegtmeyer* 1975; *Reed* et al. 1976; *Khoury* and *May* 1977). One possibility was for T antigen to act as a regulatory factor that interacts directly with the host RNA polymerase to inhibit early SV40 transcription. Alternatively, T antigen could catalyze a transient modification of some chromatin component in order to inactivate the template for early viral transcription. A third possibility was that T antigen could bind directly to the DNA template and act as a classical repressor to inhibit transcription. The specific DNA binding properties of T antigen led most workers in the field to favor this last possibility. The repressor model seemed particularly attractive because of the similarities between the T-antigen binding sites (*Tjian* 1978b) and features of the triple operator sites found in bacteriophage lambda (*Maniatis* and *Ptashne* 1973; *Meyer* et al. 1975; *Ptashne* et al. 1980). However, there was no direct evidence to indicate that interaction of T antigen to its three binding sites actually led to repression of SV40 early RNA synthesis.

It became clear that the most direct way to determine the mechanism of autoregulation was to devise an in vitro transcription system that would be capable of selectively initiating transcription at the SV40 promoters and would be sensitive to the action of T antigen. Recently two cell-free transcription systems have been shown to initiate RNA from the adenovirus late promoter (*Manley* et al. 1980; *Weil* et al. 1979). Subsequently, these transcription systems have been adapted for synthesis of RNA directed by other viral and cellular promoters (*Rio* et al. 1980; *Proudfoot* et al. 1980; *Corden* et al. 1980; *Yamamoto* et al. 1980). Thus it was shown that SV40 DNA can direct the synthesis of discrete "run off" products corresponding to transcripts initiating from the viral early and late promoters (*Rio* et al. 1980; *Handa* et al. 1981; *Mathis* and *Chambon* 1981). Next it was shown that binding of either D2 protein or T antigen to template DNA containing the binding sites specifically inhibits transcription of SV40 early RNA without affecting late RNA synthesis (*Rio* et al. 1980; *Rio* and *Robbins;* personal communication; *Hansen,* personal communication). In addition, cloned SV40 template DNA lacking sequences for T-antigen binding sites I, or I and II but containing an intact early promoter continue to direct the transcription of early RNA even in the presence of T antigen (*Rio* et al. 1980). These in vitro transcription studies provide direct biochemical evidence that the synthesis of early SV40 RNA is specifically repressed by binding of the SV40 T antigen to its triple recognition sites.

A graphic representation of the interaction between T antigen and SV40 DNA to repress early transcription is shown in Figure 4. The location of the T-antigen binding sites was determined by a combination of DNAse protection, DMS methylation, and direct electron microscopy (*Tjian* 1978a; *Tjian* 1978b; *Myers* et al. 1981c; *Myers* et al. 1981a). Although a bona fide RNA polymerase II binding site has not been defined, the promoter region required for SV40 early transcription can be deduced from a composite of in vivo (*Benoist* and *Chambon* 1980; *Benoist* and *Chambon* 1981; *Gruss* and *Khoury,* pers. comm.) and in vitro (*Rio* et al. 1980; *Rio,* personal communication) deletion mapping data. There is general agreement from in vivo mapping data that a region between 106 and 180 containing one of the 72 base-pair repeats in SV40 DNA is required for A gene expression (see review by *Shenk* in this volume). A similar putative promoter sequence (from 70–160) has also been found to be required for transcription in vitro (*Rio* et al. 1980; *Rio,* personal communication). The small discrepancy in the sequences required for in vivo and in vitro transcription of SV40 early genes is not understood.

Unlike other cases of eukaryotic promoter sequences, deletion of the "TATA" box located 40–45 bases to the left of the putative SV40 early promoter has no apparent affect on the level of synthesis of transcripts in vitro (*Rio* et al. 1980). This result is consistent with the finding that A gene expression is unaltered by "TATA" deletion mutants in vivo (*Benoist* and *Chambon* 1980). Neither the in vivo nor in vitro results rule out the possibility that the "TATA" box has a quantitative affect on the capping and processing of the A gene mRNA (*Mathis* and *Chambon* 1981; *Dynan,* personal communication). The data do, however, suggest that transcription from the SV40 early promoter does not require the "TATA" canonical sequence.

The SV40 early transcriptional "promoter" region lies distal to binding sites I and II but close to, and may actually overlap, sequences of binding site III (*Myers* et al. 1981a). This arrangement of binding sites and promoter suggests that the mechanism of transcriptional repression may involve binding of T antigen at site III to directly inhibit initiation of transcription rather than attenuation of RNA polymerase movement along the template DNA. As a test of this model, it was shown that T-antigen binding sites

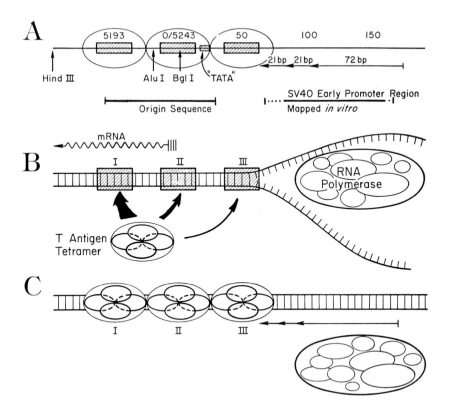

Fig. 4A–C. A schematic representation depicting potential interactions between T antigen, RNA polymerase and SV40 regulatory sequences. *A* Depicts the relative location of T-antigen binding sites (large hatched boxes and ellipses), restriction endonuclease cleavage sites (↑), "TATA" box (small hatched box), repeated sequences (leftward arrows ←); origin of DNA replication and putative early transcriptional promoter region mapped by in vivo and in vitro analysis. The nucleotide numbers at the top are in accordance with the BBB system (*Tooze* 1980). *B* A diagram depicting derepressed SV40 early RNA synthesis is shown as starting from a position to the right of the T-antigen binding sites and the duplex template DNA is shown in an unwound configuration with a molecule of RNA polymerase II holoenzyme (large ellipse with many subunits) positioned to transcribe early SV40 RNA. The small ellipses (containing four isologous subunits) represents T-antigen tetramers and the arrows with different thicknesses represent sequential and cooperative binding of T antigen to its three recognition sites (hatched boxes). The early SV40 mRNA is shown as a wavy arrow with several 5′-capped ends represented by vertical lines. *C* A diagram depicting the repression of SV40 early RNA synthesis by T antigen. All three T-antigen binding sites are filled and RNA polymerase is unable to transcribe SV40 early RNA. The arrows pointing leftward represent the location of the 21 and 72 base-pair repeated sequences in SV40

placed downstream from the adenovirus late promoter are not able to block the transcription of adenovirus RNA synthesis even when all binding sites are saturated with T antigen (*Myers* et al. 1981a). One possibility is for T antigen to repress initiation of transcription by competing for a site that partially overlaps the RNA polymerase binding sequence. Alternatively, binding of T antigen to its sites may stabilize the double stranded configuration of the template DNA thereby preventing RNA polymerase from unwinding DNA to form a transcriptional initiation complex.

It is worthwhile to note that deletion mutants lacking site I or I and II are no longer able to be repressed by T antigen even though site III is intact (*Rio* et al. 1980). A similar result was recently obtained with repression-defective mutants of early transcription in vivo (*Nathans,* personal communication). This is consistent with the finding that binding to site III may be dependent on a cooperative binding interaction between sites I and II. Thus, it appears that the mechanism of autoregulation may indirectly involve the cooperative binding of T antigen to all three sites. In addition, binding of T antigen to site III may play an active role in repressing transcription by directly preventing RNA polymerase from initiating at the SV40 early promoter.

These studies provide a molecular mechanism for the regulation of early SV40 transcription but do not help explain why late viral RNA synthesis is quiescent at early times and becomes maximally activated only after the onset of SV40 DNA replication. There have been numerous experiments both in vivo (*Cowan* et al. 1973; *Reed* et al. 1976; *Alwine* et al. 1977) and with preinitiated transcriptional complexes in vitro (*Birkenmeier* et al. 1977; *Birkenmeier* et al. 1979; *Ferdinand* et al. 1977) that have been designed to address the problem of late viral transcriptional control. However, the results of these studies have sometimes been controversial and this area of viral gene expression remains ill defined. It is, at present, not even clear whether late SV40 transcription is under negative or positive control. For instance, it was known for some time that mutations mapping in the genes encoding virion proteins exhibited an aberrant late transcriptional pattern (*Avila* et al. 1976; *Cole* et al. 1977). Several recent reports have presented data that supports the idea that late RNA synthesis at early times during infection is suppressed or attenuated by the binding of virion protein to a site on the DNA (*Laub* et al. 1979; *Llopic* and *Stark,* pers. comm.). However, these results are inconsistent with the finding that transcription of late RNA is inhibited at early times even when naked DNA is transfected into the cell (*Parker* and *Stark* 1979). An alternative possibility is for late transcription to be blocked by a cellular DNA binding protein that becomes released after viral DNA replication (*Alwine* and *Khoury* 1980).

A second major model confers the control of late viral RNA synthesis to the positive action of T antigen either directly or indirectly. At present, there is no evidence to implicate T antigen as a direct positive modulator of viral transcription. However, its role as an indirect activator of late transcription via DNA replication and induction of cellular genes has long been a popular model. An alternative simple possibility was recently suggested by the finding that, in vitro, the late promoter becomes active only at high concentrations of template DNA (*Rio* et al. 1980). This apparent differential efficiency of transcription from early and late promoters in vitro suggests that in vivo the early to late switch may also be due to differences in promoter strength. Thus, it is conceivable that the template concentration-dependent activation of late RNA synthesis, working together with the T-antigen mediated repression of early transcription, may contribute to the switch from early to late expression after the onset of DNA replication. However, the ability of cycloheximide to activate late gene transcription is a curious finding (*Handa* and *Sharp* 1980) that does not support the gene dosage model. Thus it is apparent that further investigation will be required to sort out the mechanism of late SV40 transcriptional regulation.

6 T Antigen Binding and Viral Replication

So far, we have analyzed the interaction of T antigen with its binding sites as a means of regulating viral transcription. However, it is clear from the genetics of A mutants that T antigen is also involved in initiating SV40 DNA replication (*Tegtmeyer* 1972; *Chou* and *Martin* 1974). Unfortunately, there is at present, no in vitro cell-free system that will initiate DNA synthesis at the origin of SV40 replication. Therefore, the studies that have addressed the mechanism of viral replication are incomplete. Nevertheless, the analysis of origin mutants together with specific DNA binding studies have provided some important information concerning the relationship between T-antigen binding to the origin region of SV40 and viral replication.

Deletion mapping of viable SV40 mutants have established that a sequence of approximately 70–80 bp between nucleotides 5185 and 35 are required for viral replication (SV coordinates; *Tooze* 1980; *Subramanian* and *Shenk* 1978; *Gluzman* et al. 1980a, b; *Myers* and *Tijan* 1980; Learned et al. 1981). In addition, a number of elegant studies analyzing the phenotype of base-substitution mutants at the origin of SV40 DNA replication provide compelling evidence that sequences overlapping T-antigen binding site II contain information that determines the rate of viral replication (*Shortle* and *Nathans* 1978, 1979, 1979a). These findings indicate that at least sequences in site II and possible portions of site I are involved in viral DNA synthesis. There appears to be some question whether sequences in site I are actually required for replication because in at least a few cases, mutations in site I have little effect on DNA replication (*Myers* and *Tijan* 1980; *McKay* and *diMaio,* personal communication). Thus, it is possible that site I does not play a direct role in viral replication but may, instead, be indirectly involved by virtue of cooperative binding interactions between site I and site II. This idea assumes that binding of T antigen to its recognition sites is at least necessary for initiating DNA synthesis. There are several independent lines of evidence to support this hypothesis.

First, it was shown that some pseudorevertants of origin mutants contain second-site mutations that actually map in the SV40 A gene (*Shortle* et al. 1979). Second, mutant T antigens such as the SV80 protein display a defective phenotype for viral replication (*Gish* and *Botchan,* personal communication) and a corresponding defect in DNA binding affinity for T-antigen recognition sites (*Myers* et al. 1981a). Finally, analysis of cloned wild-type and mutant SV40 origin sequences revealed a strong correlation between the efficiency of T antigen to bind DNA in vitro and the ability to replicate in monkey cells (*Myers* and *Tijan* 1980; *McKay* and *diMaio,* personal communication). Mutant DNA lacking $1/3$ of site I binds T antigen and replicates as efficiently as wild type SV40 DNA. By contrast, a deletion missing $3/4$ of site I binds T antigen less efficiently and also replicates poorly in transfected monkey cells. Similarly, mutants deleted in all of site I but retaining an intact site II are completely defective for replication and bind T antigen with very poor affinity. Finally, deletion mutants that lack only a few bases of site II and retain an intact site I and III are unable to replicate but bind T antigen as well as wild-type DNA. These results suggest that all of site II and part of site I are required for efficient binding of T antigen and viral replication. Moreover, binding of T antigen to SV40 appears necessary but not sufficient to initiate viral replication. It is intriguing that portions of site I, the strongest binding site, have an influence on the replication of SV40 DNA. In view of the cooperative binding between site I and II (*Myers* et al. 1981a), it is attractive to suggest that binding of T antigen to site I coordinates the interaction of T antigen to site II. This would explain why mutants that lower the affinity of T antigen to bind site I have an indirect affect on the efficiency of viral replication. In any case, these findings taken together strongly suggest that a direct interaction between T antigen and SV40 DNA is required for initiating viral replication.

7 Induction of Cellular DNA Synthesis and Gene Expression

There is an abundance of data that suggests the SV40 A gene product is either directly or indirectly involved with turning on cellular DNA replication (*Tegtmeyer* 1972; *Graessmann* and *Graessmann* 1976; *Tjian* 1978a) and activating specific host-gene expression (*Tooze* 1980). We have described the types of regulatory mechanisms that appear to operate during the regulation of viral gene expression. Perhaps similar regulatory T-antigen binding sites exists in the cellular genome. One way to test this idea is to isolate cellular DNA sequences that behave like origins of replication and determine whether they also bind T antigen specifically. This type of experiment has recently been attempted (*Conrad* and *Botchan*, personal communication) and a class of human, cellular DNA sequences were obtained that hybridize strongly to cloned SV40 origin region. Preliminary studies indicate that some of these sequences do indeed appear to behave with the biological properties expected of origins and/or promoters. Thus, hybrid plasmid vectors containing the specific cross-hybridizing human DNA origin sequences and a cloned TK gene are found to transform TK⁻ cells with much greater efficiency than TK gene plasmids alone. The transformed cells also appear to contain free circular plasmid DNA. In addition, preliminary studies indicate that at least some of these cellular sequences are bound selectively by T antigen (*Myers* and *Tjian*, personal communication). However, the enhanced transformation frequency provided by the cloned human origin-like sequences appear not to be dependent on the SV40 A gene product. A more complete characterization of these cellular sequences and their interaction with T antigen will be required to determine the role of the A gene in turning on cellular replication.

8 Enzymatic Properties of T Antigen

How does the binding of T antigen to site I and II induce viral replication? This question will very likely not be fully answered until an in vitro system is developed that can direct the initiation of viral DNA replication. There are, however, some properties of the SV40 large T antigen that have encouraged speculation with respect to mechanisms of viral DNA replication. For instance, it was discovered several years ago that, in addition to binding DNA, T antigen also catalyzes the hydrolysis of ATP → ADP + Pi (*Tjian* and *Robbins* 1979; *Giacherio* et al. 1979). In contrast to an associated protein kinase activity that is sometimes found in preparations of T antigen (*Tjian* and *Robbins* 1979; *Griffin* et al. 1979; *Tjian* et al. 1979), the ATPase activity is intrinsic to purified wild-type SV40 T antigen, D2 protein, and the SV80 protein (*Tjian* et al. 1979; *Clark* et al. 1980). Apparently, the lesion located at the carboxyl portion of the SV80 protein does not affect the ATPase activity of this mutant protein. The amino-terminal portion of T antigen is also unnecessary for enzyme activity because the D2 protein is an active ATPase. To map the ATPase function more accurately within the central portion of the A gene, it was shown that monoclonal antibodies raised against either the amino or carboxyl regions of T antigen have no effect on enzyme activity whereas antibodies directed against a region between 0.37 and 0.29 map units are strongly inhibitory (*Clark* and *Lane,* personal communication).

Although the raison d'être of the ATPase has yet to be revealed, it was not unreasonable to speculate that this property of T antigen is in some way connected with the replication functions of the A gene product. One popular hypothesis was that the DNA binding and ATPase activities are coupled so that the region of DNA bound by T antigen could be locally unwound to allow initiation of bidirectional DNA synthesis. This model was particularly attractive because DNA binding proteins that have ATPase activity are often associated with multienzyme complexes that are involved with initiating DNA replication in bacterial and phage systems (*Kornberg* 1980).

A number of sensitive assays have been developed to detect small changes in the superhelical density of DNA induced by unwinding proteins (*Wang* et al. 1977). One assay utilizes gel electrophoresis to resolve DNA molecules differing by one in their topological winding number (*Keller* 1975; *Pulleybank* et al. 1975). A second assay makes use of the property that unwinding proteins bind supercoiled DNA with greater affinity than relaxed double-stranded molecules.

An initial study recently reported that the SV80 protein is associated with an ATPase independent DNA unwinding activity (*Giacherio* and *Hager* 1980). However, under conditions where specific DNA binding occurs, several purified T antigens were shown to have no DNA unwinding activity (*Myers* et al. 1981b). First, using the gel electrophoresis assay, it was found that neither SV80 protein, D2 protein nor SV40 T antigen unwind SV40 DNA, plasmid DNA, or plasmid DNA containing three copies of the SV40 origin sequence. As a control, *E. coli* RNA polymerase, a known DNA unwinding protein, was shown to change the topology of template DNA under identical conditions. In addition, it was shown that the efficiency of binding T antigen to the viral origin is not influenced by the topological state of the DNA. Thus, supercorted, relaxed circular and linear SV40 DNA bind T antigen and compete for T antigen equally well. These results taken together provide compelling evidence that the SV40 A gene product is not a specific unwinding protein. However, it is still possible that in the cell T antigen acts in concert with host proteins to form a multisubunit complex possessing unwinding activity. T antigen could function by binding to the origin of viral replication and directing host unwinding proteins to this site. Alternatively, T antigen may first bind to one or more host proteins to form an active complex and subsequently orient the "holoenzyme" on the SV40 genome by binding to its recognition sequences. In either case, T antigen would act primarily as a signal or recognition subunit to direct other proteins to the SV40 origin. Consequently, DNA unwinding may still be a prerequisite involved in the mechanism by which T antigen initiates viral DNA replication. However, it appears that the SV40 A gene product alone is unable to cause helix destabilization.

There is some recent evidence to support the idea that T antigen may be bound to specific cellular proteins. A stable complex between T antigen and a cellular 53,000 dalton phosphoprotein was first detected with antiserum raised against large T that specifically coprecipitated a host 53K protein from lysates of rodent cells transformed by SV40 (*Lane* and *Crawford* 1979; *Linzer* and *Levine* 1979; *McCormick* and *Harlow* 1980). Conversely, antiserum raised against the 53K protein from mouse cells coprecipitates T antigen. In addition, purified T antigen was shown to bind specifically to the cellular 53K polypeptide in an in vitro reconstitution experiment (*McCormick* et al. 1981). Recently, it was shown that T antigen may also be weakly associated with a cellular protein in permissive monkey cells (*Harlow* et al. 1980). Presently, there is no evidence to indicate the biological function of these specific viral-cellular protein complexes. It is not even clear whether the complex is involved with transformation or lytic functions of the virus. Perhaps the isolation and characterization of the T antigen-53K complex will shed some light on its function.

9 Summary

The SV40 A gene product is a phosphoprotein with an apparent molecular weight of 96,000. Under physiological conditions, the large T polypeptide forms oligomers consisting of dimers, tetramers, and higher order aggregates such as dodecamers. The predominant species is a tetramer which is able to bind DNA specifically at three closely spaced sites (I, II, and III) located in a region of the SV40 genome containing both the origin of viral replication and the early promoter. Binding of T antigen to these sites occurs in a sequential and cooperative manner with binding to site I facilitating binding to site II and III. The contacts made between subunits of T antigen and the DNA have a two-fold symmetry and are predominantly in the major groove of the duplex DNA. Regulation of both viral replication and transcription appears to involve a direct T antigen-DNA interaction. The entire sequence within binding site II is required for DNA replication while site III lies adjacent to and may overlap the SV40 early promoter region. Analysis of deletion mutants of the SV40 origin region indicate that the cooperative binding of T antigen to sites I and II is correlated with viral DNA synthesis. A similar deletion analysis in vitro of early SV40 promoter mutants suggests that the mechanism of autoregulation involves a repressor type interaction at the three T-antigen binding sites. However, site III is probably the actual site of action where T antigen binds and directly blocks the initiation of viral early transcription by the host RNA polymerase II.

In addition to binding DNA, T antigen also catalyzes the hydrolysis of ATP and has the ability to bind specifically to a 53,000 dalton cellular protein. The precise mechanism by which T antigen initiates viral replication remains unknown and the function of the ATPase and T antigen-53K complex are not understood.

References

Alwine JC, Khoury G (1980) Control of simian virus 40 gene expression at the level of RNA synthesis and processing: thermally induced changes in the ratio of the simian virus 40 early mRNAs and proteins. J Virol 35:157–164

Alwine JC, Reed SI, Stark GR (1977) Characterization of the autoregulation of simian virus 40 gene A. J Virol 24:22–27

Avila J, Saral R, Martin RG, Khoury G (1976) The temperature-sensitive defect in SV40 group D mutants. Virology 73:89–95

Benoist C, Chambon P (1980) Deletions covering the putative promoter region of early mRNA of SV40 do not abolish T antigen expression. Proc Natl Acad Sci USA 77:3865–3869

Benoist C, Chambon P (1981) In vivo sequence requirements of the SV40 early promoter region. Nature 290:304

Birkenmeier, EH, May E, Salzman NP (1977) Characterization of simian virus 40 tsA58 transcriptional intermediates at restrictive temperatures: relationship between DNA replication and transcription. J Virol 22:702–710

Birkenmeier EH, Chiu N, Radonovich MF, May F, Salzman NP (1979) Regulation of simian virus 40 early and late gene transcription without viral DNA replication. J Virol 29:983–989

Black PH, White BJ (1967) In vitro transformation by the Ad2-SV40 hybrid viruses. J Exp Med 125:629–646

Black PH, Rowe WP, Turner HC, Heubner RJ (1963) A specific complement-fixing antigen present in SV40 tumor and transformed cells. Proc Natl Acad Sci USA 50:1148–1156

Bouck N, Beales N, Shenk T, Berg P, diMayorca G (1978) New region of the simian virus 40 genome required for efficient viral transformation. Proc Natl Acad Sci USA 75:2473–2477

Brugge JS, Butel JS (1975) Role of simian virus 40 gene A function in maintenance of transformation. J Virol 15:619–635

Carroll RB, Hager L, Dulbecco R (1974) Simian virus 40 T antigen binds to DNA. Proc Natl Acad Sci USA 71:3754–3757

Chou JY, Martin RG (1974) Complementation analysis of simian virus 40 mutants. J Virol 13: 1101–1109

Clark R, Robbins A, Tjian R (1980) Intrinsic and associated enzymatic activities of SV40 large T antigen. FMI-EMBO Workshop on Protein Phosphorylation and Bio-Regulation. Karger, Basel, pp 209–218

Cole CN, Landers T, Goff SP, Manteuil-Brutlag S, Berg P (1977) Physical and genetic characterization of deletion mutants of simian virus 40 constructed in vitro. J Virol 24:277–294

Corden J, Wasylyk B, Buchwalder A, Sassone-Corsi P, Kedinger C, Chambon P (1980) Promoter sequence of eukaryotic protein-coding genes. Science 209:1406–1414

Cowan K, Tegtmeyer P, Anthony DD (1973) Relationship of replication and transcription of simian virus 40 DNA. Proc Natl Acad Sci USA 70:1927–1930

Crawford LV, Cole CN, Smith AE, Paucha E, Tegtmeyer P, Rundell K, Berg P (1978) Organization and expression of early genes of simian virus 40. Proc Natl Acad Sci USA 75:117–121

Danna KJ, Nathan D (1972) Bidirectional replication of simian virus 40. Proc Natl Acad Sci USA 69:3097–3100

Fareed GC, Salzman NP (1972) Intermediate in SV40 DNA chain growth. Nature (New Biol) 238: 274–277

Fareed GG, Garon CF, Salzman NP (1972) Origin and direction of simian virus 40 deoxyribonucleic acid replication. J Virol 10:484–491

Ferdinand F-J, Brown M, Khoury G (1977) Synthesis and characterization of late lytic simian virus 40 RNA from transcriptional complexes. Virology 78:150–161

Fiers W, Contreras R, Haegeman G, Rogiers R, Van de Voorde A, Van Heuverswyn H, Van Herreweghe J, Volckaert G, Ysebaert M (1978) Complete nucleotide sequence of SV40 DNA. Nature 273:113–120

Friedmann T, Esty A, LaPorte P, Derringer P (1979) The nucleotide sequence and genome organization of the polyoma early region. Cell 17:715–724

Giacherio D, Hager LP (1979) A poly(dT)-stimulated ATPase activity associated with Simian Virus 40 large T antigen. J Biol Chem 254:8113–8116

Giacherio D, Hager LP (1980) A specific DNA unwinding activity associated with SV40 large T-antigen. J Biol Chem 255:8963–8966

Gluzman Y, Frisque RJ, Sambrook J (1980a) Origin-defective mutants of SV40. Cold Spring Harbor Symp Quant Biol 44:293–300

Gluzman Y, Sambrook J, Frisque RJ (1980b) Expression of early genes of origin-defective mutants of SV40. Proc Natl Acad Sci USA 77:3898–3902

Graessmann M, Graessmann A (1976) "Early" simian-virus-40-specific RNA contains information for tumor antigen formation and chromatin replication. Proc Natl Acad Sci USA 73:366–370

Graessmann A, Graessmann M, Guhl E, Mueller C (1978) Quantitative correlation between SV40 T-antigen synthesis and late viral gene expression in permissive and non-permissive cells. J Cell Biol 77:R1–R8

Griffin JD, Light S, Livingston DM (1978) Measurements of the molecular size of the simian virus 40 large T antigen. J Virol 27:218–226

Griffin JD, Spangler G, Livingston DM (1979) Protein kinase activity associated with simian virus 40 T antigen. Proc Natl Acad Sci 76:2610–2614

Handa H, Sharp PA (1980) Expression of early and late SV40 transcripts in the absence of protein synthesis. J Virol 34:592–597

22   Robert Tjian

Handa H, Kaufman RJ, Manley J, Gefter M, Sharp P (1981) Transcription of SV40 DNA in a Hela whole cell extract. J Biol Chem 256:478–482

Harlow EE, Pim D, Crawford LV (1980) The complex of SV40 large T-antigen and host 53K protein in monkey cell. J Virol 37:564–573

Hassell JA, Lukanidin E, Fey G, Sambrook J (1978) The structure and expression of two defective adenovirus 2/simian virus 40 hybrids. J Mol Biol 120:209–247

Jackson AH, Sugden B (1972) Inhibition by α-amanitin of SV40 specific RNA synthesis in nuclei of infected monkey cells. J Virol 10:1086–1089

Jaenisch P, Mayer A, Levine A (1971) Replicating SV40 molecules contain closed circular template DNA strands. Nature (New Biol) 233:72–75

Jessel D, Hudson J, Landau T, Tenen D, Livingston DM (1975) Interactions of partially purified simian virus 40 T antigen with circular viral DNA molecules. Proc Natl Acad Sci USA 72: 1960–1964

Jessel D, Landau T, Hudson J, Lalor T, Tenen D, Livingston DM (1976) Identification of regions of the SV40 genome which contain preferred SV40 T antigen-binding sites. Cell 8:535–545

Keller W (1975) Determination of the number of superhelical turns in SV40 DNA by gel electrophoresis. Proc Natl Acad Sci USA 72:4876–4880

Kelly TJ Jr, Nathans D (1977) The genome of SV40. Adv Virus Res 21:85–173

Khoury G, May E (1977) Regulation of early and late simian virus 40 transcription: overproduction of early viral RNA in the absence of a functional T-antigen. J Virol 23:167–176

Khoury G, Martin MA, Lee THN, Danna KJ, Nathans D (1973) A map of SV40 transcription sites expressed in productively infected cells. J Mol Biol 78:377–389

Khoury G, Martin MA, Lee TN, Nathans D (1975) A transcriptional map of the SV40 genome in transformed cell lines. Virology 63:263–272

Kimura G, Dulbecco R (1972) A temperature-sensitive mutant of simian virus 40 affecting transforming ability. Virology 52:529–534

Kornberg A (1980) DNA Replication. Freeman

Lane DP, Crawford LV (1979) T antigen is bound to a host protein in SV40-transformed cells. Nature 278:261–263

Laub O, Bratosin S, Horowitz M, Aloni Y (1979) The initiation of transcription of SV40 DNA at late times after infection. Virology 92:310–323

Lewis AM Jr, Rowe WP (1970) Isolation of 2 plaque variants from the Ad2-SV40 hybrid population which differ in their efficiency in yielding SV40 virus. J Virol 5:413–420

Learned RM, Myers RM, Tjian R (1981) Replications in monkey cells of plasmid DNA containing the minimal SV40 origin; structure and DNA protein interactions of replication origins. Academic Press, New York (in press)

Lewis AM Jr, Levin MJ, Wiese WH, Crumpacker CS, Henry PH (1969) A nondefective (competent) adenovirus-SV40 hybrid isolated from the Ad2-SV40 hybrid population. Proc Natl Acad Sci USA 63:1128–1135

Linzer DIH, Levine AJ (1979) Characterization of a 54K dalton cellular SV40 tumor antigen present in SV40-transformed cells and uninfected embryonal carcinoma cells. Cell 17:43–52

Livingston DM, Henderson IC, Hudson J (1974) SV40 T antigen: Partial Purification and Properties. Cold Spring Harbor Symp Quant Biol 39:283–289

Maniatis T, Ptashne M (1973) Multiple repressor binding at the operators in bacteriophage Lambda. Proc Natl Acad Sci USA 70:1531–1535

Manley JL, Fire A, Cano A, Sharp PA, Gefter ML (1980) DNA-dependent transcription of adenovirus genes in a soluble whole-cell extract. Proc Natl Acad Sci USA 77:3855–3859

Mann K, Hunter T (1980) Phosphorylation of SV40 large T-antigen in SV40 nucleoprotein complexes. Virology 107:526–532

Martin RG (1981) The transformation of cell growth and transmogrification of DNA synthesis by SV40. Adv Cancer Res 34:1–68

Martin RG, Chou JY (1975) Simian virus 40 functions required for the establishment and maintenance of malignant transformation. J Virol 15:599–612

Martin RG, Setlow VP, Chepelinsky AB, Seif R, Lewis AM Jr, Scher CD, Stiles CD, Avila J (1979) Roles of the tumor antigens in transformation by SV40. Cold Spring Harbor Symp Quant Biol 44:311–324

Mathis D, Chambon P (1981) The SV40 early region TATA box, but not the upstream sequences is required for accurate in vitro initiation of transcription. Nature 290:310

McCormick F, Harlow E (1980) Association of a murine 53,000 dalton phosphoprotein with simian virus 40 large-T antigen in transformed cells. J Virol 34:213–224

McCormick F, Chaudry F, Harvey RS, Rigby PWJ, Paucha E, Smith AE (1980) T antigens of SV40-transformed cells. Cold Spring Harbor Symp Quant Biol 44:171–178

McCormick F, Clark R, Harlow EE, Tjian R (1981) Specific binding of SV40 T antigen to a cellular 53,000 dalton protein in vitro. Nature (in press)

Meyer BJ, Kleid DG, Ptashne M (1975) Repressor turns off transcription of its own gene. Proc Natl Acad Sci USA 72:4785–4789

Myers R, Tjian R (1980) Construction and analysis of SV40 origins defective in T antigen binding and DNA replication. Proc Natl Acad Sci USA 77:6491–6495

Myers RM, Rio D, Robbins A, Tjian R (1981a) SV40 gene expression is modulated by the cooperative binding of T-antigen to DNA. Cell (in press)

Myers R, Kligman M, Tjian R (1981b) Does SV40 T antigen unwind DNA? J Biol Chem (in press)

Myers RM, Williams R, Tjian R (1981c) Oligomeric structure of D2 protein in free form and as bound to SV40 DNA. J Mol Biol 148 (in press)

Oren M, Winocour E, Prives C (1980) Differential affinities of SV40 large T-antigen for DNA. Proc Natl Acad Sci USA 77:220–224

Osborn M, Weber K (1974) SV40: T antigen, the A function, and transformation. Cold Spring Harbor Symp Quant Biol 39:267–281

Osborn M, Weber K (1975) Simian virus 40 gene A function and maintenance of transformation. J Virol 15:636–644

Parker BA, Stark GR (1979) Regulation of simian virus 40 transcription: sensitive analysis of the RNA species present early in infections by virus or viral DNA. J Virol 31:360–369

Paucha E, Mellor A, Harvey R, Smith AE, Hewick RM, Waterfield MD (1978) Large and small T antigens from SV40 have identical amino termini mapping at 0.65 map units. Proc Natl Acad Sci USA 75:2165–2169

Prives C, Gluzman Y, Winocour E (1978) Cellular and cell-free synthesis of simian virus 40 T-antigens in permissive and transformed cells. J Virol 25:587–595

Proudfoot WJ, Shander M, Manley JL, Gefter ML, Maniatis T (1980) Structure and in vitro transcription of human globin genes. Science 209:1329–1336

Ptashne M, Jeffrey A, Johnson AD, Maurer R, Meyer Pabo CO, Roberts TM, Sauer RT (1980) How the repressor and cro work. Cell 19:1–11

Pulleybank DE, Shure M, Tang D, Vinograd J, Vosberg HP (1975) Action of nicking-closing enzyme on supercoiled and nonsupercoiled closed circular DNA: formation of a Boltzmann distribution of topological isomers. Proc Natl Acad Sci USA 72:4280–4284

Reddy VB, Thimmappaya B, Dhar R, Subramanian KN, Zain BS, Pan J, Ghosh PK, Celma ML, Weissman SM (1978) The genome of simian virus 40. Science 200:494–502

Reed SI, Ferguson J, Davis RW, Stark GR (1975) T antigen binds to simian virus 40 DNA at the origin of replication. Proc Natl Acad Sci 72:1605–1609

Reed SI, Stark GR, Alwine JC (1976) Autoregulation of simian virus 40 gene A by T antigen. Proc Natl Acad Sci 73:3083–3087

Reiser J, Renart J, Crawford LV, Stark GR (1980) Specific association of simian virus 40 tumor antigen with simian virus 40 chromatin. J Virol 33:78–87

Rio D, Robbins A, Myers R, Tjian R (1980) Regulation of SV40 Early Transcription in vitro by a Purified T Antigen. Proc Natl Acad Sci USA 77:5706–5710

Rundell K, Collins JK, Tegtmeyer P, Ozer H, Lai C-J, Nathans D (1977) Identification of SV40 protein A. J Virol 21:636–646

Sambrook J, Sugden B, Keller W, Sharp PA (1973) Transcription of Simian virus 40. III. Mapping of "early" and "late" species of RNA. Proc Natl Acad Sci 70:3711–3715

Segawa M, Sugano S, Yamaguchi N (1980) Association of simian virus 40 T antigen with replicating nucleoprotein complexes of simian virus 40. J Virol 35:320–330

Seif I, Khoury G, Dhar R (1979) The genome of human papovavirus BKV. Cell 18:963–977

Shalloway D, Kleinberger T, Livingston DM (1980) Mapping of SV40 DNA replication origin binding sites for the SV40 T antigen by protection against exonuclease III digestion. Cell 20:411–422

Shortle D, Nathans D (1978) Local mutagenesis: a method for generating viral mutants with base substitutions in preselected regions of the viral genome. Proc Natl Acad Sci USA 75:2170–2174

Shortle D, Nathans D (1979) Regulatory mutants of simian virus 40: constructed mutants with base substitution at the origin of DNA replication. J Mol Biol 131:801–817

Shortle D, Nathans D (1979) Mutants of SV40 with base substitutions at the origin of DNA replication. Cold Spring Harbor Symp Quant Biol 43:663–668

Shortle D, Margolskee RF, Nathans D (1979) Mutational analysis of the simian virus 40 replicon: pseudorevertants of mutants with a defective replication origin. Proc Natl Acad Sci 76:6128–6131

Sleigh MJ, Topp WC, Hanich R, Sambrook JF (1978) Mutants of SV40 with an altered small t protein are reduced in their ability to transform cells. Cell 14:79–83

Soeda E, Arrand J, Smolar N, Griffin BE (1979) Polyoma virus DNA: sequence from the early region that contains the origin of replication and codes for small, middle and large T antigens. Cell 17:357–370

Steinberg B, Pollack R, Topp W, Botchan M (1978) Isolation and characterization of T antigen-negative revertants from a line of transformed rat cells containing one copy of the SV40 genome. Cell 13:19–32

Su RT, DePamphilis ML (1976) In vitro replication of SV40 DNA in a nucleoprotein complex. Proc Natl Acad Sci 73:3466–3470

Subramanian KN, Shenk T (1978) Definition of the boundaries of the origin of DNA replication in simian virus 40. Nucleic Acids Res 5:3635–3642

Tegtmeyer P (1972) Simian virus 40 deoxyribonucleic acid synthesis: the viral replicon. J Virol 10:591–598

Tegtmeyer P (1975) Function of simian virus 40 gene A in transforming infection. J Virol 15:613–618

Tegtmeyer P, Schwartz M, Collins JK, Rundell K (1975) Regulation of tumor antigen synthesis by simian virus 40 gene A. J Virol 16:168–178

Thummel C, Burgess T, Tjian R (1981a) Properties of SV40 small T antigen overproduced in bacteria. J Virol 37:683–697

Thummel C, Tjian R, Grodzicker T (1981b) Expression of SV40 T Antigen under control of adenovirus promoters. Cell 23:825–836

Tjian R (1978a) The binding site on SV40 DNA for a T antigen related protein. Cell 13:165–179

Tjian R (1978b) Protein-DNA interactions at the origin of Simian virus 40 DNA replication. Cold Spring Harbor Symp Quant Biol 43:655–662

Tjian R (1980) Binding of D2 protein to specific papovavirus sequences. Mechanistic studies of DNA replication and genetic recombination. Academic Press, New York, p 45

Tjian R, Robbins A (1979) Enzymatic activities associated with a purified SV40 T antigen related protein. Proc Natl Acad Sci USA 76:610–614

Tjian R, Robbins A, Clark R (1979) Catalytic properties of the SV40 large T antigen. Cold Spring Harbor Symp Quant Biol 44:103–111

Tooze J (1980) DNA tumor viruses, molecular biology of tumor viruses, part 2, 2nd edn. Cold Spring Harbor Laboratory, Cold Spring Harbor

Varshavsky AJ, Sundin O, Bohn M (1979) A stretch of "late" SV40 viral DNA about 400 bp long which includes the origin of replication is specifically exposed in SV40 minichromosomes. Cell 16:453–466

Walter G, Flory PJ Jr (1979) Phosphorylation of SV40 large T antigen. Cold Spring Harbor Symp Quant Biol 44:165–169

Wang JC, Jacobsen JH, Saucier JM (1977) Physicochemical studies on interactions between DNA and RNA polymerase. Unwinding of the DNA helix by Escherichia coli RNA polymerase. Nucleic Acid Res 4:1225–1241

Weil PA, Luse DS, Segall J, Roeder RG (1979) Selective and accurate initiation of transcription at the Ad2 major late promoter in a soluble system dependent on purified RNA polymerase II and DNA. Cell 18:469–484

Yamamoto T, deCrombrugghe B, Pastan I (1980) Identification of a functional promoter in the long terminal repeat of rous Sarcoma virus. Cell 22:787–797

Yang RC, Wu R (1978) BK virus DNA: sequence map and sequence analysis. Proc Natl Acad Sci USA 75:2150–2154

Transcriptional Control Regions: Nucleotide Sequence Requirements for Initiation by RNA Polymerase II and III

Thomas Shenk*

1   Introduction.   25
2   Transcription by RNA Polymerase III   26
2.1 Cell-free Transcription by RNA Polymerase III   26
2.2 Polymerase III Transcriptional Control Regions   27
2.3 Regulation of Polymerase III Transcription   29
3   Transcription by RNA Polymerase II   31
3.1 Initiation Sites and Cap Sites   31
3.2 Cell-free Transcription by RNA Polymerase II   32
3.3 Polymerase II Transcriptional Control Regions   33
3.4 Regulation of Polymerase II Transcription   38
4   Conclusions.   39
References   40

1 Introduction

Until recently, the nucleotide sequences involved in the initiation of transcription within eukaryotic cells remained a mystery. Now, thanks to a variety of technological advances, it is possible to identify these sequences and appreciate their functions in the transcription process. Cloning technology enables one to isolate and study genes individually. Rapid DNA and RNA sequencing procedures facilitate nucleotide sequence analysis of both the genes and the RNAs they encode. A variety of in vitro mutagenesis protocols makes it possible to direct deletions and single base-pair changes to specific nucleotide sequences. Selection procedures are available to return genes which have been manipulated in vitro to cells for analysis. And, finally, in vitro systems have been developed which accurately transcribe either RNA polymerase II- or polymerase III-type genes. Genes can now be isolated, sequenced, mutated, and their transcription studied both in vivo and in vitro. As a result, specific functions in the transcription process can be related to specific nucleotide sequences.

The purpose of my review is to explore current efforts to relate nucleotide sequence to specific functions required for initiation of transcription in eukaryotic cells. I emphasize viral models, especially adenovirus and papovaviruses, but include relevant information gleaned from a variety of cellular genes.

---
* Department of Microbiology, Health Sciences Center, State University of New York, Stony Brook, New York 11794, USA

I will follow the lead of *Sakonju* et al. (1980) and avoid use of the term promoter when describing polymerase II and III control regions. *Pribnow* (1975) suggests that in prokaryotes a promoter is composed of three functional regions at which polymerase interacts with DNA: a recognition site, a binding site, and an initiation site. There is ample evidence for these interactions in prokaryotes (*Gilbert* 1976; *Brown* et al. 1978; *Simpson* 1979; *Siebenlist* et al. 1980). Since it is not yet clear where the eukaryotic polymerases interact with their templates, the term control region will be utilized to describe sites within genes at which mutations alter expression.

2 Transcription by RNA Polymerase III

RNA polymerase III is responsible for the synthesis of 5S ribosomal RNA, tRNAs, and a variety of small cellular and viral RNAs including the adenovirus VAI and VAII (virus-associated) RNAs. Polymerase III from animal cells is inhibited by high levels (10–25 μg/ml for 50% inhibition) of α-amanitin, distinguishing it from polymerase I which is insensitive and polymerase II which is sensitive to low levels (0.01–0.05 μg/ml for 50% inhibition) of the toxin (reviewed by *Roeder* 1976). tRNAs are processed at their 5′-ends after transcription, but 5S and VA RNAs do not undergo a post-transcriptional cleavage. Tetraphosphate residues are released from the 5′-ends of 5S RNA (*Denis* and *Wegnez* 1973) and VA RNAs (*Price* and *Penman* 1972; *Celma* et al. 1977), and VA RNAs can be labeled with β-^{32}P nucleotide triphosphates in isolated nuclei (*Soderlund* et al. 1976). Also, 5S and VA RNAs are synthesized in cell-free reactions with no evidence of a precursor transcript (*Birkenmeier* et al. 1978; *Wu* 1978; *Ng* et al. 1979; *Weil* et al. 1979b; *Fowlkes* and *Shenk* 1980). Transcription of 5S and VA RNA genes should, therefore, be initiated at the position to which their 5′-ends have been mapped.

2.1 Cell-free Transcription by RNA Polymerase III

A major breakthrough in our understanding of polymerase III-mediated transcription came with the development of cell-free systems. Nuclear (*Birkenmeier* et al. 1978; *Korn* et al. 1979) and whole cell (*Ng* et al. 1979) extracts of *Xenopus* oocytes were shown to accurately transcribe cloned, *Xenopus* 5S RNA genes. Cytoplasmic extracts prepared from human KB cells (*Wu* 1978; *Weil* et al. 1979b), mouse plasmacytoma cells, and *Xenopus* oocytes (*Weil* et al. 1979b) selectively transcribe cloned 5S, tRNA, and VA RNA genes. These cytoplasmic extracts contain the bulk (65–90%) of cellular polymerase III activity (*Weil* et al. 1979b). The polymerase and other components apparently leak out of the nucleus during the fractionation procedure. Multiple factors are required for accurate transcription by polymerase III. *Segall* et al. (1980) have separated a KB cell extract into four different protein-containing fractions by chromatography on phosphocellulose. Two fractions plus polymerase III are required for transcription of VAI and tRNA genes. These same two fractions plus a third are required for transcription of 5S RNA genes.

2.2 Polymerase III Transcriptional Control Regions

Telford et al. (1979) isolated a *Xenopus laevis* DNA fragment containing a tRNA^{met} coding sequence and only 22 base pairs preceding the 5′-end of the transcript. This DNA was actively transcribed when injected into centrifuged oocytes, placing the boundary of the DNA sequence required for initiation of transcription by polymerase III not more than 22 base pairs before the 5′-end of the coding sequence. Curiously, when this gene was cut into halves (*Kressmann* et al. 1979) neither the 5′- nor 3′-portion was transcribed upon injection into oocytes. Thus it seemed that something other than the tRNA^{met} gene 5′-flanking sequence was required for its transcription.

   D.D. Brown and his co-workers demonstrated that the polymerase III control region for a *Xenopus* 5S RNA gene was contained within its coding region (*Sakonju* et al. 1980; *Bogenhagen* et al. 1980). Deletions were generated by in vitro manipulation of a 5S RNA gene which was cloned in the plasmid pBR322. The altered genes were then used as templates in cell-free extracts to assess the effect of the deletion mutations. One set of deletions extended from the 5′-side of the gene, through its 5′-flanking sequences and into the coding region. Deletions within the 5′-flanking sequences altered the specific initiation site in some cases, but did not prevent transcription of the gene. In fact, it was possible to delete to position +50 (+1 is the first nucleotide of the coding region, –1 is the first nucleotide of the 5′-flanking region) without preventing transcription. When the 5′-end of the coding region was removed, transcription was initiated within pBR322 sequences to produce a hybrid plasmid-5S transcript of approximately normal size. When the deletion extended from the 5′-end to position +55 or further, little or no transcript was synthesized. Therefore, the 5′-boundary of the polymerase III control region lies between position +50 and +55 within the coding region of the 5S RNA gene. A similar set of deletions extending from the other side of the gene fixed the 3′-boundary of the control region between +80 and +83. The location of the control region was confirmed by excising the DNA segment encoding positions +41 to +87 within the 5S transcript and recloning it into pBR322. This small DNA segment directed specific initiation of transcription by polymerase III at an upstream site within plasmid sequences. Thus, the 5′-flanking sequences, the normal initiation site, and the first 50 base pairs of the coding region are not essential. Brown and his colleagues called the critical segment within the coding region of the 5S RNA gene an intragenic control region.

   Engelke et al. (1980) identified and purified a 37K dalton polypeptide from *Xenopus* oocytes which is required for transcription of the 5S gene. These workers monitored the activity of this factor by its ability to facilitate transcription of exogenous 5S RNA genes in unfertilized *Xenopus* egg extracts which are otherwise incompetent for 5S RNA transcription. The purified factor binds specifically to the 5S RNA genes. "Footprinting" analyses (method of *Galas* and *Schmitz* 1978) demonstrated that the factor interacts with nucleotides +45–+96 within the coding region of the 5S RNA gene – almost precisely the location of the intragenic control region defined by deletion mutagenesis. Although this factor is essential for transcription of the *Xenopus* 5S RNA gene in cell-free extracts, it is not required for transcription of either a *Xenopus* tRNA or the adenovirus VAI RNA gene. The function of the 37K dalton polypeptide in the initiation of transcription is not yet clear. Since it recognizes and binds to the intragenic control region of the 5S RNA gene its function might be to guide the polymerase to an appropriate initiation site in a manner somewhat analogous to the sigma factor of *E. coli* RNA polymerase. The availability of this polypeptide could also regulate the expression of the class of RNA polymerase III genes which requires this factor (5S RNA) independently of other genes (tRNAs).

Even though tRNA and VA RNA genes do not require the 37K polypeptide to be transcribed, it is nevertheless clear that they too contain intragenic control regions. *De Franco* et al. (1980) have found that two Drosophila tRNA^{lys} genes do not require their 5'-flanking sequences to be transcribed in vitro. *Koski* et al. (1980) have isolated a mutant containing a single base-pair change within the coding region of the yeast SUP4 tRNA^{tyr} gene which prevents its transcription in vitro. Also, *Fowlkes* and *Shenk* (1980), and *Guilfoyle* and *Weinmann* (1981) have shown that the adenovirus 2 and 5 VA RNA genes contain intragenic control regions. Sequences between +10 and +69 within the coding region of the VAI RNA gene are required for its transcription in cytoplasmic extracts of HeLa cells. Again, deletions within the 5'-flanking sequences did not prevent transcription, but could influence the precise initiation site (see also *Thimmappaya* et al. 1979).

Fowlkes and *Shenk* (1980) have identified two sequences within the adenovirus VAI RNA intragenic control region which appear to be conserved in a variety of different genes transcribed by polymerase III (Fig. 1). The first homologous sequence is near the 5'-end of the control region and reads 5'-GTGGPyNNPuGTGG-3'. The second is near the 3'-boundary of the control region and reads 5'-GGGTTCGAANCC-3'. Similar sequences are present in the EBER (Epstein-Barr virus encoded RNA) genes (*Lerner* et al. 1981; *M. Rosa* and *J. Steitz*, personal communication), tRNA genes (both eukaryotic and prokaryotic), the mouse and hamster 4.5S genes (*Peters* et al. 1977; *Jelinek* and *Leinwand* 1978; *Harada* and *Ikawa* 1979; *Harada* et al. 1979), genes such as A36 which are human Alu family (*Houck* et al. 1979) polymerase III transcriptional units (*Duncan* et al. 1981), and the *Xenopus* 5S RNA gene. The VAI sequences are not represented perfectly in each gene, but the substantial homology together with their relatively constant location within these genes indicates that they are likely to be of critical importance. Indeed, if several base pairs are removed from either sequence in the VAI RNA gene, the mutant template is no longer transcribed in vitro (*Fowlkes* and *Shenk* 1980; *Guilfoyle* and *Weinmann* 1981). Further, single base-pair changes within these sequences in the yeast SUP4 tRNA^{tyr} gene can drastically affect its transcription in vitro (*Koski* et al. 1980). A change at position +56 (numbered according to *Sprinzl* et al. 1980) prevented detectable initiation of transcription, while changes at +15 and +21 enhanced in vitro transcription. The alteration at +56 is within the 3'-region and that at +15 within the 5'-region of homology.

It is curious that the conserved sequences noted in Figure 1 are present in both eukaryotic and prokaryotic tRNAs (*Fowlkes* and *Shenk* 1980). Assuming that the promoters for prokaryotic tRNAs are always located 5' to their coding region, it appears plausible that these sequences have been conserved to accommodate tRNA functions and not necessarily functions involved in the synthesis of the tRNA. One might speculate that tRNAs evolved in an organism where transcriptional control resided in a flanking region of the gene. As tRNAs were perfected certain regions became invariant. Then, one might guess, as eukaryotes appeared, these constant regions developed a second function as part of a control region for a eukaryotic RNA polymerase. Alternatively, one could reverse the rationale and argue that the intragenic control region is the more primitive regulatory arrangement. Thus, as prokaryotes moved this function to the 5'-flanking region of tRNA genes, one of several original functions of the coding region was lost.

Polymerase III-type genes can be divided into at least two groups. The first group as

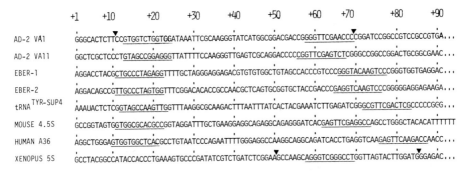

Fig. 1. Partial nucleotide sequence of a variety of genes transcribed by RNA polymerase III. Sequences are the same sense as the RNA encoded and +1 marks the 5′-end of the primary transcript. Arrowheads mark the intragenic control region boundaries of the VAI (*Fowlkes* and *Shenk* 1980; *Guilfoyle* and *Weinmann* 1981) and 5S genes (*Bogenhagen* et al. 1980; *Sakonju* et al. 1980). The conserved sequences within the control region are underlined. The sources for the sequences are as follows: Ad-2 VAI and VAII (*Akusjärvi* et al. 1980), EBER 1 and EBER 2 (*M.D. Rosa* and *J.A. Steitz*, personal communication), tRNA[tyr-sup4] (*Koski* et al. 1980), mouse 4.5S (*Harada* and *Kato* 1980), human A36 (*Duncan* et al. 1981), *Xenopus* 5S (*Korn* and *Brown* 1978)

yet includes only the 5S RNA gene; the second class consists of tRNA and VA RNA genes and very likely the other viral and cellular genes included in Figure 1. This grouping is based on several observations. First, the 5S RNA gene requires the 37K polypeptide for its transcription in vitro (*Engelke* et al. 1980; *Segall* et al. 1980) while tRNA and VA RNAs do not. Second, the intragenic control region of the 5S gene is in a different position relative to the 5′-end of the transcript (+50–+83) than is the VAI control region (+10–+69). Thus there must be a difference in the mechanism utilized to measure from the control sequences to the initiation sites of these two genes. The different measurements probably derive from the fact that different polypeptides interact with the control region of these genes. Finally, the 5S gene shows no evidence of a sequence corresponding to the 5′-homology shared by the other genes listed in Figure 1. This is not surprising given the fact that the region which would contain the homology is not included within the control region of the 5S RNA gene. The similarities and differences between various genes transcribed by polymerase III may simply reflect their evolutionary relatedness. However, as mentioned above, the differences do provide an attractive mechanism for coordinately regulating the expression of subgroupings of these genes.

2.3 Regulation of Polymerase III Transcription

A variety of mechanisms are apparent which serve to regulate transcription by polymerase III at the level of initiation. Several lines of evidence indicate that the 5′-flanking sequences of polymerase III-type genes serve to modulate the efficiency with which they are transcribed. *De Franco* et al. (1980) isolted two *Drosophila* tRNA[lys] genes with identical coding regions, but different 5′-flanking sequences. The two genes were transcribed with very different efficiencies in nuclear extracts of *Xenopus* oocytes. When the 5′-

flanking sequences of the less efficiently transcribed gene were replaced by pBR322 sequences, the modified template directed the synthesis of substantially increased amounts of product. When the 5'-flanking sequences of the two tRNA genes were switched, the reconstructed genes displayed the characteristic of the gene from which the flanking sequences were derived. It seems clear that the 5'-flanking sequence is modulating the expression of the tRNA genes. A similar effect was observed for the VAI RNA gene by *Fowlkes* and *Shenk* (1980). Mutant templates carrying deletions in their 5'-flanking sequences were transcribed in vitro less efficiently than genes with a wild-type flanking sequence. Finally, *Sprague* et al. (1980) found that a truncated silkworm tRNA[ala] gene which contained only 11 nucleotides of its normal 5'-flanking sequence was not transcribed at detectable levels in silkworm cell-free extracts. Curiously, the truncated gene was transcribed as well as the wild-type gene in *Xenopus* oocyte extracts.

The mechanism by which the flanking sequences modulate transcription is not yet clear. These regions from a variety of genes do exhibit sequence similarities (*Korn* and *Brown* 1978, and it is quite likely that the polymerase interacts here during initiation of transcription since alterations can influence the precise initiation site (*Thimmappaya* et al. 1979; *Sakonju* et al. 1980; *Fowlkers* and *Shenk* 1980; *Guilfoyle* and *Weinmann* 1981). If the polymerase contacts these sequences during initiation of transcription, it is not surprising that their composition modulates its function.

A second mechanism has been described which undoubtedly regulates transcription of the *Xenopus* 5S RNA gene (*Honda* and *Roeder* 1980; *Pelham* and *Brown* 1980). 5S RNA is stored in the oocyte as a 7S ribonucleoprotein complex, and the major protein component of the 7S particle is the 37K dalton polypeptide which also binds to the intragenic control region of the 5S gene. When 5S RNA is added to a *Xenopus* cell-free extract, transcription of the 5S gene is inhibited, presumably because the RNA competes with its template for the 37K polypeptide. Thus the product inhibits its own transcription. This type of feedback inhibition might also function for other genes transcribed by polymerase III. For example, both VA and EBER RNAs (Fig. 1) exist in cells as ribonucleoprotein particles, and they can both be precipitated by a particular class of sera, designated anti-La, from patients with systemic lupus erythematosis (*Lerner* et al. 1980; 1981). Conceivably, the VA and EBER ribonucleoprotein particles contain a common polypeptide which binds to their intragenic control regions and is required for their transcription.

Transcription by polymerase III may also be controlled at the level of chromatin structure. *Louis* et al. (1980) studied nucleosome phasing in the 5S RNA cluster of drosophila. They prepared nucleosome monomers by digestion of *Drosophila* chromatin with micrococcal nuclease, extracted the monomeric DNA fragments, and recut them with a restriction endonuclease which cuts only once within the 5S repeat unit. A specific cleavage pattern was generated, leading to the conclusion that nucleosomes can be positioned on the 5S gene in one of two possible phases (if nucleosome position was random relative to the DNA sequence, the restriction endonuclease would have generated a smear of random-sized fragments). In one phase, the center of the gene is exposed in the linker region and in the second phase the 5'-flanking sequences are located in this region. Both of these regions of the *Drosophila* 5S gene presumably contain key regulatory sequences. Perhaps the linker sequences which are accessible to micrococcal nuclease are equally accessible to transcriptional control factors, while sequences associated with the nucleosome are not. If this is true, nucleosome phasing could play an important role in the regulation of 5S gene expression.

It appears that much of the regulation of polymerase III-type genes is accomplished by relatively simple means. These include gene copy number (e.g. there are many more copies of 5S gene than individual tRNA genes), the efficiency with which the gene is transcribed (modulation by 5'-flanking sequences), and by feedback inhibition (5S RNA binds the very factor required for its transcription). There are other levels of regulation, however, which remain obscure. A case in point is the switch during *Xenopus* development from production of oocyte-type to somatic-type 5S RNA (reviewed in *Ford* and *Brown* 1976). This type of regulation may be mediated by polypeptides which have yet to be identified (discussed in *Honda* and *Roeder* 1980).

3 Transcription by RNA Polymerase II

RNA polymerase II is responsible for the synthesis of heterogeneous nuclear RNA which is processed to mRNAs. The post-transcriptional processing events include capping, methylation, splicing, cleavage, and polyadenylation. Available data suggest that unlike polymerase III, the polymerase II control regions are located in a more "conventional" position. That is, the control sequences generally precede and include the 5'-ends of transcripts, as is the case for prokaryotes.

3.1 Initiation Sites and Cap Sites

In order to discuss the control regions for polymerase II transcription, it is necessary to know the site at which transcripts are initiated. The 5'-ends of eukaryotic mRNAs usually occur in the form of a cap structure with the general formula $m^7GpppNm$ (*Shatkin* 1976). Generally, but not always, a purine nucleotide is found in the 5'-penultimate position. Does the penultimate nucleotide represent the site at which transcription is initiated? This of course depends on the mechanism of cap formation. Generally, capping involves the transfer of a GMP residue from GTP to a 5'-di- or triphosphate-terminated RNA molecule (*Groner* and *Hurwitz* 1975; *Furuichi* and *Shatkin* 1976; *Furuichi* et al. 1976; *Moss* et al. 1976; *Winicov* and *Perry* 1976; *Wei* and *Moss* 1977). Thus primary transcripts with a 5'-terminal triphosphate represent ideal substrates for capping. But, if an RNA molecule with a 5'-terminal monophosphate can be converted within the cell to a 5'-triphosphate-terminated species, then cap sites need not reflect initiation sites. A primary transcript could be cleaved and the newly exposed 5'-end capped. In fact, vaccinia virus cores contain a 5'-phosphate-polyribonucleotide kinase which facilitates just such a reaction (*Spencer* et al. 1978).

Despite the potential for capping at internal cleavage sites on primary transcripts, a variety of biochemical experiments using defined viral and cellular templates indicate that cap sites generally are in close proximity to transcription-initiation sites. The initiation site of the adenovirus 2 late transcriptional unit has been located on the viral genome by a variety of analyses, including nascent chain mapping (*Weber* et al. 1977; *Ziff* and *Evans* 1978), uv mapping (*Goldberg* et al. 1977), and mapping by means of DRB (5, 6 dichloro-1-β-D-ribofuranosylbenzimidazole, a nucleoside analogue)-induced termination of transcription (*Fraser* et al. 1978; 1979). These methods rely on the isolation of short, 5'-proximal RNA fragments which are radioactively labeled. The RNAs are hybridized to restriction endonuclease-generated DNA fragments to position the shortest fragments on the viral genome and thereby locate the initiation site of the transcriptional unit. The initiation site for the adenovirus major late transcriptional unit lies at 16.5 map units. The capped 5′-terminus of the late transcript was also mapped to this site by aligning T_1 ribonuclease-generated oligonucleotides from nuclear RNA with the DNA sequence of this region (*Ziff* and *Evans* 1978). Similar results were obtained when the capped 5′-end was synthesized in isolated nuclei (*Manley* et al. 1979; *Baker* and *Ziff* 1980) or in cell-free extracts (*Weil* et al. 1979a; *Manley* et al. 1980). In all cases no oligonucleotides were evident corresponding to RNA sequences immediately upstream of the cap site. Similar experiments indicate that the initiation sites and capped 5′-termini of early adenovirus transcripts lie in close proximity (*Berk* and *Sharp* 1977; *Evans* et al. 1977; *Berk* and *Sharp* 1978; *Baker* et al. 1979; *Chow* et al. 1979; *Sehgal* et al. 1979; *Wilson* et al. 1979; *Baker* and *Ziff*, 1981).

The relationship between late SV40 initiation and cap sites has been particularly worrisome because the cap sites are heterogeneous and are spread over a distance of about 300 base pairs (discussed in detail below). Nevertheless, nascent chain mapping indicates that late transcription is initiated in this region (*Ford* and *Hsu* 1978; *Laub* et al. 1979), and cell-free transcription generates RNAs with 5′-ends which map to the same general region as those produced in intact cells with no evidence for precursor molecules (*Honda* et al. 1980). Using another approach, *Contreras* and *Fiers* (1981) analyzed nascent RNA synthesized in permeabilized cells in the presence of β-^{32}P-labeled nucleoside triphosphates. In the presence of β-^{32}P-ATP, only GpppA cap cores were labeled (in the β-position), and in the presence of β-^{32}P-GTP, only GpppG cap cores were labeled (again in the β-position). Contreras and Fiers concluded that the β-phosphate in the cap is derived from the 5′-terminal polyphosphate of the RNA, and therefore late SV40 mRNA caps are added directly to the 5′-ends of primary transcripts.

Finally, initiation and cap sites also appear to coincide for transcripts encoded by the mouse β-major globin gene. Nascent chain mapping in isolated nuclei (*Hofer* and *Darnell* 1981) places the major initiation site for this transcription unit very near to the location of the mRNA cap site in the β-globin gene sequence (*Konkel* et al. 1978). Also, cell-free transcription of the β-globin gene generates an RNA initiated at the normal cap site, with no evidence for transcription of RNA sequences immediately upstream of this site (*Luse* and *Roeder* 1980).

All available evidence suggests that initiation and cap sites are either very close or coincide. Therefore, for the remainder of this discussion I will assume that cap sites correspond to initiation sites for polymerase II-mediated transcription.

3.2 Cell-free Transcription by RNA Polymerase II

Shortly after cell extracts capable of polymerase III transcription became available, similar extracts were developed for polymerase II. *Weil* et al. (1979a) supplemented a KB cell cytoplasmic extract with purified calf thymus polymerase II, and obtained accurate initiation at the adenovirus 2 major late control site. The transcript was judged to be correctly initiated both by sizing "run off" products generated by cleavage of the DNA template with a variety of restriction endonucleases, and by comparing the T_1 ribonuclease-generated oligonucleotides from the 5′-end of the in vitro-synthesized transcript to those generated by cleavage of the RNA produced within cells. The fingerprints were identical. Further, no oligonucleotides were observed from sequences immediately upstream of the cap site. This cell-free extract also initiated specifically at the cap site of the mouse β-globin gene (*Luse* and *Roeder* 1980). *Matsui* et al. (1980) fractionated the KB cell extract and identified four fractions required for accurate and specific initiation by polymerase II at the adenovirus major late control site. *Manley* et al. (1980) prepared a concentrated extract of HeLa cells which can initiate transcription specifically at a variety of adenovirus polymerase II control regions. This extract does not require supplementation with polymerase as does the extract utilized by *Weil* et al. (1979a). The HeLa cell extract is also capable of transcribing both early and late SV40 RNA species which appear to have 5′-ends analogous to those generated in vivo (*Honda* et al. 1980).

At first consideration it seems paradoxical that uninfected cell extracts can efficiently initiate transcription at late viral control regions. However, it is now clear that both the adenovirus major late control region (*Chow* et al. 1979; *Lewis* and *Mathews* 1980; *Shaw* and *Ziff* 1980) and papovavirus late transcriptional units (*Ferdinand* et al. 1977; *Parker* and *Stark* 1979; *Piper* 1979) are active at early times after infection. The early to late switch in the viral growth cycle must be mediated at least in part by events which follow the initiation of transcription.

3.3 Polymerase II Transcriptional Control Regions

The control region which regulates transcription appears to reside in the 5′-flanking sequences of polymerase II-type genes. A good variety of these genes have been sequenced and the 5′-ends of the mRNAs they encode have been located. The 5′-flanking regions of several viral and cellular genes are displayed in Figure 2. Asterisks identify mRNA cap sites. It is quite common for a gene to encode multiple cap sites (e.g. SV40 early mRNA, Fig. 2), and there is a clear hierarchy of cap-site preferences: A>G>>U>C (*Baker* and *Ziff* 1981). Portions of the flanking sequences which appear to be conserved in a variety of genes are underlined in Figure 2. *D. Hogness* and *M. Goldberg* were the first to recognize such a conserved sequence, an A-T stretch which is generally found near position –25 to –35 (preceding the start site) of polymerase II-type genes. This sequence is generally referred to as the "TATAA" box. It is remarkably similar in sequence to the Pribnow box (TATAAT) located about ten base pairs upstream from the initiation site of prokaryotic transcription units (*Pribnow* 1975), but the sequences probably serve quite different functions in prokaryotes and eukaryotes. A second homology occurs in the –70 to –80 region. The model sequence at this location is $5'-GG_T^CCAATCT-3'$ (*Benoist* et al. 1980; *Corden* et al. 1980; *Efstratiadis* et al. 1980). The widespread occurrence of these two homologies and their comparatively constant locations relative to cap sites suggests they probably play important roles in transcription. Some, but not all, of the genes contain regions of partial (hyphenated) twofold symmetry around the start sites for transcription (e.g. Ad2 Ela, –11 to +9, CTCAAGAGGC/CACTCTTGAG: mouse β-globin, –17 to –2, AGGATCAG/TTGCTCCT; ovalbumin, –7 to +7, TGTCTGT/-ACATACA; Fig. 2) (*Gannon* et al. 1979). Hyphenated symmetries are found in prokaryotic operators and at other regulatory sites which interact with proteins (e.g. *Gilbert* 1976), and could serve similar functions in eukaryotic control regions.

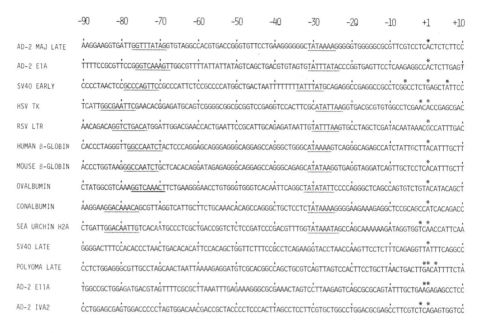

Fig. 2. Partial nucleotide sequence of a variety of genes transcribed by RNA polymerase II. Sequences are the sense of the RNA encoded and asterisks (+1) mark the capped 5′-ends of mRNAs. The first nucleotide of the 5′-flanking sequences is-1. Conserved sequences within the 5′-flanking sequences are underlined. The sources for the sequences and 5′-cap sites are as follows: Ad-2 E1A cap site (*Baker* and *Ziff* 1981), Ad-5 sequence (*Van Ormondt* et al. 1978), herpes simplex virus thymidine kinase (*McKnight* 1980), SV40 early cap sites (*Reddy* et al. 1979; *Thompson* et al. 1979; *Haegeman* and *Fiers* 1980), SV40 sequence (*Fiers* et al. 1978; *Reddy* et al. 1978b), Rous sarcoma virus long terminal repeat (*Yamamoto* et al. 1980a, b), human β-globin (*Efstratiadis* et al. 1980), mouse β-globin (*Konkel* et al. 1978), ovalbumin (*Gannon* et al. 1979; *Benoist* et al. 1980), conalbumin (*Cochet* et al. 1979), sea urchin H2A cap sites (*Hentschel* et al. 1980), sea urchin H2A sequence (*Busslinger* et al. 1980), SV40 late cap sites (*Ghosh* et al. 1978; *Haegeman* and *Fiers* 1978; *Reddy* et al. 1978a; *Canaani* et al. 1979), polyoma late cap sites (*Flavell* et al. 1979; 1980), polyoma sequence (*Soeda* et al. 1980), Ad-2 EIIA (*Baker* et al. 1979; *Baker* and *Ziff* 1981), Ad-2 IVA 2 (*Baker* and *Ziff* 1981)

Several viral genes have been identified which do not contain TATAA-box sequences in their –25 to –35 region. These include the SV40 late, polyoma late, and adenovirus 2 EIIA and IVA2 transcription units. These genes nevertheless share short regions spread through positions –40 to –80 homologous both with each other and with genes which contain TATAA boxes (*Contreras* and *Fiers* 1981).

What are the functions of the conserved sequences identified in Figure 2? A variety of experiments using cell-free extracts to monitor the effects of alterations constructed in vitro suggest that the TATAA box and its surrounding sequences are the only critical components of the polymerase II control region. Deletions extending from an upstream position toward the cap site of the conalbumin gene to position –44 or from a downstream position to –10 did not prevent in vitro initiation (*Corden* et al. 1980; *Wasylyk* et al. 1980b). However, a single base-pair change within the TATAA box (TATA to TAGA) reduced the efficiency of initiation in the cell-free extract ten-fold (*Wasylyk* et al. 1980a). Similar results were obtained with the adenovirus 2 major late control region (*Corden* et al. 1980; *Hu* and *Manley* 1981). The adenovirus control region functioned, provided the sequences between –12 and –32 remained intact. In this case deletions between –12 and +3 reduced the efficiency of initiation. Significantly, a cloned segment containing the adenovirus TATAA box (–12 to –32) directed initiation by polymerase II in cell-free extracts (*Corden* et al. 1980). There is one case in which removal of the TATAA box did not prevent transcription in vitro. *Rio* et al. (1980) deleted this sequence from the SV40 early gene, and it was still transcribed in HeLa cell extracts.

In general, the TATAA box is not essential for transcription in vivo. *Benoist* and *Chambon* (1980) constructed an SV40 deletion mutant, HS6, which lacks 58 base pairs, including the TATAA box preceding the early transcription unit (Fig. 3; the bottom stand is the sense of early mRNAs, cap sites are indicated by arrowheads, TATAA box is underlined, HS6 deletion indicated by brackets). Two observations indicate that the mutant is capable of synthesizing early mRNAs. First, T antigen is produced in monkey cells transfected by HS6 DNA, and second, the mutant DNA can transform rat cells. A more direct and quantitative analysis of HS6 early transcription was not possible since the viral origin of DNA replication was inactivated by the mutation. Similar results were obtained when the TATAA box preceding the polyoma virus early transcription unit was deleted (*Bendig* et al. 1980). In this case the viral replication origin still functioned, and the mutants synthesized normal levels of early mRNAs. Finally, the TATAA box preceding the sea urchin H2A transcription units is not essential for in vivo function (*Grosschedl* and *Birnstiel* 1980). In this instance mutant genes were assayed for function by injection into *Xenopus* oocyte nuclei. A 54 base-pair deletion which included the TATAA box reduced (five-fold) but did not prevent transcription. Thus, in contrast to the in vitro situation, there is considerable evidence that the TATAA box is not an essential component of the polymerase II control region when assayed in vivo.

The adenovirus E1A transcription unit may be an exception to this generalization. *Osborne* et al. (1981) cloned the E1A gene into pBR322, mutated the clone in vitro and then tested for its ability to complement an adenovirus 5 deletion mutant lacking this gene (*dl*312, *Jones* and *Shenk* 1979a). The yield of *dl*312 after transfection of HeLa cells was increased about 50-fold by adding the plasmid. Deletion of sequences preceding position –38 in the E1A gene within the plasmid (see Fig. 2) had no effect on its complementing activity. But, if the deletion was extended to position –23, removing the TATAA box, there was a significant reduction in complementing activity. Perhaps the TATAA box functions differently in the transcriptional control region of the E1A gene than in the SV40, polyoma, and sea urchin histone genes discussed above. Alternatively, the plasmid sequences may not be controlled like genes on the viral chromosome in this experiment. Conceivably, chromatin structure is very important for regulation of polymerase II transcription (discussed below), and the plasmid DNA is not fully assembled into such a structure before it is first transcribed. This could explain the fact that it appears to be regulated like naked DNA added to cell-free extracts.

Assuming that the TATAA box, in general, is not essential for transcription in vivo, what is its function? *Gluzmann* et al. (1980) isolated several SV40 mutants which are relevant to this question. These mutants lack the Bgl I cleavage site centered at nucleotide 0/5243 on the SV40 genome (Δ9, lacks nine base pairs; Δ58, lacks 58 base pairs, Fig. 3). Δ9 is located between the TATAA box and initiation sites for early mRNAs, Δ58 deletes the major initiation sites. Both of these mutants synthesize early mRNAs and can

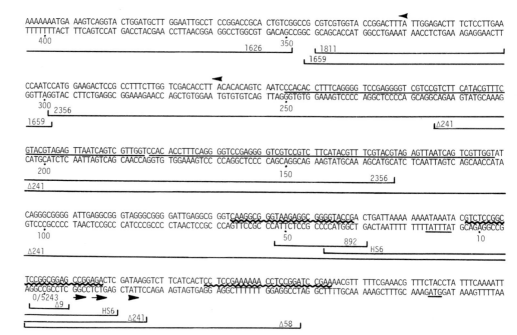

Fig. 3. Sequence of the SV40 genome which encodes the early and late transcriptional control regions. Sequence is from *Fiers* et al. (1978), *Reddy* et al. (1978b), and *Van Heuverswyn* and *Fiers* (1979). The sequence is numbered according to the SV-system (*Buchman* et al. 1980). The upper strand is the sense of late mRNAs and the lower strand the sense of early mRNAs. Cap sites for mRNAs are indicated by arrowheads (early: *Reddy* et al. 1979; *Thompson* et al. 1979; *Haegeman* and *Fiers* 1980; only two of many late caps are shown: *Ghosh* et al. 1978; *Haegeman* and *Fiers* 1978; *Reddy* et al. 1978a; *Canaani* et al. 1979). Wavy lines between base pairs indicate T-antigen binding sites as determined by *Tjian* (1979). Straight lines between base pairs highlight the 72 base-pair tandem repeat. The early strand TATAA box and translational initiation codon are underlined. Deletions are indicated by brackets: *dl*1626 and 1659 (*Subramanian* 1979), *dl*1811 (*Haegeman* et al. 1979) *dl*2356 (*Gruss* et al. 1981), △241, △58 and △9 (*Gluzman* et al. 1980), *dl*892 (*Shenk* et al. 1976; *Subramanian* and *Shenk* 1978), HS6 (*Benoist* and *Chambon* 1980).

transform rat cells. *Ghosh* et al. (1981) located the 5′-ends of the early viral mRNAs synthesized by these mutants in transformed cells. The 5′-ends were displaced downstream from the wild-type start sites. In fact, they were displaced by distances approximately equal to the size of each deletion. This suggested a measurement was made across the region containing the deletions. Another mutant, *dl*892 (*Shenk* et al. 1976; *Subramanian* and *Shenk* 1978), was also examined. This mutant lacks 19 base pairs upstream from the TATAA box and generates wild-type mRNAs. Thus, the measurement is made from a site located downstream from *dl*892 and upstream from △9 and △58. This region includes the TATAA box. Apparently, the TATAA box helps to specify the precise start site for transcription. Perhaps the polymerase contacts this site which serves to align it with a specific point at which to initiate transcription. Consistent with this notion, *Grosschedl* and *Birnstiel* (1980) find that multiple initiation sites are utilized in vivo (instead of the normal unique site) when the TATAA box is deleted from the sea urchin H2A gene.

However, lack of this sequence does not necessitate substantial heterogeneity in initiation sites as is evidenced by the adenovirus 2 EIIA and IVA2 genes (*Baker* et al. 1979; *Baker* and *Ziff* 1981; Fig. 2).

What sequences are essential for initiation of transcription by polymerase II in vivo? One obvious candidate is the conserved sequence located near –70 to –80 preceding the initiation site (Fig. 2). However, there is as yet no evidence that this sequence is essential. In fact, *Grosschedl* and *Birnstiel* (1980) found that a 55 base-pair deletion which included this sequence increased the level of transcription of the sea urchin H2A gene in vivo. The essential site seems to lie even further upstream in SV40 within a 72 base-pair sequence which is tandemly repeated (nucleotide 107–178/179–250, Fig. 3). *Gruss* et al. (1981) found that one copy of this tandem repeat could be removed with no effect on early transcription, but when most of both copies were deleted (*dl*2356, –172 base pairs, Fig. 3) the early control region did not function. Their conclusion was based on the fact that *dl*2356 failed to complement tsA28 (an early mutant), and no viral mRNA or T antigen could be detected in cells infected with the mutant DNA. *Gluzman* et al. (1980) also isolated a mutant which failed to express early functions. This mutant contains a deletion which extends from the early mRNA cap site upstream through the tandem repeats (Δ241, –241 base pairs, Fig. 3).

The component of the early SV40 polymerase II control region essential for in vivo transcription lies at least 112 base pairs upstream from the mRNA cap site. Mutants with similar phenotypes have also been isolated far upstream from the polyoma virus cap site (*M. Fried* and *E. Reeley,* personal communication). Furthermore, polyoma mutants have been isolated which, unlike the wild-type virus, can grow in undifferentiated teratocarcinoma cells (*Katinka* et al. 1980; *Sekikawa* and *Levine* 1981). Infection of these cells with wild-type virus produces very small amounts of viral RNA; the mutants produce more RNA. They all contain alterations in a region about 200 base pairs upstream from the major early mRNA initiation site (and about 80 nucleotides upstream from minor initiation sites), again suggesting that a critical element of the early transcriptional control region lies far upstream. Finally, a mutation which is located 184 base pairs upstream from the sea urchin mRNA initiation site reduced the level of transcription of this gene 15-fold in *Xenopus* occytes (*Grosschedl* and *Birnstiel* 1980).

There are several ways in which this upstream site might function in the initiation of transcription. Possibly, polymerase II spans a large region on the template and actually contacts this far upstream region (preceding –112, taking the SV40 early control region as an example) as well as sites at –30 and +1. This is not unlikely when one considers that the smaller. *E. coli* polymerase contacts an 80 base-pair region (*Schmitz* and *Galas* 1979). When the supercoiling of the DNA template in chromatin is considered (about 75–80 base pairs per superhelical turn of B-form DNA, *Felsenfeld* 1978), polymerase II could very likely interact directly with sites on the template quite far removed in sequence from the initiation site. Alternatively, a regulatory protein which is not part of the polymerase could interact with the far upstream sequence. This protein could act to direct the polymerase to its downstream initiation site or it could function to phase the chromatin structure of the 5′-flanking region of the transcription unit (*Minty* and *Newmark* 1980; discussed below).

The in vivo and in vitro descriptions of critical control regions appear to be in conflict. Since the same mutations in the same genes have not been studied both in vivo and in vitro, it is conceivable that no conflict exists and the data reflect several different classes of polymerase II control regions. The more likely explanation is that the cell-free extracts are not yet faithfully reflecting control mechanisms operative in vivo. The extracts may lack critical regulatory components. It is also likely that the super structure of the DNA template is critical for its proper regulation. Normally, transcription units are "packaged" in chromatin, while naked DNA is supplied to extracts and may or may not be assembled into chromatin.

Very little is known about the transcriptional control regions of polymerase II-type genes which lack TATAA boxes (Fig. 2). Examples of this type of gene are all viral and fall into two groups. One group consists of two adenovirus 2 transcription units, EIIA and IVA2. These genes appear to initiate transcription at a relatively unique location (*Baker* et al. 1979; *Baker* and *Ziff* 1981). The second group consists of the SV40 and polyoma virus late transcription units. Transcription of these genes is initiated at a wide variety of sites spread over several hundred base pairs (*Ghosh* et al. 1978; *Haegeman* and *Fiers* 1978; *Reddy* et al. 1978a; *Canaani* et al. 1979; *Flavell* et al. 1979, 1980; *Piatak* et al. 1981). The major initiation site for SV40 late mRNAs is at position 325 in Figure 3; an additional seven or more sites each represent 1–20% of the total. *Contreras* and *Fiers* (1981) have pointed out that extensive sequences homologies exist between the sequences upstream of many of these start sites; the homologies also extend to genes which contain TATAA boxes.

It is clear that critical elements of the late SV40 control region lie upstream (toward the origin of DNA replication) of the unique HpaII cleavage site (position 330–333, Fig. 3), since foreign genes cloned at this site can be expressed under late viral control (*Hamer* and *Leder* 1979; *Gruss* and *Khoury* 1981). Several mutants have been described which alter transcription of the late SV40 genes. *dl*2356 removes most of the 72 base-pair repeat within the SV40 control regions (*Gruss* et al. 1981; Fig. 3). As discussed above, this mutant fails to express early functions and, therefore, marks a critical element of the SV40 early control region. This mutant also fails to express late functions and therefore might also locate a component of the late control region. However, a straightforward interpretation of this mutant's phenotype is not yet possible since its effect on late transcription could be indirect, resulting from primary effects on early expression or DNA replication. Mutants have been described which delete the major late 5'-cap site (*dl*1811, –40 base pairs; *Haegeman* et al. 1979; *dl*1659, –48 base pairs; *Subramanian* 1979; *Piatak* et al. 1981; Fig. 3). The mutants are viable and produce mRNAs with new cap sites. *Piatak* et al. (1981) determined that *dl*1659 directs the production of mRNAs with 5'-ends downstream from the normal major 5'-initiation site. These investigators also examined a second mutant (*dl*1626, –99 base pairs; *Subramanian* 1979; Fig. 3). This mutation does not disturb the sequence encoding the major late cap site, but deletes a segment of DNA encoding the major 19S and 16S mRNA leader sequences. Curiously, this mutant produces mRNAs whose 5'-ends lie upstream from the normal, major initiation site. The most striking new mRNA is a major 19S species initiated several hundred base pairs upstream from the normal, major initiation site. Analysis of additional mutants should clarify what is now a confusing picture of papovavirus late transcriptional control regions.

3.4 Regulation of Polymerase II Transcription

Positive and negative regulatory polypeptides almost certainly play a significant role in regulation of polymerase II initiation. There is considerable in vivo evidence leading to the conclusion that the SV40 early gene product regulates its own synthesis (*Tegtmeyer* 1974; *Tegtmeyer* et al. 1975; *Reed* et al. 1976; *Alwine* et al. 1977; *Khoury* and *May* 1977), and does so most likely by binding to the control region for early mRNA synthesis (*Reed* et al. 1975; *Jessel* et al. 1976; *Tjian* 1978). This autoregulation has recently been demonstrated to occur in vitro and to operate at the level of initiation (*Rio* et al. 1980). These investigators demonstrated that the D2 protein (a hybrid polypeptide containing a short N-terminal fragment of an adenovirus 2 polypeptide fused to the majority of the SV40 T antigen) inhibits synthesis of the SV40 early transcript in HeLa cell extracts while synthesis of SV40 or adenovirus 2 late transcripts was not affected. There are several adenovirus early gene products which also appear to regulate transcription in vivo. For example, an E1A gene product appears to be a positive regulator of other early regions (*Berk* et al. 1979; *Jones* and *Shenk* 1979b) and the EIIA gene product may be a negative regulator of EIV transcription (*Nevins* and *Winkler* 1980). Cell-free extracts may facilitate analysis of the mechanisms by which these gene products regulate transcription as was the case for the SV40 T antigen.

Initiation of transcription by polymerase II is also likely to be regulated at the level of chromatin structure. Several types of experiments indicate that genes which are actively transcribed have a different chromatin conformation than those which are silent. Genes which are actively transcribed within a cell (e.g., globin genes in a reticulocyte cell) are preferentially transcribed when *E. coli* or eukaryotic RNA polymerases are added to cellular chromatin, suggesting they are more accessible (*Axel* et al. 1973; *Gilmour* and *Paul* 1973; *Barrett* et al. 1974; *Steggles* et al. 1974). The same genes are also more accessible to digestion by DNase I (*Garel* and *Axel* 1976; *Weintraub* and *Groudine* 1976). This type of experiment, of course, must be interpreted cautiously when building regulatory models, since the altered chromatin conformation could be either the cause or effect of active transcription. Recently, *Wu* (1980) and *Keene* et al. (1981) have demonstrated that the 5'-ends of *Drosophila* heat-shock genes are hypersensitive to DNase I digestion. This focuses the altered chromatin structure to potential polymerase II initiation sites. There is an analogous "open" region on SV40 chromatin which, intriguingly, maps to the region including early and late transcriptional control regions (*Scott* and *Wigmore* 1978; *Varshavsky* et al. 1978; *Waldeck* et al. 1978; *Sundin* and *Varshavsky* 1979; *Varshavsky* et al. 1979; *Jakobovits* et al. 1980). Finally, there have recently been reports which indicate that nucleosomes are not arranged randomly on DNA, but exhibit a phase relationship with respect to DNA sequence (*Musich* et al. 1977; *Ponder* and *Crawford* 1977; *Chao* et al. 1979; *Wittig* and *Wittig* 1979; *Levy* and *Noll* 1980; *Louis* et al. 1980). Phasing could represent an important means of regulating initiation of transcription by positioning critical control sequences in locations within chromatin which are more or less accessible to polymerase and other regulatory factors.

4 Conclusions

The broad outlines of RNA polymerase II and III control regions are now evident. Construction of additional mutants and evaluation of their in vivo and in vitro functions will serve to refine these outlines. Two polypeptides (37K which binds the 5S RNA gene and SV40 T antigen) which interact with transcriptional control elements have already been identified and have provided insights into the mechanism and regulation of transcriptional initiation. Clearly much will be learned as additional components of cell-free extracts are purified and the sites on DNA templates with which they interact are identified. Finally, there are tantalizing hints that chromatin structure may play an important role in transcription. As the structure of chromatin is more thoroughly probed in the vicinity of transcriptional control regions, potential regulatory functions should become more evident.

Acknowledgments. I thank *Mary Fils-Aime* for her capable assistance in the preparation of this manuscript. Thanks are also due my colleagues who kindly sent preprints of their most recent work, and *Pat Hearing* and *John Logan* for critical reading of the review. I am an Established Investigator of the American Heart Association.

References

Akusjärvi G, Mathews MB, Andersson P, Vennstrom B, Pettersson U (1980) Structure of genes for virus-associated RNA$_I$ and RNA$_{II}$ of adenovirus type 2. Proc Natl Acad Sci USA 77:2424–2428

Alwine C, Reed SI, Stark GR (1977) Characterization of the autoregulation of SV40 gene A. J Virol 24:22–27

Axel R, Cedar H, Felsenfeld G (1973) Synthesis of globin RNA from duck-reticulocyte chromatin in vitro. Proc Natl Acad Sci USA 70:2029–2032

Baker CC, Ziff EB (1980) Biogenesis, structures, and sites of encoding of the 5′ termini of adenovirus-2 mRNAs. Cold Spring Harbor Symp Quant Biol 44:415–428

Baker CC, Ziff EB (1981) Promoters and heterogeneous 5′ termini of the messenger RNAs of adenovirus-2. J Mol Biol (in press)

Baker CC, Herisse J, Courtois C, Galibert F, Ziff E (1979) Messenger RNA for the Ad2 DNA binding protein: DNA sequences encoding the first leader and heterogeneity at the mRNAs 5′ end. Cell 18:569–580

Barrett T, Maryanka D, Hamlyn PH, Gould HJ (1974) Nonhistone proteins control gene expression in reconstituted chromatin. Proc Natl Acad Sci USA 71:5057–5061

Bendig MM, Thomas T, Folk WR (1980) Regulatory mutants of polyoma virus defective in DNA replication and the synthesis of early proteins. Cell 20:401–409

Benoist C, Chambon P (1980) Deletions covering the putative promoter region of early mRNAs of simian virus 40 do not abolish T antigen expression. Proc Natl Acad Sci USA 77:3865–3869

Benoist C, O'Hare K, Breathnach R, Chambon P (1980) The ovalbumin gene-sequence of putative control regions. Nucleic Acids Res 8:127–142

Berk AJ, Sharp PA (1977) Ultraviolet mapping of the adenovirus 2 early promoters. Cell 12:45–55

Berk AJ, Sharp PA (1978) Structure of the adenovirus 2 early mRNAs. Cell 14:695–711

Berk AJ, Lee F, Harrison T, Williams J, Sharp PA (1979) Pre-early Ad5 gene product regulates synthesis of early viral mRNAs. Cell 17:935–944

Birkenmeier EH, Brown DD, Jordan E (1978) A nuclear extract of Xenopus laevis oocytes that accurately transcribes 5S RNA genes. Cell 15:1077–1086

Bogenhagen DF, Sakonju S, Brown DD (1980) A control region in the center of the 5S RNA gene directs specific initiation of transcription: II. The 3′ border of the region. Cell 19:27–35

Brown KD, Bennett GN, Lee F, Schweingruber ME, Yanofsky C (1978) RNA polymerase interaction at the promoter-operator region of the tryptophan operon of *E. coli S. typhimurium*. J Mol Biol 121:153–177

Buchman AR, Burnett L, Berg P (1980) In: Tooze J (ed) DNA tumor viruses. Cold Spring Harbor Laboratory, New York, pp 799–829

Busslinger M, Portmann R, Irminger JC, Birnstiel M (1980) Ubiquitous and gene-specific regulatory 5′ sequences in a sea urchin histone DNA clone coding for histone protein variants. Nucleic Acids Res 8:957–978

Canaani D, Kahana C, Mukamel A, Groner Y (1979) Sequence heterogeneity at the 5′ termini of late simian virus 40 19S and 16S mRNAs. Proc Natl Acad Sci USA 76:3078–3082

Celma ML, Pan J, Weissman SM (1977) Studies of low molecular weight RNA from cells infected with adenovirus 2. II. Heterogeneity at the 5′ end of VA-RNA I. J Biol Chem 252:9043–9046

Chao MV, Gralla J, Martinson HG (1979) DNA sequence directs placement of histone cores on restriction fragments during nucleosome formation. Biochemistry 8:1068–1074

Chow LT, Broker TR, Lewis JB (1979) Complex splicing patterns of RNAs from the early regions of adenovirus-2. J Mol Biol 134:265–303

Cochet M, Gannon F, Hen R, Maroteaux L, Perrin F, Chambon P (1979) Organization and sequence studies of the 17-piece chicken conalbumin gene. Nature 282:567–574

Contreras R, Fiers W (1981) Initiation of transcription by RNA polymerase II in permeable, SV-40-infected or noninfected CV1 cells: evidence for multiple promotors of SV40 late transcription. Nucleic Acids Res 9:215–236

Corden J, Wasylyk B, Buchwalder A, Sassone-Corsi P, Kedinger C, Chambon P (1980) Promoter sequences of eukaryotic protein-coding genes. Science 209:1406–1414

DeFranco D, Schmidt O, Soll D (1980) The control regions for eukaryotic tRNA gene transcription. Proc Natl Acad Sci USA 77:3365–3368

Denis H, Wegnez M (1973) Recherches biochimiques sur l'oogenese. 7. Synthese et maturation du RNA 5S dans les petis oocytes de Xenopus laevis. Biochimie 55:1137–1151

Duncan CH, Jagadeeswaran P, Wang RRC, Weissman SM (1981) Alu family RNA polymerase III transcriptional units interspersed in human beta-like globin genes: structural analysis of templates and transcripts. Gene 13:185–196

Efstratiadis A, Posakony J, Maniatis T, Lawn R, O'Connell C, Spiritz R, DeRiel J, Forget B, Weissman S, Slightom J, Blechl A, Smithies O, Baralle F, Shoulders C, Proudfoot N (1980) The structure and evolution of the human β-globin gene family. Cell 21:653–668

Engelke DR, Ng S-Y, Shastry BS, Roeder RG (1980) Specific interaction of a purified transcription factor with an internal control region of 5S RNA genes. Cell 19:717–728

Evans R, Fraser N, Ziff E, Weber J, Wilson M, Darnell J (1977) The initiation sites for RNA transcription in Ad2 DNA. Cell 12:733–739

Felsenfeld G (1978) Chromatin. Nature 271:115–121

Ferdinand FJ, Brown M, Khoury G (1977) Characterization of early SV40 transcriptional complexes: late transcription in the absence of detectable DNA replication. Proc Natl Acad Sci USA 74:5443–5447

Fiers W, Contreras R, Haegeman G, Rogiers R, Van de Voorde A, Van Heuverswyn H, Van Herreweghe J, Volckaert G, Ysebaert M (1978) Complete nucleotide sequence of SV40 DNA. Nature 273:113–120

Flavell A, Cowie A, Legon S, Kamen R (1979) Multiple 5′-terminal cap structures in late polyoma virus RNA. Cell 16:357–371

Flavell AJ, Cowie A, Arrand JR, Kamen R (1980) Localization of three major capped 5′ ends of polyoma virus late mRNAs within a single tetranucleotide sequence in the viral genome. J Virol 33:902–908

Ford PJ, Brown DD (1976) Sequences of 5S ribosomal DNA from Xenopus mulleri and the evolution of 5S gene-coding sequences. Cell 8:485–493

Ford JP, Hsu M-T (1978) Transcription pattern of in vivo-labeled late simian virus 40 RNA: equimolar transcription beyond the mRNA 3′ terminus. J Virol 28:795–801

Fowlkes DM, Shenk T (1980) Transcriptional control regions of the adenovirus VAI RNA gene. Cell 22:405–413

Fraser NW, Sehgal PB, Darnell JE (1978) DRB-induced premature termination of late adenovirus transcription. Nature 272:590–593

Fraser NW, Sehgal PB, Darnell JE (1979) Multiple discrete sites for premature RNA chain termination late in adenovirus-2 infection: enhancement by 5, 6-dichloro-β-D-ribofuranosylbenzimidazole. Proc Natl Acad Sci USA 76:2571–2575

Furuichi Y, Shatkin A (1976) Differential synthesis of blocked and unblocked 5′ termini in reovirus mRNA: effect of pyrophosphate and pyrophosphatase. Proc Natl Acad Sci 73:3448–3452

Furuichi Y, Muthukrishnan S, Tomasz J, Shatkin AJ (1976) Mechanism of formation of reovirus mRNA 5′-terminal blocked and methylated sequence, m^7GpppG^mpC. J Biol Chem 251:5043–5053

Galas DJ, Schmitz A (1978) DNAase footprinting: a simple method for the detection of protein-DNA binding specificity. Nucleic Acids Res 5:3157–3170

Gannon F, O'Hare K, Perrin F, LePennec JP, Benoist C, Cochet M, Breathnach R, Royal A, Garapin A, Cami B, Chambon P (1979) Organization and sequences at the 5' end of a cloned complete ovalbumin gene. Nature 278:428–434

Garel A, Axel R (1976) Selective digestion of transcriptionally active ovalbumin gene from oviduct nuclei. Proc Natl Acad Sci USA 73:3966–3970

Ghosh PK, Lebowitz P, Frisque RJ, Gluzman Y (1981) Identification of a promoter component involved in positioning the 5'-termini of the simian virus 40 early mRNAs. Proc Natl Acad Sci USA 78:100–104

Ghosh P, Reddy V, Swinscoe J, Lebowitz P, Weissman S (1978) The heterogeneity and 5'-terminal structures of the late RNAs of SV40. J Mol Biol 126:813–846

Gilbert W (1976) In: Losick R, Chamberlin M (eds) RNA polymerase. Cold Spring Harbor Laboratory, New York, pp 193–205

Gilmour RS, Paul J (1973) Tissue-Specific transcription of the globin gene in isolated chromatin. Proc Natl Acad Sci USA 70:3440–3442

Gluzman Y, Sambrook JF, Frisque RJ (1980) Expression of early genes of origin-defective mutants of SV40. Proc Natl Acad Sci USA 77:3898–3902

Goldberg S, Weber J, Darnell JE (1977) The definition of a large viral transcription unit late in Ad2 infection of HeLa cells: mapping by effect of ultraviolet irradiation. Cell 10:617–621

Groner Y, Hurwitz J (1975) Synthesis of RNA containing a methylated blocked 5' terminus by HeLa nuclear homogenates. Proc Natl Acad Sci USA 72:2930–2934

Grosschedl R, Birnstiel ML (1980) Identification of regulatory sequences in the prelude sequences of an H2A histone gene by the study of specific deletion mutants in vivo. Proc Natl Acad Sci USA 77:1432–1436

Gruss P, Dhar R, Khoury G (1981) The SV40 tandem repeats as an element of the early promoter. Proc Natl Acad Sci USA 78:943–947

Gruss P, Khoury G (1981) Expression of SV40 rat preproinsulin recombinants in monkey kidney cells: use of preproinsulin RNA processing signals. Proc Natl Acad Sci USA 78:133–137

Guilfoyle R, Weinmann R (1981) The control region for adenovirus VA RNA transcription. Proc Natl Acad Sci USA (in press)

Haegeman G, Fiers W (1978) Localization of the 5' terminus of late SV40 mRNA. Nucleic Acids Res 5:2359–2371

Haegeman G, Fiers W (1980) Characterization of the 5'-terminal cap structures of early simian virus 40 mRNA. J Virol 35:955–961

Haegeman G, Van Heuverswyn H, Gheysen D, Fiers W (1979) Heterogeneity of the 5' terminus of late mRNA induced by a viable SV40 deletion mutant. J Virol 31:484–493

Hamer DH, Leder P (1979) Expression of the chromosomal mouse β-major-globin gene cloned in SV40. Nature 281:35–40

Harada F, Ikawa Y (1979) A new series of RNAs associated with the genome of spleen focus forming virus (SFFV) and poly(A)-containing RNA from SFFV-infected cells. Nucleic Acids Res 7:895–908

Harada F, Kato N, Hoshino H (1979) Series of 4.5S RNAs associated with poly(A)-containing RNAs of rodent cells. Nucleic Acids Res 7:909–917

Harada S, Kato N (1980) Nucleotide sequences of 4.5S RNA associated with polyA-containing RNAs of mouse and hamster cells. Nucleic Acids Res 8:1273–1285

Hentschel C, Irminger JC, Bucher P, Birnstiel M (1980) Sea urchin histone mRNA termini are located in gene regions downstream from putative regulatory sequences. Nature 285:147–151

Hofer E, Darnell JE (1981) The primary transcription unit of the mouse β-major globin gene. Cell 23:585–593

Honda BM, Roeder RG (1980) Association of a 5S gene transcription factor with 5S RNA and altered levels of the factor during cell differentiation. Cell 22:119–126

Honda H, Kaufman RJ, Manley J, Gefter M, Sharp PA (1980) Transcription of SV40 in a HeLa whole cell extract. J Biol Chem 256:478–482

Houck CM, Rinehart FP, Schmid CW (1979) A ubiquitous family of repeated DNA sequences in the human genome. J Mol Biol 132:289–306

Hu S-L, Manley J (1981) DNA sequence required for initiation of transcription in vitro from the major promoter of adenovirus-2. Proc Natl Acad Sci USA 78:820–824

Jakobovits EB, Bratosin S, Aloni Y (1980) A nucleosome-free region in SV40 minichromosomes. Nature 285:263–265

Jelinek W, Leinwand L (1978) Low molecular weight RNAs hydrogen-bonded to nuclear and cyto-plasmic poly(A)-terminated RNA from cultured chinese hamster ovary cells. Cell 15:205-214

Jessel D, Landau T, Hudson J, Lalor T, Tenen D, Livingston DM (1976) Identification of regions of the SV40 genome which contain preferred SV40 T antigen-binding sites. Cell 8:535-545

Jones N, Shenk T (1979a) Isolation of Ad5 host range deletion mutants defective for transformation of rat embryo cells. Cell 17:683-689

Jones N, Shenk T (1979b) An adenovirus type 5 early gene function regulates expression of other early viral genes. Proc Natl Acad Sci USA 76:3665-3669

Katinka M, Yaniv M, Vasseur M, Blangy D (1980) Expression of polyoma early functions in mouse embryonal carcinoma cells depends on sequence rearrangements in the beginning of the late region. Cell 20:393-399

Keene MA, Corces V, Lowenhaupt K, Elgin SRB (1981) DNase I hypersensitive sites in *Drosophila* chromatin occur at the 5'-ends of regions of transcription. Proc Natl Acad Sci USA 78:143-146

Khoury G, May E (1977) Regulation of early and late SV40 transcription: overproduction of early viral RNA in the absence of a functional T antigen. J Virol 77:167-176

Konkel D, Tilghman S, Leder P (1978) The sequence of the chromosomal mouse β-globin major gene: homologies in capping, splicing and poly A sites. Cell 15:1125-1132

Korn LJ, Birkenmeier EH, Brown DD (1979) Transcription initiation of Xenopus 5S ribosomal RNA genes in vitro. Nucleic Acids Res 7:947-958

Korn LT, Brown DD (1978) Nucleotide sequence of Xenopus borealis oocyte 5S DNA: comparison of sequences that flank several related eukaryotic genes. Cell 15:1145-1156

Koski RA, Clarkson SG, Kurjan J, Hall BD, Smith M (1980) Mutations of the yeast SUP4 tRNA^{Tyr} locus: Transcription of the mutant genes in vitro. Cell 22:415-425

Kressmann A, Hofstetter H, DiCapua E, Grosschedl R, Birnstiel ML (1979) A tRNA gene of Xeno-pus Laevis contains at least two sites promoting transcription. Nucleic Acids Res 7:1749-1763

Laub O, Bratosin S, Horowitz M, Aloni Y (1979) The initiation of transcription of SV40 DNA at late time after infection. Virology 92:310-323

Lerner MR, Andrews NC, Miller G, Steitz JA (1980) Two small RNAs encoded by Epstein-Barr virus and complexed with protein are precipitated by antibodies from patients with systemic lupus erythematosus. Proc Natl Acad Sci USA 78:805-809

Lerner MR, Boyle JA, Hardin JA, Steitz JA (1981) Two novel classes of small ribonucleoproteins detected by antibodies associated with lupus erythematosus. Science 211:400-402

Levy A, Noll M (1980) Multiple phases of nucleosomes in the hsp 70 genes of *Drosophila melano-gaster*. Nucleic Acids Res 8:6959-6968

Lewis J, Mathews M (1980) Control of adenovirus early gene expression: a class of immediate early products. Cell 21:303-313

Louis C, Schedl P, Sanmal B, Worcel A (1980) Chromatin structure of the 5S RNA genes of *D. melanogaster*. Cell 22:387-392

Luse DS, Roeder RG (1980) Accurate transcription initiation on a purified mouse β-globin DNA fragment in a cell-free system. Cell 20:691-699

Manley JL, Fire A, Cano A, Sharp PA, Gefter ML (1980) DNA-Dependent transcription of adeno-virus genes in a soluble whole-cell extract. Proc Natl Acad Sci USA 77:3855-3859

Manley JL, Sharp PA, Gefter ML (1979) RNA synthesis in isolated nuclei in vitro: initiation of the Ad2 major late mRNA precursor. Proc Natl Acad Sci USA 76:160-164

Matsui T, Segall J, Weil PA, Roeder RG (1980) Multiple factors required for accurate initiation of transcription by purified RNA polymerase II. J Biol Chem 255:11992-11996

McKnight SL (1980) The nucleotide sequence of the herpes simplex thymidine kinase gene. Nucleic Acids Res 8:5949-5964

Minty A, Newmark P (1980) Gene regulation: new, old and remote controls. Nature 288:210-211

Moss B, Gershowitz A, Wei C-M, Boone R (1976) Formation of the guanylylated and methylated 5'-terminus of vaccinia virus mRNA. Virology 72:341-351

Musich PR, Maio JJ, Brown FL (1977) Interactions of a phase relationship between restriction sites and chromatin subunits in African green monkey and calf nuclei. J Mol Biol 117:637-655

Nevins JR, Winkler JJ (1980) Regulations of early adenovirus transcription: a protein product of early region 2 specifically represses region 4 transcription. Proc Natl Acad Sci USA 77:1893-1897

Ng SY, Parker CS, Roeder RG (1979) Transcription of cloned Xenopus 5S RNA genes by X. laevis

RNA polymerase III in reconstituted systems. Proc Natl Acad Sci USA 76:136–140

Osborne TF, Schell RE, Burch-Jaffe E, Berget SJ, Berk AJ (1981) Mapping a eukaryotic promoter: a DNA sequence required for in vivo expression of adenovirus pre-early functions. Proc Natl Acad Sci USA 78:1381–1385

Parker BA, Stark GR (1979) Regulation of SV40 transcription: sensitive analysis of the RNA species present early in infections by virus or viral DNA. J Virol 31:360–369

Pelham HRB, Brown DD (1980) A specific transcription factor that can bind either the 5S RNA gene or 5S RNA. Proc Natl Acad Sci USA 77:4170–4174

Peters GG, Harada F, Dahlberg JE, Panet A, Haseltine WA, Baltimore D (1977) Low-molecular-weight RNAs of Moloney Murine Leukemia Virus: identification of primer for RNA-directed DNA synthesis. J Virol 21:1031–1041

Piatak M, Subramanian KN, Roy P, Weissman SM (1981) Late mRNA production by viable SV40 mutants with deletions in the leader region. J Mol Biol (in press)

Piper PW (1979) Polyoma virus transcription early during productive infection of mouse 3T6 cells. J Mol Biol 131:399–407

Ponder BAJ, Crawford LV (1977) The arrangement of nucleosomes in nucleoprotein complexes from polyoma virus and SV40. Cell 11:35–49

Pribnow D (1975) Bacteriophage T7 early promoters: nucleotide sequences of two RNA polymerase binding sites. J Mol Biol 99:419–443

Price P, Penman S (1972) A distinct RNA polymerase activity, synthesizing 5.5S, 5S and 4S RNA in nuclei from Ad2-infected HeLa cells. J Mol Biol 70:435–450

Reddy VB, Ghosh PK, Lebowitz P, Weissman SM (1978a) Gaps and duplicated sequences in the leaders of SV40 16S RNA. Nucleic Acids Res 5:4195–4214

Reddy VB, Thimmappaya B, Dhar R, Subramanian KN, Zain S, Pan J, Ghosh PK, Celma ML, Weissman SM (1978b) The genome of SV40. Science 200:494–502

Reddy VB, Ghosh P, Lebowitz P, Piatak M, Weissman SM (1979) Simian virus 40 early mRNAs: genomic localization of 3' and 5' termini and two major splices in mRNA from transformed and lytically infected cells. J Virol 30:279–296

Reed S, Ferguson J, Davis RW, Stark GR (1975) T-Antigen binds to SV40 DNA at the origin of DNA replication. Proc Natl Acad Sci USA 72:1605–1609

Reed SI, Stark GR, Alwine JC (1976) Autoregulation of SV40 gene A by T antigen. Proc Natl Acad Sci USA 73:3083–3087

Rio D, Robbins A, Myers R, Tjian R (1980) Regulation of simian virus 40 early transcription in vitro by a purified tumor antigen. Proc Natl Acad Sci USA 77:5706–5710

Roeder RG (1976) Eukaryotic nuclear RNA polymerase. In: Losick R, Chamberlin M (eds) RNA Polymerase, Cold Spring Harbor, New York

Sakonju S, Bogenhagen DF, Brown DD (1980) A control region in the center of the 5S RNA gene directs specific initiation of transcription: I. The 5' border of the region. Cell 19:13–25

Schmitz A, Galas DJ (1979) The interaction of RNA polymerase and lac repressor with the lac control region. Nucleic Acids Res 6:111–137

Scott WA, Wigmore DJ (1978) Sites in simian virus 40 chromatin which are preferentially cleaved by endonucleases. Cell 15:1511–1518

Shatkin AJ (1978) Capping of eukaryotic mRNAs. Cell 9:646–653

Segall J, Matsui T, Roeder RG (1980) Multiple factors are required for the accurate transcription of purified genes by RNA polymerase III. J Biol Chem 255:11986–11991

Sehgal PB, Fraser NW, Darnell JE (1979) Early Ad2 transcription units: only promoter-proximal RNA continues to be made in the presence of DRB. Virology 94:185–191

Sekikawa K, Levine AJ (1981) Isolation and characterization of polyoma host range mutants that replicate in multipotential embryonal carcinoma cells. Proc Natl Sci USA 18:1100–1104

Shaw AR, Ziff EB (1980) Transcripts from the adenovirus-2 major late promoter yield a single family of 3' coterminal mRNAs during early infection and five families at late times. Cell 22:905–916

Shenk TE, Carbon J, Berg P (1976) Construction and analysis of viable deletion mutants of SV40. J Virol 18:664–671

Siebenlist U, Simpson RB, Gilbert W (1980) E. coli RNA polymerase interacts homologously with two different promoters. Cell 20:269–281

Simpson RB (1979) Contacts between E. coli RNA polymerase and thymines in the lac UV5 promoter. Proc Natl Acad Sci USA 76:3233–3237

Soderlund H, Pettersson U, Venstrom B, Philipson L, Mathews MB (1976) A new species of virus-coded low molecular weight RNA from cells infected with Ad2. Cell 7:585–593

Soeda E, Arrand JR, Smolar N, Walsh JE, Griffin BE (1980) Coding potential and regulatory signals of the polyoma virus genome. Nature 283:445–453

Spencer E, Loring J, Hurwitz J, Monroy G (1978) Enzymatic conversion of 5′-phosphate-terminated RNA to 5′-di- and triphosphate-terminated RNA. Proc Natl Acad Sci USA 75:4793–4797

Sprague KU, Larson D, Morton D (1980) 5′ flanking sequence signals are required for activity of silkworm alanine tRNA genes in homologous in vitro transcription systems. Cell 22:171–178

Sprinzl M, Grueter F, Spelzhaus A, Gauss DH (1980) Compilation of tRNA sequences. Nucleic Acids Res 8:r1-r22

Steggles AW, Wilson GN, Kantor JA, Picciano DJ, Falvey AK, Anderson WF (1974) Cell-free transcription of mammalian chromatin: transcription of globin mRNA sequences from bone-marrow chromatin with mammalian RNA polymerase. Proc Natl Acad Sci USA 71:1219–1223

Subramanian KN (1979) Segments of simian virus 40 DNA spanning most of the leader sequences of the major late viral mRNA are dispensable. Proc Natl Acad Sci USA 76:2556–2560

Subramanian K, Shenk T (1978) Definition of the boundaries of the SV40 origin of DNA replication. Nucleic Acids Res 5:3635–3642

Sundin O, Varshavsky A (1979) Staphylococcal nuclease makes a single non-random cut in the simian virus 40 minichromosome. J Mol Biol 132:535–546

Tegtmeyer P (1974) Altered patterns of protein synthesis in infection by SV40 mutants. Cold Spring Harbor Symp Quant Biol 39:9–16

Tegtmeyer P, Schwartz M, Collins JK, Rundell K (1975) Regulation of tumor antigen synthesis by simian virus 40 gene A. J Virol 16:168–178

Telford JL, Kressmann A, Koski RA, Grosschedl R, Muller F, Clarkson SG, Birnstiel ML (1979) Delimitation of a promoter for RNA polymerase III by means of a functional test

Thimmappaya B, Jones N, Shenk T (1979) A mutation which alters initiation of transcription by RNA polymerase III on the Ad5 chromosome. Cell 18:947–954

Thompson JA, Radonovich MF, Salzman NP (1979) Characterization of the 5′-terminal structure of SV40 early mRNAs. J Virol 31:437–446

Tjian R (1978) The binding site on SV40 DNA for a T antigen-related protein. Cell 13:165–179

Tjian R (1979) Protein-DNA interactions at the origin of SV40 DNA replication. Cold Spring Harbor Symp Quant Biol 43:655–662

Van Heuverswyn H, Fiers W (1979) Nucleotide sequence of the *Hind-C* fragment of SV40 DNA. Eur J Biochem 100:51–60

Van Ormondt H, Maat J, DeWaard A, Van der Eb AJ (1978) The nucleotide sequence of the transforming HpaI-E fragment of adenovirus type 5 DNA. Gene 4:309–328

Varshavsky AJ, Sundin OH, Bohn MJ (1978) SV40 viral minichromosome: preferential exposure of the origin of replication as probed by restriction endonuclease. Nucleic Acids Res 5:3469–3478

Varshavsky AJ, Sundin O, Bohn M (1979) A stretch of "late" SV40 viral DNA about 400 bp long which includes the origin of replication is specifically exposed in SV40 minichromosomes. Cell 16:453–466

Waldeck W, Fohring B, Chowdhurg K, Gruss P, Sauer G (1978) Origin of DNA replication in papovavirus chromatin is recognized by endogenous endonuclease. Proc Natl Acad Sci USA 75:5964–5968

Wasylyk B, Derbyshire R, Guy A, Molko D, Roget A, Teolue R, Chambon P (1980a) Specific in vitro transcription of conalbumin gene is drastically decreased by a single-point mutation in TATA box homology sequence. Proc Natl Acad Sci USA 77:7024–7028

Wasylyk B, Kedinger C, Corden J, Brinson O, Chambon P (1980b). Specific in vitro initiation of transcription on conalbumin and ovalbumin genes and comparison with adenovirus-2 early and late genes. Nature 285:367–373

Weber J, Jelinek W, Darnell JE (1977) The definition of a large viral transcription unit late in Ad2 infection of HeLa cells: mapping of nascent RNA molecules labeled in isolated nuclei. Cell 10:611–616

Wei C-M, Moss B (1977) 5′ terminal capping of RNA by guanylyltransferase from HeLa cell nuclei. Proc Natl Acad Sci USA 74:3758–3762

Weil PA, Luse DS, Segall J, Roeder RG (1979a) Selective and accurate initiation of transcription at the Ad2 major late promoter in a soluble system dependent on purified RNA polymerase II and DNA. Cell 18:469-484

Weil PA, Segall J, Harris B, Ng S-Y, Roeder RG (1979b) Faithful transcription of eukaryotic genes by RNA polymerase III in systems reconstituted with purified DNA templates. J Biol Chem 254:6163-6173

Weintraub H, Groudine M (1976) Chromosomal subunits in active genes have an altered conformation. Science 93:848-858

Wilson MC, Fraser NW, Darnell JE (1979) Mapping of RNA initiation sites by high doses of UV irradiation: evidence for three independent promoters within the left 11% of the Ad2 genome. Virology 94:175-184

Winicov I, Perry RP (1976) Synthesis, methylation and capping of nuclear RNA by a subcellular system. Biochemistry 15:5039-5046

Wittig B, Wittig S (1979) A phase relationship associates tRNA structural gene sequences with nucleosome cores. Cell 18:1173-1183

Wu C (1980) The 5' ends of *Drosophila* heat shock genes in chromatin are hypersensitive to DNase I. Nature 286:854-860

Wu GJ (1978) Adenovirus DNA-directed transcription of 5.5S RNA in vitro. Proc Natl Acad Sci USA 75:2175-2179

Yamamoto T, Jay G, Pastan I (1980b) Unusual features in the nucleotide sequence of a cDNA clone derived from the common region of avian sarcoma virus mRNA. Proc Natl Acad Sci USA 77: 176-180

Yamamoto T, deCrombrugghe B, Pastan I (1980a) Identification of a functional promoter in the long terminal repeat of Rous sarcoma virus. Cell 22:787-797

Ziff E, Evans R (1978) Coincidence of the promoter and capped 5' terminus of RNA from the adenovirus-2 major late transcription unit. Cell 15:1463-1475

Splicing and the Regulation of Viral Gene Expression

S.J. FLINT*

1   The Structure and Synthesis of Spliced Viral mRNA Species 47
1.1   Spliced Viral mRNA Species Which Share Translated Sequences 48
1.1.1 mRNA Structure 48
1.1.2 Mechanism of mRNA Synthesis 55
1.2   Spliced Viral mRNA Species that Do not Share Translated Sequences   56

2   The Mechanism of Splicing. 64
2.1   Splicing Signals in Viral RNA 64
2.2   Components of the Splicing Machinery   67

References   70

1 The Structure and Synthesis of Spliced Viral mRNA Species

Spliced viral mRNA species are synthesized in permissive cells infected by several viruses that possess DNA genomes, such as the parvoviruses, papovaviruses, and adenoviruses, or by those whose life cycle depends on synthesis of a double-stranded DNA copy of an RNA genome, the retroviruses. Splicing also seems to play a part in the expression of at least one gene included in the genome of a conventional RNA virus, influenza A. Splicing of colinear products of transcription of viral genetic information constructs mRNA species from sequences complementary to noncontiguous regions in the genome. In this sense, splicing of viral and of cellular mRNA precursors are completely analogous. However, transcripts of viral genes, when spliced, always seem to be able to follow alternative processing pathways, each characterized by a unique splicing event. In general, then, splicing permits the synthesis of more than one mRNA species from each product of transcription of viral genetic information.

Two distinct patterns of posttranscriptional processing of viral RNA species, each with quite different consequences, may be distinguished within this framework. Splicing of a processing intermediate may occur within potential protein coding sequences; alternatively, it may serve to join small sets of sequences located at or near the 5'-end of the primary transcript, so-called leaders, to optional sets of coding sequences, which are themselves usually continuous. The first mechanism creates overlapping mRNA species that share some, but not all, of their coding sequences. By contrast, mRNA species tailored by the second kind of splicing mechanism possess short 5'-terminal sequences in common, but, in principle, need not share any additional sequences. The spliced viral mRNA species whose structures have been elucidated fall into one or other of these two

* Princeton University, Dept. of Biochemical Sciences, Princeton, New Jersey 08540, USA

categories, which will be considered separately to facilitate comparisons among different viral systems.

1.1 Spliced Viral mRNA Species Which Share Translated Sequences

1.1.1 mRNA Structure

Viruses suffer some constraints upon the physical size of their genomes (usually considered to be the result of packing limitations) and frequently provide striking examples of efficient molecular organization: very little of the available nucleotide sequence is not informational in one way or another. Some prokaryotic viruses appear to have successfully evolved an additional degree of molecular efficiency, the use of two reading frames in the same stretch of nucleic acid sequence to specify two unrelated polypeptides. This device has been adopted by viruses that possess either DNA (*Barrell* et al. 1976; *Sanger* et al. 1977) or RNA (*Atkins* et al. 1979; *Beremond* and *Blumenthal* 1979; *Model* et al. 1979) genomes. Among animal viruses, posttranscriptional splicing, which may or may not lead to a shift in the frame in which an RNA species is translated, can elicit a similar outcome.

The early region of the SV40 genome, 0.66–0.154 map units (see Fig. 1A), for example, encodes two polypeptides of apparent molecular weights 94–100,000 daltons and 15–17,000 daltons, large and small T antigens. These polypeptides can be immunoprecipitated from extracts of SV40-infected or -transformed cells or from the products of in vitro translation of SV40 early mRNA by sera from animals bearing SV40-induced tumors (*Prives* et al. 1977; *Paucha* et al. 1977). The two T antigens possess in common methionine-containing tryptic peptides (*Crawford* et al. 1978; *Smith* et al. 1978) located at their N-termini (*Paucha* et al. 1978; *Mellor* and *Smith* 1978; *Simmons* and *Martin* 1978, *Linke* et al. 1979). The mRNA species from which the large and small T antigens are translated must therefore share some coding sequences. Both proteins, however, also generate unique peptides upon trypsin digestion and therefore cannot share all their coding sequences. The arrangement of SV40 early coding sequences shown in Figure 1 was deduced from the observation that SV40 mutants carrying deletions within the region 0.59–0.54 map units synthesize perfectly normal large T antigen, but either fail to synthesize any small T antigen or specify polypeptides of decreased size (*Crawford* et al. 1978; *Sleigh* et al. 1978). Clearly, then, sequences between 0.59 and 0.54 units in the genome cannot contribute to the amino acid sequence of large T antigen, but must be expressed in small T antigen. The arrangement of SV40 early coding sequences must therefore be that shown in Figure 1: the two SV40 T-antigen polypeptides are translated from mRNA species that differ in the ways in which they are spliced (*Berk* and *Sharp* 1978a; *Reddy* et al. 1979a; *Thompson* et al. 1979).

As illustrated in Figure 1.1, both SV40 early mRNA species contain sequences complementary to two common sets of genomic sequences, from their 5′-termini at 0.66–0.60 units and from 0.533 units to their shared poly(A) site at 0.154, or in the SV40 DNA sequence as numbered by *Buchman* et al. (1980), (in which numbering proceeds from the centremost nucleotide of the 27 base-pair palindromic sequence containing the one *Bgl* 1 site at 0.67 units in a clockwise direction) nucleotides 5163–4918 inclusive and nucleotides 4571–2586, a polyadenylation site. The smaller mRNA contains only these se-

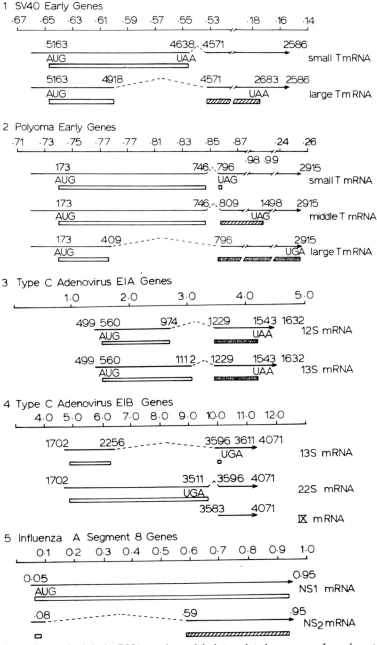

Fig. 1. Coterminal viral mRNA species and their translated sequences. In each part of the figure, the viral genome is represented as the topmost horizontal line divided into map units. The mRNA species are drawn as continuous lines, with arrowheads in the direction of transcription. Sequences deleted from primary products of transcription by splicing are indicated by the caret symbols. The sequences actually translated from each mRNA are represented by the boxes drawn below each mRNA species. To illustrate the frames used for translation, the frame read in the 5′-part of the mRNA is open whereas frames shifted by one or two nucleotides relative to the first are shown as stippled and cross-hatched respectively. The sources of these data, and the systems by which the genomic sequences are numbered, are given in the text

quences and is therefore spliced from nucleotide 4918 to nucleotide 4571. In this case, splicing removes 346 nucleotides (4917–4572, inclusive) including A-T rich segments and the region 0.547–0.534 where termination codons block all three reading frames (*Thimmappaya* and *Weissman* 1977; *Volckaert* et al. 1978). Before the splice point at 0.60 units, one reading frame is open from an AUG initiation codon at nucleotide 5146 to the splice point and beyond it; a second frame, shifted by one nucleotide, is open throughout the remainder of the early region to the terminating UAA codon at nucleotide 2693, a total of 705 amino acid codons (*Dhar* et al. 1977; *Thimmappaya* and *Weissman* 1977; *Reddy* et al. 1978a; *Fiers* et al. 1978). This smaller early mRNA species must therefore encode large T antigen. The second mRNA is not spliced at 0.60 units but rather retains sequences from this point to a second donor splice site at 0.564 units, nucleotide 4638 (see Fig. 1.1). This latter nucleotide is joined to the same splice acceptor site at 0.533 units, nucleotide 4571, used in the synthesis of large T-antigen mRNA. Splicing of this larger SV40 early mRNA species thus removes only 66 nucleotides (4637–4572 inclusive) from SV40 early precursor RNA. Moreover, this splicing has no effect upon translation, for such small T-antigen mRNA retains an UAA termination codon, 4635–4638, immediately before the splice point. As a result, the small and large T-antigen polypeptides share N-terminal sequences, but possess unique C-terminal sequences, which neither overlap nor are read in the same frame (see Fig. 1.1).

Not surprisingly, a similar arrangement in which multiple mRNA species share some, but not all, of their coding sequences, is exhibited by the products of the early region of the genome of the related papovavirus, polyoma. The overall organization of the genomes of these two viruses is similar. However, the early region of polyoma DNA encodes not two, but three tumor antigens: that unique to polyoma exhibits an apparent molecular weight of 55–63,000 daltons and has therefore been termed middle T antigen (*Ito* et al. 1977a; *Smart* and *Ito* 1978; *Hutchinson* et al. 1978; *Simmons* et al. 1979). Peptide mapping reveals that all three polyoma T antigens have N-terminal sequence in common, that small and middle T antigens also share a second set of peptides, and that each protein includes unique peptides. Thus, the three T antigens must share some coding sequences, middle and small T antigens must share sequences not represented in large T antigen, and each of the three must contain some archetypal coding sequences. The arrangement of the coding sequences for these three polyoma early products and the structures of the mRNA species from which they are translated have been deduced from the DNA sequence of the polyoma early region (*Friedman* et al. 1979; *Soeda* et al. 1979; 1980), the effects of deletions within the early region upon synthesis of the T antigens in deletion mutant infected cells (*Silver* et al. 1978; *Schaffhausen* et al. 1978; *Ito* et al. 1977b, 1980), and analysis of the size and structure of polyoma mRNA species (*Hunter* et al. 1978; *Kamen* et al. 1980a).

The polyoma large and small T-antigen mRNAs are fashioned in a manner similar, but not completely analogous, to their SV40 counterparts. The smallest polyoma mRNA species encodes large T antigen and is spliced from nucleotide 409 in the DNA sequence (numbered according to *Soeda* et al. 1980 from zero at the point at the centre of the *Hpa* II site at 0.71 units, in a clockwise direction), to nucleotide 795. Splicing to contrive polyoma large T-antigen mRNA species thus removes 385 nucleotides, 410–794 inclusive and shifts the reading frame by one nucleotide beyond the splice point site. To the 5′-side of the splice point, one reading frame, designated frame 1, is open from nucleotide 173 to the splice site; beyond it, frame 2 is open for translation throughout the early region to a termination codon at 2913 (see Fig. 1.2). Thus, polyoma large T-antigen mRNA contains codons for 785 amino acid residues. As with SV40, the polyoma small T-antigen mRNA is not spliced at the same donor site as the large T mRNA, but contains sequences from the common 5′-end of the early mRNA species to a second donor site at nucleotide 746, which is ligated to the 795 acceptor site (see Fig. 1B). Only 48 nucleotides are therefore removed during biogenesis of small T-antigen mRNA. Moreover, this splice does not result in a change of reading frame and small T-antigen mRNA can be read in small T-antigen mRNA, frame 1 before and after the splice point. In this frame a termination codon is encountered at nucleotide 805. Thus, only three amino acid residues are actually encoded beyond the splice point in polyoma small T-antigen mRNA. In this respect, the SV40 and polyoma small T-antigen coding sequences differ slightly; the SV40 small T-antigen mRNA is also spliced, but no information beyond the splice point is actually translated.

A much more substantial difference between the early regions of the polyoma and SV40 genomes is the inclusion of coding sequences for middle T antigen in the former but not the latter DNA. Middle T antigen shares N-terminal sequences with the large and small T-antigen polypeptides, but its mRNA is uniquely spliced, most probably from nucleotide 746 to nucleotide 809, to remove the frame 1 termination codon at which translation of small T antigen halts. Such a splicing event would also result in a shift in the reading frame of two nucleotides, to frame 3 (see Fig. 1.2), as it removes 62 nucleotides. Thus, all three reading frames of the polyoma early region are used to generate three early polypeptides that are cognate, but partially unique.

It is clear from the preceding discussion that splicing of RNA transcripts of the early regions of the genomes of these two papovaviruses mediates a limited realignment of coding sequences such that the DNA sequence is not expressed in simple colinear fashion. The resulting gene products have some amino acid sequences in common, but others are unique. It is easy to infer the advantages of this kind of arrangement, the synthesis of two gene products from one DNA sequence. It would seem reasonable that the papovavirus early gene products perform different functions, for each has a unique primary sequence and consequently higher-order structure. This does indeed seem to be the case: the small T antigen of SV40, for example, is not absolutely required for reproduction of the virus (*Shenk* et al. 1976), whereas large T antigen is (*Lai* and *Nathans* 1975; *Cole* et al. 1977). The various T antigens also appear to fulfill separate roles in transformation, although the precise nature of these is not yet fully appreciated (*Kelly* and *Nathan* 1977; *Schlegel* and *Benjamin* 1978; *Sleigh* et al. 1978; *Martin* et al. 1979; *Seif* and *Martin* 1979; *Lewis* and *Martin* 1979; *Fluck* and *Benjamin* 1979; *Seif* 1980; *Ito* et al. 1980).

Similar consequences follow posttranscription splicing of RNA species transcribed from the genomes of at least two other groups of animal viruses, the adenoviruses and the orthomyxoviruses. The structures of mRNA species complementary to the five regions of the type 2 adenovirus genome, expressed at high frequency during the early phase of productive infection, have been determined by both electron microscopic examination of hybrids formed between adenoviral early RNA and DNA (*Kitchingman* et al. 1977; *Chow* et al. 1979; *Kitchingman* and *Westphal* 1980) and the nuclease S1-assay (*Berk* and *Sharp* 1978b). As illustrated in Figure 2, each of the five regions is expressed in two or more mRNA species and quite complex patterns of mRNA products are evident. Most striking are those complementary to regions E3 and E4; in each case six or seven individual mRNA species that share different extents and regions of the DNA sequence.

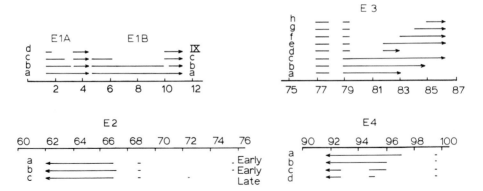

Fig. 2. Multiple mRNA species encoded by adenoviral early genes. For each of the five adenoviral early regions shown, viral DNA is represented as a solid horizontal line divided into map units. The mRNA species complementary to each region are depicted as horizontal arrows, drawn in the direction of transcription. Sequences deleted during splicing are indicated by gaps. The sources of these data are given in the text. In addition to the mRNA species shown, other minor forms have been described (*Chow* et al. 1979). Those complementary to region 2 include (i) forms of E2a and E2c with a small splice at 66.3 units, (ii) minor forms with a 5′-leader at 86.2–86.7 units, and (iii) very rare forms that carry both early and late leader sequences. Those transcribed from region E3 include unspliced forms of E3a and E3c, whereas minor species with variant splices are also complementary to region E4

No one E3 and E4 mRNA comprises a majority among the populations depicted in Figure 2 (*Chow* et al. 1979), suggesting that the number of distinct polypeptides specified by these two early regions may be quite substantial. Multiple viral polypeptides have been assigned to each of regions E3 and E4 (*Lewis* et al. 1976; *Persson* et al. 1978; *Wold* and *Green* 1979; *Ross* et al. 1980), but fewer polypeptides than mRNA species encoded by each region have been identified so far. At the present time, E3 and E4 polypeptides described have neither been ascribed to individual mRNA species, nor analysed for their sequence relationships. Nevertheless, analogy with the arrangement of papovavirus early coding sequences strongly suggests that splicing of primary transcripts of the adenoviral E3 and E4 genes generates several partially related mRNA species, and therefore polypeptides, from the original colinear RNA product; adenoviral E3 and E4 genes simply appear to present a rather extreme example of this phenomenon.

In considering early region 1 of the group C (serotypes 2 and 5) adenoviral genome, we return to a pattern of viral mRNA species more akin to that of the papovaviruses. As depicted in Figure 1.3, early region E1A, 0.8–4.4 units, like E3 and E4, encodes several mRNA species but these exhibit a simple relationship to one another; they are both 3′- and 5′-coterminal and differ in the amount of internal information removed when they are spliced. This family of adenoviral early mRNA species, as well as those complementary to early region E1B, 4.6–11.3 units, thus resemble the papovaviral early RNAs.

The major mRNA species complementary to region E1A made at early times during productive infection, which exhibit sedimentation coefficients of 13S and 12S (*Spector* et al. 1978; *Wilson* et al. 1978), have been sequenced from cloned cDNA copies (*Perricaudet* et al. 1979). The precise arrangements of coding sequences has been deduced from comparison of mRNA sequences with that of the left-hand end of type C adenovirus DNA (*van Ormondt* et al. 1978; *Maat* and *van Ormondt* 1979). The two major type C adenoviral E1A mRNA species share sequences from nucleotide 499 (*Baker* and *Ziff* 1980) (the sequence being numbered from left to right, from the left-hand end) to nucleotide 974. The 13S mRNA also includes sequences from nucleotide 975 to nucleotide 1112, but these are absent from the smaller early mRNA. Both splice donor sites, at nucleotides 975 and 1112, are joined to an acceptor site at nucleotide 1229 and the two mRNAs are then colinear to a polyadenylation site at nucleotide 1632. Thus, splicing removes from both E1A early mRNA species RNA copies of the region 1113–1228 nucleotides which, like some of the sequences spliced out of SV40 transcripts, are rich in A-T residues and contains many translational termination codons. These splicing events remove 116 and 254 nucleotides to create the 13S and 12S mRNAs respectively, and thus induce a change in reading frame beyond the splice point in both cases (see Fig. 1.3); nevertheless, the same reading frame is translated in the 3′-segment of the two mRNA species. Their polypeptide products therefore differ only by the presence of an additional, internal set of 45 amino acids, specified by residues 974–1111 inclusive, in the protein specified by the larger mRNA species. The organization of the major early mRNA species specified by regions E1A of the type 12 and type 7 adenoviruses (members of subgroups A and B respectively) appear to be quite similar to that of adenovirus type 2 or 5, although the smaller Ad12 mRNA has its donor splice site shifted 45 nucleotides to the right compared to its type C adenovirus counterpart (*Perricaudet* et al. 1980b; *Yoshida* and *Fujinaga* 1980; *Sugisaki* et al. 1980).

It has been appreciated for some time that region E1A in the adenoviral genome encodes several (four to six) related polypeptides (*Lewis* et al. 1976; *Harter* and *Lewis* 1978; *Halbert* et al. 1979; *van der Eb* et al. 1980). These exhibit apparent molecular weights of 42–53,000 Mr, much greater than the coding capacities of the E1A 13S and 12S mRNA species, calculated to be 32,000 and 26,000 Mr respectively (*Perricaudet* et al. 1979). This discrepancy might reflect posttranslational modification of the proteins or their aberrant migration in SDS-polyacrylamide gels, the result of an unusually high content of proline and glutamic acid residues. Some mutations have been introduced specifically into E1A sequences expressed only in the 13S mRNA (*N. Jones,* personal communication), but the polypeptides of E1A have not yet been assigned functional roles. It is clear, however, that the products of this early region participate in several steps of the productive cycle, including synthesis of viral DNA and expression as stable mRNA species of other early genes (*Harrison* et al. 1977; *Graham* et al. 1978; *Jones* and *Shenk* 1979a and b; *Berk* et al. 1979), and play a role in transformation (*Graham* et al. 1978; *Jones* and *Shenk* 1979a). It does not seem unreasonable to suppose that the various E1A products perform different tasks, although this remains to be demonstrated.

A similar approach, sequencing of cloned cDNA copies of early mRNA species (*Perricaudet* et al. 1980b), has established the arrangement of E1B coding sequences, which specify two major polypeptides, 55–60,000 Mr and 15–17,000 Mr (*Lewis* et al. 1976; *Halbert* et al. 1979; *van der Eb* et al. 1980), translated from spliced mRNA species of 22S and 13S (*Kitchingman* et al. 1977; *Spector* et al. 1978; *Berk* and *Sharp* 1978b; *Chow* et al. 1979; *Spector* et al. 1980; *Kitchingman* and *Westphal* 1980). The structures deduced are summarized in Figure 1.4. The two mRNA species include common sequences from their 5′-termini at nucleotide 1702 (*Baker* and *Ziff* 1980) to nucleotide 2256. The smaller mRNA species is spliced from this point to an acceptor site around nucleotide 3595, such that translation could continue from nucleotide 3596 in a frame shifted by one nucleotide relative to that open before the splice point. This second frame, however, contains a ter-

minating UGA codon at nucleotide 3611. Thus, only five amino and residues are translated from E1B 13S mRNA beyond the splice point. The 22S mRNA species includes sequences from nucleotide 2256 to a second donor splice site at 3511 and thus retains the
majority of the sequences removed from the 13S mRNA by splicing, including a region
that is rich in cysteine codons. The 22S mRNA is spliced from nucleotide 3511 to nucleotide 3596, resulting in the removal of only 84 nucleotides. Surprisingly, though, the donor
splice point in 22S E1B mRNA lies beyond a termination codon, UGA, at nucleotide
3508, so that the portion of this mRNA beyond the splice point, nucleotides 3560 to a
polyadenylation site at 4071, cannot be translated. It is clear from the illustration of these
structures in Figure 1.4 that the adenoviral E1B mRNA species closely resemble those
complementary to the SV40 early region: the two polypeptides specified by 22S and 13S
E1B mRNA species must possess common N-terminal sequences but differ completely
in their C-terminal residues. Their polypeptide products can readily be imagined to fulfill
unique functions during the growth cycle of the virus, but these, like those of individual
E1A polypeptides, remain to be identified.

The presence of any splice in E1B 22S mRNA deserves additional comment: the
splice depicted in Figure 1.4 has no effect upon the product of translation of this mRNA,
raising the question of why it is present at all. The same phenomenon, a splice to the 3'-
side of the translation termination codon, is observed in the SV40 mRNA which specifies
small T antigen (see Fig. 1.1). It has been suggested that splicing is essential to the synthesis
of stable, mature mRNA species or their transport to the cytoplasm (see Sect. 2.1).
However, stable, cellular mRNA species that are not spliced can be made [for example
histone (*Kedes* 1976) and interferon mRNAs (*Derynck* et al. 1980; *Nagata* et al. 1980; *Streu-
lie* et al. 1980)] suggesting that splicing cannot be absolutely necessary to the biosynthesis
of all eukaryotic mRNA species. Moreover, this view is difficult to reconcile with the
observation that the adenoviral mRNA encoding polypeptide IX is not spliced and overlaps the 3'-ends of the E1B mRNAs, from 3583 to 4071 nucleotides (*Alestrom* et al. 1980).
Splicing of the E1B 22S and 13S mRNA species thus eliminates the cap and promoter
sites of polypeptide IX mRNA (see Fig. 1.4), but whether this has any biological significance is not known. Of course, such a specific explanation cannot be extended to the
SV40 small T-antigen mRNA. Indeed, the whole question of why some mRNA species
should be spliced while others are not has not yet received a satisfactory explanation,
probably because an sufficient number of examples of the two types of mRNA structure
have not yet been collected.

An unexpected example of a similar arrangement of viral coding sequences has been
encountered recently. The two nonstructural proteins NS1 and NS2 synthesized in cells
infected by influenza A viruses, molecular weights 25,000 and 11,000 Mr respectively, are
both encoded by the smallest segment of the eight-part influenza genome (*Lamb* et al.
1978; *Lamb* and *Choppin* 1979; *Inglis* et al. 1979). Segment 8 is apparently unique in specifying more than a single polypeptide product and is transcribed into separate mRNA
species for the two polypeptides (*Lamb* et al. 1980). Nuclease S1 mapping of the mRNA
species transcribed from influenza segment 8 RNA, using cloned DNA copies of segment 8 RNA as probe, revealed that NS1 mRNA is 850 nucleotides in length and maps
from 0.05 to 0.95 units, whereas NS2 mRNA is complementary to the region 0.59–0.95
units and thus 3'-coterminal with the NS1 species (*Lamb* et al. 1980). However, the two
polypeptides appear to share neither methionine- nor leucine-containing tryptic peptides, suggesting that their mRNAs must be translated in different reading frames. Deter-

mination of the sequence of segment 8 genomic mRNA and the two mRNA species transcribed from it (*Lamb* and *Lai* 1980; *Porter* et al. 1980) has revealed that, in fact, the smaller NS2 mRNA is spliced, as illustrated in Figure 1.5. The 3'-ends of the NS1 and NS2 mRNA species are indeed 3'-coterminal from 0.59 units to a common polyadenylation site at 0.95 units. The NS1 mRNA is colinear with genomic segment 8 RNA from 0.05 units to this poly(A) site, some 840 nucleotides in total. The NS2 mRNA, however, includes a 473 nucleotide intervening sequence, 0.08–0.59 units. The two mRNA species are also 5'-coterminal for a short distance, 56 nucleotides. The common sequence includes an initiating AUG codon and codons for nine subsequent amino acids. The NS2 splice results in a one nucleotide shift in reading frame beyond the acceptor splice site at 0.59 units, relative to the frame in which NS1 mRNA is translated. Clearly, then, the two proteins share only ten amino acid residues at their N-termini such that two quite different polypeptides are produced from one influenza A genomic sequence. By now a familiar arrangement (see Fig. 1) among DNA viruses, this is the first example of spliced mRNA species generated from transcripts synthesized by viral RNA polymerase. In the case of influenza, transcription of genomic RNA, which is of the negative polarity, by viral RNA polymerase takes place in the infected cell nucleus (*Hay* et al. 1977; *Taylor* et al. 1977; *Barrett* et al. 1979; *Mark* et al. 1979). It is therefore quite conceivable that the polyadenylated cRNA copies of virion RNA made in this transcriptional step could be recognized by the cellular splicing machinery. The close identity of the sequences at the splice junctions of NS2 mRNA with the eukaryotic consensus sequence (*Lamb* and *Lai* 1980; see Sect. 2.1) provides considerable support for this notion.

It is clear from the preceding discussion that several viruses, whose genomes are transcribed in the nucleus of the cells they infect, rely on splicing of products of transcription to create two or more polypeptides from a single nucleotide sequence. There is considerable flexibility in the precise ways in which different alignments of potential coding sequence are created by splicing steps, including splicing coupled with a switch in reading frame (for example, influenza NS1 and NS2 mRNAs, polyoma middle and large T-antigen mRNAs), and splicing events that generate overlapping, internal deletions (for example, adenoviral E1A mRNAs) (see Fig. 1). The adaptation of splicing mechanisms by these viruses to the generation of multiple products from a single, conventional gene permits more extensive use of limited coding space. The fact that several completely unrelated viruses have evolved in a similar direction would seem to emphasize the advantages to the virus inherent in such an arrangement. It is perhaps because such constraints do not exist in eukaryotic genomes that the use of splicing to fashion multiple products from one DNA sequence is essentially restricted to viral transcripts. Whether mRNA species complementary to the genomes of other viruses that replicate in the nucleus, such as herpesviruses, are also spliced remains to be established.

1.1.2 Mechanism of mRNA Synthesis

Expression of viral genes that fall into the class described in the previous section is epitomized by adenoviral early RNA. Even in this system, however, only the bare outlines of posttranscriptional processing can be drawn and we possess no information whatsoever about the mechanism(s) that determine which of several potential splice points is used during processing of a given viral RNA chain. The primary products of transcription of each adenoviral early gene are initiated independently (*Berk* and *Sharp* 1977; *Evans* et al. 1977; *Wilson* et al. 1979; *Seghal* et al. 1979) at the cap site (*Baker* and *Ziff* 1980; *Manley* et al. 1980; *Wasylyk* et al. 1980), and extend to a site beyond the site at which poly(A) is added (*Weber* et al. 1980). Polyadenylation of adenoviral early RNAs precedes splicing (*Blanchard* et al. 1979; *Goldenberg* and *Raskas* 1979; *Weber* et al. 1980), that is, the critical processing step that determines which particular mRNA species is fashioned from a given transcript occurs last. At the present time, however, we have no understanding of the mechanism(s) that govern this critical choice, although there is considerable evidence to suggest that the choice of splice points is subject to temporal regulation during viral infection (*Spector* et al. 1978; *Chow* et al. 1979).

The synthesis of papovavirus early mRNA species appears to follow a similar pathway: transcription is initiated at the early promoter site that lies near the origin of replication at 0.67 map units (see *Shenk*, this volume) and continues through the early region, probably passing the poly(A) site at 0.154 map units (*Reed* and *Alwine* 1977; *Piper* 1979). Processing of SV40 early RNA therefore includes polyadenylation of the 3'-ends of RNA chains destined to function as mRNA, probably following cleavage, and splicing. Once again, splicing probably takes place after the precursor RNA has been polyadenylated (*May* et al. 1978).

1.2 Spliced Viral mRNA Species that Do not Share Translated Sequences

A second class of spliced viral mRNA species can be distinguished from that described in Section 1.1 by the fact that splicing does not generate different arrays of a coding sequence from an initial colinear transcript, but rather serves to release individual, unrelated coding sequences from a polygenic transcript. This phenomenon is epitomized by the mechanism by which the major late genes of adenovirus type 2, those encoded in the strand transcribed in the rightward direction to the right of position 30, are expressed. Transcription of this region by RNA polymerase form II is initiated at one promoter site, near 16.45 units (*Ziff* and *Evans* 1978; *Evans* et al. 1979; *Weil* et al. 1979; *Manley* et al. 1979a, *Baker* and *Ziff* 1980) and continues to a termination site at or near the right-hand end of the viral genome to yield large RNA molecules, up to 25 kb in length (*Bachenheimer* and *Darnell* 1975; *Weber* et al. 1977; *Goldberg* et al. 1977). The late promoter site is coincident with the cap site and capping occurs very soon after, or perhaps concomitant with, initiation of transcription (*Ziff* and *Evans* 1978; *Manley* et al. 1979a; *Babich* et al. 1980). Polyadenylic acid is added to five sites near 38, 50, 62, 78, and 91.5 units both in vivo (*Fraser* and *Ziff* 1978; *Ziff* and *Fraser* 1978; *McGrogan* and *Raskas* 1978; *Nevins* and *Darnell* 1978a) and in isolated nuclei (*Manley* et al. 1979b; *Yang* and *Flint* 1979), presumably following specific cleavage of the primary transcript. Polyadenylation, like capping, occurs before transcription is complete: RNA sequences that lie immediately to the 5'-side of each of the five poly(A) sites shown in Figure 3 are labelled at equal rates in periods of time shorter than those necessary to transcribe the complete r-strand unit (*Nevins* and *Darnell* 1978b; *Nevins* 1979). Were cleavage and polyadenylation dependent upon complete transcription of the r-strand unit, RNA sequences adjacent to distal poly(A) site would be labelled, during very short periods, before those adjacent to promoter proximal sites. Thus, it has been concluded that polyadenylation must take place before the transcriptional machinery has traversed the entire unit, that is, nascent, adenoviral late RNA is the substrate for polyadenylation. However, even when a promoter proximal poly(A) site is recognized, presumably a short time after its transcription by form II RNA polymerase, the remainder of the transcriptional unit is copied, for all viral RNA sequences complementary to the r-strand to the right of position 30 are represented in approximately equimolar amounts in pulse-labelled, late, nuclear RNA (*Nevins* and *Darnell* 1978b). Such apparent extravagance is difficult to appreciate at the present time. Such a mechanism of polyadenylation also implies the existence of some regulatory phenomenon that permits each poly(A) site to be recognized only about once every five times (*Nevins* and *Darnell* 1978b) that it is copied by the transcriptional machinery. Whether selection of poly(A) sites is under the control of an active regulatory mechanism (*Nevins* and *Darnell* 1978b) is not yet established.

Maturation of type 2 adenoviral late mRNA species from the r-strand precursor is mediated by splicing, as well as polyadenylation. These mRNAs, some 14 in number, fall into five families, designated LI to LV in Figure 3, in which the members are 3'-coterminal (*Fraser* and *Ziff* 1978; *Ziff* and *Fraser* 1978; *Nevins* and *Darnell* 1978a; *McGrogan* and *Raskas* 1978; *Chow* et al. 1977a). In addition, each late mRNA species contains the same 5'-terminal sequences, 202 nucleotides altogether (*Zain* et al. 1979; *Akusjärvi* and *Pettersson* 1979 a, b) constructed, as illustrated in Figure 3, by splicing three separate sets of sequences of precursor RNA; these lie near 16.45, 19.6 and 26.8 map units in the r-strand (*Berget* et al. 1977; *Chow* et al. 1977b; *Klessig* 1977; *Dunn* and *Hassel* 1977). The mature leader can be joined to several alternative sites within each polyadenylated, adenoviral intermediate to form the overlapping mRNA species illustrated in Figure 3. The sizes of polyadenylated intermediates (*Nevins* and *Darnell* 1978b; *Manley* et al. 1979b; *Yang* and *Flint* 1979) and the presence of intervening sequences between the first and second components of the common 5'-leader in nuclear, poly(A)-containing adenoviral RNA (*Ziff* and *Evans* 1978) suggest that polyadenylation precedes splicing. Analysis of the structures of poly(A)-lacking and -containing RNA species synthesized in nuclei isolated during the late phase of adenovirus 2 infection (*Yang* and *Flint* 1979; *Manley* et al. 1979b; *V.W. Yang* and *S.J. Flint*, unpublished observations) has confirmed that leader to mRNA body splicing depends upon polyadenylation, but also revealed that synthesis of the 5'-tripartite leader segment is independent of polyadenylation. Such a mechanism can be rationalized in the sense that it is the choice of poly(A) site and the choice of the splice acceptor site to which the tripartite leader is ligated that determine which adenoviral late mRNA species will be fashioned from a given primary transcript. As the five poly(A) sites shown in Figure 3 are apparently utilized with approximately equal efficiencies (*Nevins* and *Darnell* 1978b), it must be concluded that selection of this latter splice site is paramount in quantitative regulation of the individual late mRNA species (*Flint* and *Sharp* 1976). It should be apparent from the mechanism of adenoviral, late mRNA species shown in Figure 3 that the observed dependence of leader to body splicing upon polyadenylation is an absolute prerequisite for orderly synthesis of mature mRNA species.

Each late mRNA species contains the 5'-tripartite leader segment shown in Figure 3, implying that only one mRNA species can be processed from each primary transcriptional product, even though the latter contains the sequences of some 14 mRNAs, whose coding sequences do not overlap. This conclusion is supported by the observation that only 20% of nuclear, adenoviral RNA sequences enter the cytoplasm during the late phase of productive infection (*Flint* and *Sharp* 1976; *Nevins* and *Darnell* 1978b). It should be noted that although promoter proximal regions of the late transcriptional unit are copied more frequently than the remainder of the unit (*Weber* et al. 1977; *Nevins* and *Darnell* 1978b; *Fraser* et al. 1978, 1979; *Evans* et al. 1979), there is no evidence that such molecules provide an additional source of leader sequences.

Splicing of the 5'-end of the primary transcript to construct the 5'-tripartite leader segment proceeds by means of several intermediates; thus steady state, nuclear late RNA preparation from adenovirus infected cells (*Berget* and *Sharp* 1979) or viral RNA synthesized in nuclei isolated from adenovirus infected cells (*Yang* and *Flint* 1979) contain splices at many sites deleted in late mRNA. The most prominent of these lie at 21.6, 24.8, 25.6. 26.2, 26.4, and 26.9 map units. The structures of nuclear RNA molecules that contain such nuclear-specific splice junctions (*Berget* and *Sharp* 1979) reveal that splicing of the adenovirus 2 late transcript has 5'→3'-polarity, that is, it continues sequentially from the 5'- toward the 3'-end, apparently in discrete steps. Removal of intervening sequences in several, discrete steps has also been reported for α-2 collagen RNA (*Avvedimento* et al. 1980), but in this case a 3'→5'-polarity was observed. In yet other systems, ovalbumin and ovomucoid mRNA precursors, for example, splicing appears to be able to follow several alternative pathways, that is, there is apparently no obligate order in which the several intervening sequences must be removed (*Tsai* et al. 1980). "Pausing" during leader to body splicing is also likely to be the rule and is revealed as rare forms of late mRNA species that contain additional leader segments derived from several sites between the 3'-end of the usual leader segment and the 5'-end of the mRNA body (*Chow* and *Broker* 1978; *Dunn* et al. 1978).

Although the members of each family of adenoviral late mRNA species share extensive sets of 3'-terminal sequences (see Fig. 3), each specifies a unique polypeptide, translated from its exposed 5'-terminal sequences (*Lewis* et al. 1977; *Riccardi* et al. 1979; *Miller* et al. 1980). Thus, although the larger mRNA species of each family contain coding sequences for two or more late polypeptides, only those adjacent to the 5'-end are translated: coding sequences that are internal in the larger mRNAs are translated only from the smaller mRNA species in which they occupy the 5'-terminal position, exactly as predicted on the basis of our current understanding of the mechanism by which translation of an eukaryotic mRNA is initiated (see *Kozak*, this volume).

From one point of view, this kind of splicing regimen can be considered to be similar to that discussed in the previous section: it is the choice of splice points within polyadenylated processing intermediates that determines both the nature of the protein products ultimately translated from each transcript and the concentration of individual mRNA species in the cytoplasm. However, splicing *within* adenovirus 2 late coding sequences is rarely observed (*Chow* et al. 1977a; *Chow* and *Broker* 1978; *S.M. Berget* personal communication) and the choice of splice points, at least donor sites, is obviously much greater within the adenovirus late transcriptional product than within any of the viral RNA transcripts considered in the previous section.

It is clear that the mode of adenoviral gene expression illustrated in Figure 3 permits *posttranscriptional* determination of the nature and quantity of adenovirus late mRNA species. At the transcriptional level, expression of this block of viral late genes, which include the major structural proteins of the virus, is subject to control at only one promoter site. We must assume that such a mechanism, the use of simply one transcriptional control signal coupled with a large array of posttranscriptional processing choices, is of advantage to the virus. And this advantage must be extremely significant to offset the apparent profligacy of such a mechanism of viral gene expression: for reasons discussed

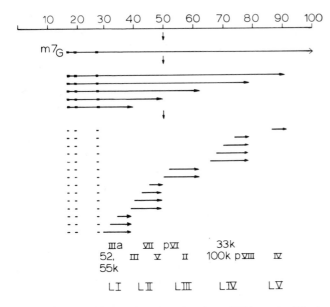

Fig. 3. Synthesis of the major adenovirus late mRNA species. The type C adenoviral genome is represented by the solid horizontal line, 0–100 units at the top of the figure. Below is shown the primary product of late transcription initiated at 16.45 units with the arrow indicating the direction of transcription and including the three sets of sequences, near 16.45, 19.6, and 26.8 units, that constitute the 5'-leader sequence common to r-strand mRNA species. Polyadenylation at the five sites shown as solid arrowheads generates the set of 5'-coterminal intermediates illustrated. Splicing fashions the 5'-terminal leader segment, and ligates it to one of several sites within each polyadenylated intermediate to generate the five families of late, r-strand mRNA species depicted at the bottom of the figure. The polypeptides translated from each of these mRNA species are also shown. The sources of the data upon which this scheme is based are given in the text

in the previous paragraphs, the great majority of the sequences of each primary transcript are not conserved in cytoplasmic mRNA. It might also be speculated that regulation of viral gene expression at the level of splicing permits more finely tuned and flexible control of synthesis of individual viral mRNA species; it is, however, difficult to argue this case with much force in the absence of an understanding of the mechanism(s) that mediate, and regulate, splicing of adenoviral late RNA. In fact, the only thing that can be safely concluded at the present time is that a mechanism like that shown in Figure 3 has some inherent advantage, for it has also been adopted by several other viruses.

A second example of this mode of expression of viral genetic information is provided by the integrated proviral DNA of retroviruses. The proviral DNA is a colinear, double-stranded copy of the genomic, positive strand RNA (30–40S) (see *Bishop* 1978, for a review) except for the presence of repeated sequences at both ends, the so-called long terminal repeats, LTRs, which include sequences from the 3'- and 5'-ends of the viral RNA (*Hughes* et al. 1978; *Hsu* et al. 1978; *Shank* et al. 1978; *Cohen* et al. 1979; *Sabran* et al. 1979; *van de Woude* et al. 1979; *Lowy* et al. 1980). Integration occurs between the two copies of the LTR in the circular proviral DNA and is therefore site-specific with respect to viral sequences. Shown in Figure 4 AB is a schematic representation of the viral mRNA species expressed from an integrated retrovirus genome, that of a nondefective, trans-

A SV40 Late mRNAs

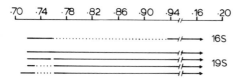

B Retrovirus mRNAs

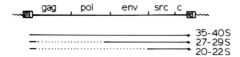

Fig. 4A, B. Structure of spliced 3′-coterminal viral mRNA species. *A SV40 late mRNA species:* the late region of the SV40 genome is represented by the solid horizontal line, divided into map units, at the top of the figure. Below are shown sequences represented in mRNA, drawn in the direction of transcription. Arrowheads indicate polyadenylation sites and sequences deleted as a result of splicing are shown as dotted lines. The 16S late mRNA species shown constitutes approximately 85% of the total. The four most common species of SV40 19S late mRNA are shown: of these the bottom two are the most abundant species in the 19S mRNA class. The sources of these data are given in the text. *B Retrovirus mRNA species:* an integrated genome of a nondefective, transforming retrovirus is represented by the solid horizontal line, upon which the locations of the four viral genes are shown approximately to scale. The long terminal repeats, 500–600 nucleotides are indicated, ■, next to cellular DNA sequences, ■. Below are shown the three major classes of retroviral mRNA species synthesized in cells infected by such a virus, drawn in the direction of transcription. Symbols employed are as in part A of the figure. The text includes the sources of this information

forming avian sarcoma virus in this example. Transcription probably initiates within the left-hand LTR, as the genome is drawn conventionally in Figure 4; all retroviral LTRs that have been sequenced to date contain sequences resembling the sites at which transcription by form II RNA polymerase is initiated in eukaryotic cells (*see* Shenk, this volume). (*Sutcliffe* et al. 1980; *Dhar* et al. 1980; *van Beveren* et al. 1980; *Shimotohno* et al. 1980; *Benz* et al. 1980). Such promoter-like sequences lie upstream from the region corresponding to the 5′-end of retroviral RNA transcribed from proviral DNA in vivo or in vitro (*Dhar* et al. 1980; *Sutcliffe* et al. 1980; *Benz* et al. 1980; *Yamamoto* et al. 1980). Each LTR also contains signals characteristic of polyadenylation sites, suggesting that integrated retroviral DNA carries all the necessary signals to specify its transcription by the host-cell transcriptional machinery. The failure to detect any rapidly labelled, nuclear RNA chains larger than genomic 30–40S RNA in retrovirus infected cells (*Haseltine* and *Baltimore* 1976; *Fan* 1977) and the observation that transcription of retroviral sequences initiates near the 3′-end of left-hand LTR (*Benz* et al. 1980; *Yamamoto* et al. 1980) support this conclusion. Thus the primary product of transcription of integrated retrovirus DNA appears to correspond to genomic RNA.

As illustrated in Figure 4, however, a polyadenylated RNA species of genomic size can also function as mRNA, directing the synthesis of the precursor to the *gag* proteins

(*Arcement* et al. 1977; *Evans* et al. 1977), whose sequences occupy the 5'-terminal position, and occasionally the precursor to reverse transcriptase. The reverse transcriptase gene, *pol*, is internal to the *gag* gene (see Fig. 4) and its translation may result from occasional read-through of the termination site at the end of the *gag* gene to produce a very large polyprotein precursor that contains both *gag* and *pol* sequences (*Oppermann* et al. 1977; *Paterson* et al. 1977; *Kopchick* et al. 1978; *Murphy* et al. 1978; *Philipson* et al. 1978). Retrovirus-infected cells also contain subgenomic, polysomal RNA species whose structure depends on the nature of the infecting virus. In the case of nondefective avian sarcoma viruses, two such species, 27–29S and 20–22S, are observed. As illustrated in Figure 4, the former comprises sequences complementary to the *env* and *src* genes, whereas the latter contains *src*-specific information; both contain the common 3'-terminal c-region adjacent to their poly(A) chains (*Hayward* 1977; *Weiss* et al. 1977; *van Zaane* et al. 1977; *Parsons* et al. 1978). Although translational read-through may occasionally take place, the retroviral mRNA species can be considered to form a 3'-coterminal family in which only 5'-terminal sequences uniquely exposed in a given mRNA can be translated, a situation entirely analogous to that described previously for each of the five families of type 2 adenoviral late mRNA.

Analogy to adenovirus late gene expression is heightened by the fact that retroviral, subgenomic mRNA species carry a common 5'-terminal leader segment, derived from sequences that lie near the 5'-end of genomic RNA, including the 5'-terminal cap (*Mellon* and *Duesberg* 1977; *Kryzek* et al. 1978; *Fan* and *Verma* 1978; *Cordell* et al. 1978; *Rothenberg* et al. 1978). The leader is 100–500 nucleotides in length (*Rothenberg* et al. 1978; *Cordell* et al. 1978) and is spliced to sites promoter proximal to *env* or *src* sequences to produce the mRNA species depicted in Figure 4. It is possible that the 30–40S RNA, at least that functioning as mRNA, might be spliced, for sequences resembling splice points (see Section 2.1) are present a short distance following the 5'-end of such RNA (*Dhar* et al. 1980). This remains to be demonstrated experimentally.

The viral mRNA species synthesized during the late phase of papovavirus infection also constitute a 3'-coterminal set, as illustrated for SV40 late mRNA in Fugure 4 A. Transcription of SV40 late sequences appears to be initiated near coordinate 0.735 (*Ford* and *Hsu* 1978; *Laub* et al. 1979) and continue for least 1000 nucleotides beyond the polyadenylation site near 0.154 units (*Ford* and *Hsu* 1978; *Lai* et al. 1978). The predominant nuclear species of SV40 specific RNA is not spliced, but carries a capped 5'-terminus and 3'-terminal poly(A) (*Lai* et al. 1978), suggesting that splicing is the final step in the processing of mature viral mRNA species from initial products of transcription. Such nuclear RNA is spliced to yield 18–19S and 16S late mRNA species that encode $VP_2 + VP_3$ and VP_1 respectively, the structural proteins of the capsid (*Hsu* and *Ford* 1977; *Aloni* et al. 1977; *Lavi* and *Groner* 1977; *Celma* et al. 1977; *Haegerman* and *Fiers* 1978; *Bratosin* et al. 1978; *Lai* et al. 1978). In this simple outline, the mode of synthesis of SV40 late mRNA species closely resembles that discussed previously for adenovirus late genes.

This resemblance is emphasized by the fact that the splicing events that fashion SV40 late mRNAs ligate a 5'-leader segment to colinear coding sequences. The regions specifying VP_1 and VP_2, and the corresponding 16S and 19S mRNA bodies begin at 0.939 and 0.765 maps units, for VP_1 and VP_2 mRNA species respectively (see. Fig. 4). However, the leader segments themselves are rather heterogeneous. The major species of SV40 16S mRNA, which comprises some 85% of the total 16S population, carries a 202 nucleotide-long leader, specified by nucleotides 325–526 inclusive (see Fig. 4), but at least eight other

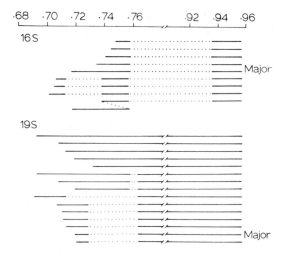

Fig. 5. Multiple leader sequences of SV40 late mRNA species. The 5'-part of the late region of the SV40 genome is depicted as the horizontal line divided into map units at the top of the figure. Below are shown the multiple forms of the late leader sequences present on SV40 16S and 19S late mRNA species (*Ghosh* et al. 1978a, b; *Reddy* et al. 1978, 1979b). Sequences present in the mRNA are drawn as solid lines, whereas those deleted during splicing are represented as dotted lines. The major species are indicated

forms of SV40 16S mRNA with variant leaders have been described (*Ghosh* et al. 1978a, b; *Reddy* et al. 1979b; *Haegerman* et al. 1979; *Bina-Stein* et al. 1979; *Canaani* et al. 1979). These, as illustrated in Figure 5, fall into three major classes: those in which the leader itself is continuous from several different starting points to nucleotide 526 (including the major 16S species), those in which the leader contains a tandem duplication as shown in Figure 5, and those in which the leader itself is discontinuous and is formed of sequences from at least three different 5'-start sites that lie between nucleotides 235 and 295 to nucleotide 295 spliced to the segment nucleotides 435 to 526. As also illustrated in Figure 5, an even more bewildering array of SV40 late 19S mRNA species bearing variant leader segments has been described. No one is predominant, but the major species in each class are shown in Figure 4. It is noteworthy that capped 5'-termini corresponding to almost all of the various leaders have been identified (*Canaani* et al. 1979). Such heterogeneity implies that RNA polymerase form II can initiate transcription at multiple sites in SV40 DNA, or that processing of SV40 late transcripts includes the generation of novel 5'-termini by specific posttranscriptional cleavage followed by capping. There is no reason to suppose that these alternatives are mutually exclusive.

The late mRNA of polyoma infected cells, in which three distinct viral species of 19S, 18S, and 16S can be distinguished (*Horowitz* et al. 1978; *Manor* et al. 1979; *Kamen* et al. 1980 a, b) also comprise a 3'-coterminal family whose individual members carry heterogeneous 5'-terminal leader sequences (*Kamen* et al. 1980; *Flavell* et al. 1979, 1980). Polyoma late leader sequences are also characterized by the presence of reiterations of sequences that are represented only once in the genome (*Legon* et al. 1979). Transcription of the polyoma late region does not terminate efficiently, but can continue to copy the viral genome several times to produce very large RNA molecules, tandem repeats of the entire viral genome (*Acheson* et al. 1971; *Rosenthal* et al. 1976; *Birg* et al. 1977; *Lev* and *Manor* 1977; *Acheson* 1978). Thus the reiterated sequences of late leader segments are believed to result from splicing together of the individual copies of the repeat present in giant transcripts. Such variations in the leader segment do not appear to affect expression of papovaviral late polypeptides, for their initiating AUG codons lie beyond the start of the mRNA bodies (*Ghosh* et al. 1978a, b; *Reddy* et al. 1978, 1979b; *Soeda* et al. 1980). Despite the eccentricities exhibited by papovavirus late leader segments, it is clear that the general organization and mode of expression of papovavirus late genes closely resembles the prototype, expression of adenoviral late genes, discussed previously.

The parvoviruses, which contain extremely small, single-stranded DNA genomes, $1.4–1.6 \times 10^6$ daltons, fall into two groups, the autonomous viruses, such as H1, Kilham rat virus, and minute virus of mice, and those that are defective and able to replicate in the presence of helper adenoviruses, adeno-associated viruses (AAV) (see *Ward* and *Tattersall* 1978, for a review). Synthesis of parvovirus mRNA in infected cells depends entirely on the hosts' biosynthetic machinery and exhibits no temporal regulation. Recent analysis of the structure of nuclear and cytoplasmic, viral RNA species made in AAV (*Laughlin* et al. 1979; *Green* and *Roeder* 1980a; *Green* et al. 1980) or autonomous parvovirus (*Tal* et al. 1979; *Green* et al. 1979) infected cells suggest that the major mRNA species are spliced from initial products of transcription. In AAV-infected cells, for example, the major viral RNA species made exhibit lengths of 4.3, 3.6, 2.6, and 2.3 kb. Of these, only the 2.6 and 2.3 kb species are found on polysomes. These four mRNA species share 3′-termini at 96 map units, but appear to possess unique 5′-termini. The 5′-ends of the 4.5 and 3.6 kb nuclear species have been mapped to 6 and 19 units respectively, whereas the cytoplasmic species begin near 38.5 units. The predominant polysomal viral RNA, 2.3 kb, carries a 55 nucleotide leader sequence encoded at this site spliced to the mRNA body, which starts near 46.5 units. Evidence that this RNA species can be expressed from a promoter site near 38.5 units, at least in vitro, has recently been obtained (*Green* and *Roeder* 1980b), perhaps hinting that the AAV genome includes overlapping transcriptional units. Cytoplasmic viral RNA species synthesized in H1- or KRV-infected cells may be derived by splicing of a large transcript complementary to some 95% of the viral genome (*Green* et al. 1979; *Tal* et al. 1979). However, the mode of transcription of such autonomous parvoviral DNAs is not yet established. Thus, while the existence of overlapping parvoviral RNA species suggests analogy to the viral RNA families discussed in preceding paragraphs of this section, it is not presently clear that such analogy extends to the mechanism of parvoviral mRNA synthesis.

Although the splicing patterns described in both this section and Section 1.1 result in the synthesis of more than one mRNA species, and thus polypeptide, from a single primary product of transcription, they do exhibit quite substantial differences. The splicing mechanisms discussed in Section 1.1 closely resemble those that fashion the mature products of many cellular genes, with the virus-specific twist of the use of alternate splicing points within coding sequences to generate two or more related, yet distinct, gene products from a single genomic sequence. The kinds of arrangement discussed in this section however, permit the expression of *unrelated* gene products from a single transcriptional unit. The latter is thus polycistronic in the original sense of the term. Only one cellular analogue of this mechanism of mRNA synthesis has been found among the cellular genes surveyed to date, posttranscriptional selection of the mRNA species encoding membrane-bound and secreted forms of immunoglobulin IgM μ chains from a common precursor (*Singer* et al. 1980; *Early* et al. 1980; *Rogers* et al. 1980).

It is of some interest to consider why the kind of mechanism of viral gene expression illustrated in Figure 4 is common to several groups of unrelated viruses. One possibility might be that the leader segments themselves fulfill some important function, common to different viral systems. The adenovirus late leader sequence, for example, although it contains no initiation codons, includes the 5′-terminal cap and sequences complementary to the 3′-end of 18S ribosomal RNA (*Akusjärvi* and *Pettersson* 1979a, b; *Zain* et al. 1979; *Zain* and *Roberts* 1979), features that appear to be of importance in ribosome binding and initiation of translation (see *Kozak*, this volume). Clearly, the adenovirus leader fulfills functions of the 5′ untranslated region of any mRNA chain, but whether it confers any unique advantage, for example leading to the preferential expression of adenoviral mRNA species during the late phase of productive infection (*Anderson* et al. 1973; *Beltz* and *Flint* 1979) remains to be established. Furthermore, this latter idea, although attractive in the context of the properties of adenovirus infection, cannot apply to the leader segments of viruses that do not inhibit host-gene expression, including the retroviruses and papovaviruses.

Similarly, the recent observation that at least one of the SV40 late leader segments, the major 16S mRNA leader, also present on some forms of 19S mRNA (see Fig. 5) can be expressed as a small polypeptide, 62 amino acid residues (*G. Khoury*, personal communication), can have no counterpart in the adenovirus leader segment, which contains no putative initiation codons. Thus, there is no obvious function, specific to viral systems, that can be ascribed to all viral leader segments. It is therefore probably reasonable to conclude that the mechanism of mRNA synthesis itself confers some advantage(s). It obviously permits post transcriptional regulation of the synthesis of individual mRNA species from the initial, multigenic primary product of transcription of viral genetic information, but, as discussed previously, we do not yet appreciate the significance of such posttranscriptional, by contrast to transcriptional, regulation. It will be of interest to learn to what extent the mechanism of expression of viral genes illustrated in Figures 3 and 4 reflects normal control mechanisms of eukaryotic cells: the recent observations on immunoglobulin IgM μ – chain mRNA synthesis mentioned previously are particularly intriguing in this regard, as are reports of posttranscriptional selection of the RNA sequences that leave the nucleus to function as mRNA during sea urchin development (*Wold* et al. 1978).

2 The Mechanism of Splicing

2.1 Splicing signals in Viral RNA

It can be deduced from the examples of spliced, viral RNA molecules included in Section 1 that the sizes of intervening sequences, those removed during splicing, vary from only tens of nucleotides (certain papovavirus mRNAs) to more than 10,000 nucleotides in the case of the promoter distal adenovirus late mRNAs. Fortunately, however, it is sequences immediately surrounding splice sites that seem to be most important to their recognition by splicing machinery.

The sequences of quite a large number of sites at which viral transcripts are spliced are now available and are listed in Figure 6. Most have been obtained by direct comparisons between genomic sequences and the sequence of cloned DNA copies of individual mRNA species. In many instances, this approach identifies splice junctions to within one or two nucleotides, the ambiguity resulting from very small repetitions at the splice sites. The sequences shown in Figure 6 have therefore been aligned to conform to the rule proposed by *Breathnach* et al. (1978), that the 5'- and 3'-ends of an intervening sequence are bounded by the dinucleotides GU and AG respectively. This feature was, in fact, the first common element detected among mRNA precursor splice junctions. As more sequences have become available, attempts have been made to deduce additional Common features (see *Seif* et al. 1979 a, b; *Lerner* et al. 1980; *Rogers* and *Wall* 1980). Shown in Figure 6, for example, are the consensus sequences for 5'- and 3'-splice junctions within an eukaryotic mRNA precursor derived by *Lerner* et al. (1980) from a consideration of some 30 unique splice junctions, including some present in papovavirus RNA species. Indeed, inspection of Figure 6 reveals that the majority of viral splice junctions shown match the consensus sequence as well as do cellular splice junction sequences. Thus, like sequences near splice sites in cellular mRNA precursors, viral intervening sequences are bounded by the dinucleotides GU and AG and contain pyrimidine-rich tracts preceding the 3'-terminal AG of the intervening sequence. The great similarity of cellular and viral mRNA precursor splicing signals strongly suggests that viral RNA chains are recognized by the cellular splicing machinery.

The results of experiments with deletion mutants of SV40 provide strong support for the notion that sequences immediately surrounding splice junctions are both necessary and sufficient for splicing. As discussed in Section 1.1, deletions that remove small T-antigen coding sequences, that is sections of the large T-antigen intervening sequence, do not impair large T-antigen synthesis or growth of the virus. Sequencing of the DNA of such SV40 deletion mutants has now established that sequences of the intervening sequence to within 10–13 nucleotides of the donor (5') and acceptor (3') sites can be removed without inhibition of splicing of large T-antigen mRNA (*Volckaert* et al. 1979; *Thimmappaya* and *Shenk* 1979; *Khoury* et al. 1979). Similarly, SV40 mutants that carry deletions or insertions in the late leader region that do not actually obliterate splice junctions induce the synthesis of late mRNA and polypeptides in infected cells (*Contreras* et al. 1979; *Villareal* et al. 1979; *Subramanian* 1979), although the forms of the leader may be altered compared to the major forms made in cells infected by wild-type virus (*Villareal* et al. 1979). It is therefore clear that intervening sequences immediately adjacent to 5'- and 3'-splice sites are sufficient to promote splicing. Nevertheless, internal sequences of an intervening sequence can influence the efficiency with which that intervening sequence is spliced from an mRNA precursor: some deletions result in aberrant ratios of spliced early or late gene products (*Khoury* et al. 1979; *Villareal* et al. 1979). In the SV40 early region, for example, deletions that do not include the small T-antigen donor splice site, that is, reside exclusively within its unique coding sequences (see Fig. 1), direct the synthesis of discrete, shortened forms of small T-antigen mRNA, whose size correlates well with the length of the deleted genomic region. However, the abundance of such variant mRNA species and of the altered polypeptides translated from them is altered relative to the amount of small T-antigen mRNA made during wild-type infections. Such observations not only imply that internal regions of an intervening sequence, somewhat removed from splice sites, can influence the efficiency of the splicing reaction (perhaps through participation in the formation of the secondary or tertiary substrate structure rec-

5' mRNA	Intervening Sequence	mRNA 3'	
UCCAGGUAAGA	UAUUCUUACAGGGCU	Large T	Py Early
UCCAAGUAAGU	UAUUCUUACAGGGCU	Small T	
UCCAAGUAAGU	UCUCCCCUAGAACG	Middle T	
AUCAAGUAAGU	UCUAUUUUAAGAGUC	Leader	Py Late
AUCAAGUAAGU	UAUUUCCCUAGGAAU	18S	
AUCAAGUAAGU	AAACUUUUAAGUGAA	19S	
AUCAAGUAAGU	UUUAAUUCUAGGGCU	16S	
CAGAGGUUUUG	UUUUUUUAUAGGUGC	Large T	BKV Early
UUAAGGUAACU	UUUUUUUAUAGGUGC	Small T	
CCUAGGUAAGU	UGUAUUUCCAGGUUC	19S	BKV Late
CCUAGGUAAGU	UUUACUUCUAGGCCU	16S	
CUAAGGUAAAT	GUGUAUUUUAGAUUU	Large T	SV40 Early
CUGAGGUAUUU	GUGUAUUUUAGAUUU	Small T	
AACUGGUAAGU	CAGCUCUCUAGGCCU	16S	SV40 Late
CGGCUGUCACG	UUUUAUUUCAGGUCC	19S	
AGAGGGUGAGG	UUUUUUAAAAGGUCC	12S	AdC E1A
CUACAGUAAGU	UUUUUUAAAAGGUCC	13S	
UACAGGUGGCU	CUGUUUUGCAGCAGC	13S	AdC E1B
UUGAGGUA UU	CUGUUUUGCAGCAGC	22S	
UUACAGUAAGU	UGUUGUUUUAGGUCC	N2S	Ad12 E1A
GGAACGUGAAG	UGUUGUUUUGAGUCC	13S	
GACAGGUACCA	UUAUCUUCAGAUUG	2.3kb	AAV
UUCAGGUAGAC	UUCUUUUCCAGGACA	NS2	Influenza 8
^A_CAGGUAAGU	UYUYYYUXCAGG		Consensus Sequence
UUGGGGUCAGU	UUUUUCCACAGCUCGC	leader 1 - 2	Ad2 Late
GAACGGUAAGA	UUGUUGUGUAGGUACU	leader 2 - 3	
GCAAGGUAGGC	AUUUACAACAGUUUCC	leader 3 - 4 (fiber)	
AGGAGGUGAGC	UAUUGUUGCAGAUGAA	leader 4 - fiber	
GCAAGGUAGGC	GUCGCCGCCAGAGGAG	leader 3 - hexon	

ognized by splicing enzymes), but also emphasize a point made previously, that the frequency with which a particular splice is made regulates viral gene expression.

When an SV40 splice junction is deleted from the genome, the corresponding mRNA does not accumulate in significant amounts (*Volckaert* et al. 1979; *Lai* and *Khoury* 1979; *Gruss* et al. 1979). In these circumstances, mutant DNA seems to be transcribed, but stable, mutant RNA does not accumulate. A similar result obtains in cells transfected with recombinant DNA molecules that lack splicing signals, for example β-globin double-stranded cDNA inserted into the SV40 late region such that the usual viral splicing signals are obliterated (*Hamer* et al. 1979). It is observations such as these that form the basis for the suggestion that splice junctions are control signals for the production of stable mRNA species and that transport of such mRNA species from the nucleus to the cytoplasm is inseparably linked to their splicing. While it does not seem likely that sequences surrounding splice junctions influence transport directly, it is quite conceivable that unspliced mRNA precursors cannot adopt the correct conformation, or RNP structure.

2.2 Components of the Splicing Machinery

As implied throughout this discussion, all available information suggests that viral RNA chains are spliced by cellular splicing systems. Thus, the splice signals present in viral RNA molecules closely resemble those of cellular gene products, regardless of the nature of the virus or its host cell (see Sect. 2.1). In this context, it is perhaps worth emphasizing that cellular mRNA precursor splice junctions are themselves strongly conserved among vertebrates and insects (see, for example, sequences summarized by *Lerner* et al. 1980; *Rogers* and *Wall* 1980). It therefore comes as no surprise that a given viral RNA product can be spliced to produce the same mRNA species in cells of different host species (*Reddy* et al. 1979a; *Sambrook* et al. 1980; *Flint* and *Beltz* 1980).

The conclusion that eukaryotic viruses rely on the cellular splicing machinery, which itself must be quite highly conserved, raises the central question, what is the physical nature of the entities (other than the substrate) that mediate splicing of mRNA precursors in eukaryotic cells? Enzymes that achieve endonucleolytic cleavage at specific sites and correct religation of the sequences conserved in mRNA must be required, but those that recognize mRNA precursors have not yet been identified. Indeed, progress in the development of in vitro systems that splice mRNA precursors has been slow. A variety of nuclear systems that splice adenoviral or SV40 RNA sequences with different degrees of efficiency have been described (*Blanchard* et al. 1979; *Manley* et al. 1979a; *Yang* and *Flint*

Fig. 6. Sequences at viral RNA splice junctions. All sequences are given in the 5′ → 3′ direction. The dashed vertical lines represent boundaries between mRNA and intervening sequences. Where small direct repetitions lead to ambiguity in precise location of splice junctions, the sequences have been aligned to follow the GU . . . AG rule (see text). Sequences that are underlined are identical to the sequence listed immediately above and represent donor or acceptor splice sites that are used in the generation of more than one mRNA species. The eukaryotic consensus sequences, in which Y = a pyrimidine, X = any nucleotide, of *Lerner* et al. (1980) is included for comparison. The Ad2 late RNA sequences are listed separately for reasons discussed in the text. The sequences shown are from the following sources: Polyoma, *Soeda* et al. 1980; BK virus, *Seif* et al. 1979a, b; SV40, *Ghosh* et al. 1978a, b; *Reddy* et al. 1978, 1979b; *Buchman* et al. 1980; Ad type 2 E1A, *Perricaudet* et al. 1979a; Ad type 2 E1B, *Perricaudet* et al. 1980; Ad type 12 E1A, *Perricaudet* et al. 1980; Influenza Segment 8, *Lamb* and *Lai* 1980; Ad2 late sequences, *Akusjärvi* and *Pettersson* 1979a, b; *Zain* et al. 1979

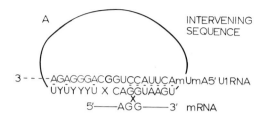

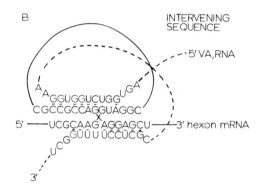

Fig. 7A, B. Roles for small nuclear RNAs in mRNA splicing. *A* Possible interaction between the 5'-end of U1 RNA and an mRNA precursor containing the consensus splice junction sequence. Adapted from *Lerner* et al. (1980). *B* Possible interaction between VA₁ RNA and an Ad2 hexon mRNA precursor. The mRNA precursor sequences (solid line) shown are those around the splice sites at the end of the third leader segment and the body of the hexon sequences (see Fig. 3). The VA₁ RNA chain is represented by the dashed line. Adapted from *Murray* and *Holliday* (1979). In both parts of the figure, the splice site is indicated by the crossover in the precursor and Watson-Crick base pairs are indicated by the dots

1979; *Hamada* et al. 1980). Such systems represent no more than a first step in the identification and isolation of splicing activities. They have, however, proved valuable in testing one hypothesis about the constitution of the splicing machinery, that small RNA molecules participate in splicing reactions (*Lerner* et al. 1980; *Rogers* and *Wall* 1980).

One member of the set of most abundant, small, nuclear RNAs, U1 RNA, bears at its 5'-end a sequence that is a close complement of the consensus splice sequences (*Lerner* and *Steitz* 1979; *Lerner* et al. 1980). This class of RNA molecules exist in the nucleus associated with proteins to form small, nuclear ribonucleoprotein particle, snRNPs and in this form are recognized by antibodies from some patients with systemic lupus erythematosus, SLE (*Lerner* and *Steitz* 1979). U1 snRNP exhibits a number of properties consistent with a role in RNA processing, including conservation among eukaryotic species (*Lerner* et al. 1980), highest abundance in metabolically active tissues (*Lerner* et al. 1980), and cosedimentation with structures containing mRNA precursors (*Zieve* and *Penman* 1976; *Diemel* et al. 1977; *Howard* 1978; *Lerner* et al. 1980). As illustrated in Figure 7A, U1 RNA could form base pairs with sequences within each end of a typical intervening sequence to form a structure in which the residues to be ligated during splicing are closely aligned (*Lerner* et al. 1980; *Rogers* and *Wall* 1980). As this model predicts, SLE antibodies that recognize U1 snRNP, when added to isolated nuclei, inhibit the splicing of adenoviral early RNA species complementary to regions E1 and E2 (*Yang* et al. 1981). SLE antibodies that recognize other classes of snRNP, or small cytoplasmic RNP structures, have no effect on splicing of viral RNA sequences transcribed in isolated nuclei. This observation, then, implies a critical role for U1 snRNP in splicing of these adenoviral early RNA transcripts and almost certainly of cellular mRNA precursors; adenoviral early splice junctions closely resemble those of cellular transcripts. The nature of this role, however, remains to be elucidated. U1 snRNP could include all necessary splicing components, the RNA to fashion the correct substrate structure, the protein components to provide the necessary enzymatic activities. An RNA processing enzyme of *E. coli*, RNAase P, exhibits just such a form, a small, discrete RNA molecule associated with several polypeptides (*Stark* et al. 1978). Alternatively, U1 snRNP could simply serve as the scaffold upon which the appropriate substrate structure is constructed. In this case the protein components of U1 snRNP might contribute to stabilization of the interaction between U1 RNA and sequences near splice sites. The resolution of this question awaits the development of soluble splicing systems.

In the light of our meagre knowledge of the splicing apparatus, it is not surprising that we remain in complete ignorance of mechanisms that regulate splicing. It has been mentioned frequently during this discussion that, in the viral systems described, it is the choice of one of several alternate splice sites that determines the final cytoplasmic concentrations of individual viral mRNA species, and the nature of the products translated from them. However, we do not appreciate what determines the frequencies with which different splice sites within an mRNA precursor are utilized. In principle, the frequency of recognition could simply be a property inherent to each splice site, that is, determined by its sequence and/or higher order structure, or it could be controlled actively by some governing mechanism. The former idea has the virtue of simplicity, and perhaps some experimental support. When, for example, the most commonly utilized splice junctions present in SV40 late RNA species are obliterated by insertion or deletion of DNA, sequences that are normally recognized only rarely can be used at higher frequency (*Villareal* et al. 1979; *Haegerman* et al. 1979). Similarly, a hybrid mRNA species made in cells infected by the nondefective adenovirus type 2-SV40 hybrid virus, Ad2$^+$ ND$_4$, is fashioned using a novel SV40 acceptor splice site at 0.46 units in the SV40 genome. Such a site is not apparently employed in SV40 infected cells, and a fraction of the Ad2$^+$ ND$_4$ population lacks the normal SV40 early splicing sites (*Khoury* et al. 1980). Both these observations can be interpreted in terms of the recognition of weaker splice sites only in the absence of strong signals. Thus, they might imply the existence of a hierarchy of splice sites, differing in the efficiency with which they are recognized and utilized by the splicing machinery. More subtle experiments, for example specific in vitro alterations of splicing signals, will be required to test this notion.

Whether or not viruses can modify the splicing systems of their host cells also remains an open question. It has, for example, been suggested that small, virus-specific RNAs, VA-RNA, synthesized by form III RNA polymerase in adenovirus infected cells might play a role splicing of adenoviral late gene products (*Murray* and *Holliday* 1979), analogous to that described for U1 RNA. This hypothesis stems from the fact that 19 nucleotides of the major VA-RNA, VA$_1$-RNA, located at two separate sites in the VA RNA chain can form a base-paired structure with sequences at the ends of the intervening sequence between the 3'-end of the tripartite leader segment and the 5'-end of hexon mRNA body sequences. Such an interaction, illustrated in Figure 7B, would include 10 G:C and 4 G:U base pairs. There is some evidence to suggest that VA RNA species can indeed form short duplexes with adenoviral late nuclear RNA or with cloned DNA copies of the fiber mRNA that include the entire leader segment as well as the 5'-end of the gene (*Mathews* 1980), but a critical test of this hypothesis has yet to be performed.

A major difference between the postulated base pairing of U1 RNA and the consensus splice junction sequences (Fig. 7A) and that of VA_1 RNA to hexon precursor RNA (Fig. 7B) is that the latter includes interactions between nucleotides retained in mature mRNA and the so-called "splicer" RNA, whereas the former does not. It can be imagined that such interaction between VA_1 RNA and sequences of the mature message confers additional specificity upon the RNA:RNA interaction. Further experimental information, such as the sequences of additional junctions between intervening sequences and adenovirus 2 late mRNA bodies, is required to evaluate this idea. It may be significant that the fiber sequence corresponding to that shown at the bottom of Figure 7B for hexon mRNA includes only one base change, compared to the hexon sequence, in the region postulated for base-pair formation with VA_1 RNA (see Fig. 6).

If VA RNA does indeed function as a "splicer", then some more specific interaction of the kind postulated would seem to be essential. The type 2 adenoviral late splice junction sequences that are known do not differ radically from the consensus sequences, except in the low probability of a G-residue immediately adjacent to the 3'-end of the intervening sequence (see Fig. 6). Thus, any interactions specific to viral RNA precursors would have to rely upon sequences surrounding splice junctions other than those of the intervening sequence. The similarity between the adenovirus late splice junction sequences and those of other viral and cellular transcripts raises an additional interesting question, namely, why it should be necessary for adenovirus to encode its own, unique "splicer" RNA, specific for late transcripts, when it is clear that U1 RNA can mediate splicing of adenoviral early RNA species. An intriguing possibility is that this change in "splicer" as infection continues may be related to adenoviral inhibition of cellular gene expression, which is mediated at a posttranscriptional level (*Beltz* and *Flint* 1979) during the late phase of infection.

It has recently been discovered that SV40-infected cells synthesize, during the late phase of infection, a small, 65 nucleotide-long RNA species transcribed from the late strand near 0.21 units (*Alwine* et al. 1980). Such an RNA species must be complementary to sequences near the 3'-end of early region transcripts, but no evidence that this small SV40 RNA species influences expression of SV40 early genetic information has been obtained.

At the present time, virus-induced modification of cellular splicing systems remains a tantilizing possibility, with several interesting implications for splicing mechanisms in general and the ways in which a virus might influence expression of the genetic information of its host cell. Undoubtedly, this idea will receive further attention.

References

Acheson NH (1978) Polyoma virus giant RNAs contain tandem repeats of the nucleotide sequences of the entire viral genome. Proc Natl Acad Sci USA 75:4754–4758

Acheson NH, Buetti E, Scherrer K, Weil R (1971) Transcription of the polyoma virus genome: synthesis and cleavage of giant, late polyoma-specific RNA. Proc Natl Acad Sci USA 68:2231–2235

Akusjärvi G, Pettersson U (1979a) Sequence analysis of adenovirus DNA: complete nucleotide sequence of the spliced 5′ non-coding region of adenovirus 2 hexon messenger RNA. Cell 16:841–850

Akusjärvi G, Pettersson U (1979b) Nucleotide sequence at the junction between the coding region of the adenovirus 2 hexon mRNA and its leader sequence. Proc Natl Acad Sci USA 75:5822–5826

Alestrom P, Akusjärvi G, Perricaudet M, Mathews MB, Klessig DF, Pettersson U (1980) The gene for polypeptide IX of adenovirus by type 2 and its unspliced messenger RNA. Cell 19:671–681

Aloni Y, Dhar R, Laub O, Horowitz M, Khoury G (1977) Novel mechanism for RNA maturation: the leader sequences of SV40 mRNA are not transcribed adjacent to the coding sequences. Proc Natl Acad Sci USA 74:3686–3690

Alwine JC, Dhar R, Khoury G (1980) A small RNA induced late in SV40 infection can associate with early viral mRNAs. Proc Natl Acad Sci USA 77:1379–1383

Anderson CW, Baum PR, Gesteland RF (1973) Processing of adenovirus 2 induced proteins. J Virol 12:241–252

Arcement LJ, Karshin WL, Naso RB, Arlinghaus RB (1977) "Gag" polyprotein precursors of Rauscher murine leukemia virus. Virology 81:284–287

Atkins JF, Steitz JA, Anderson CW, Model P (1979) Binding of mammalian ribosomes to MS2 phage RNA reveals an overlapping gene encoding a lysis function. Cell 18:247–256

Avvedimento VE, Vogeli G, Yamada Y, Maizel JV, Pastan I, de Crombrugghe B (1980) Correlation between splicing sites within an intron and their sequence complementarity with U1RNA. Cell 21:689–696

Babich A, Nevins JR, Darnell JE (1980) Early capping of transcripts from the adenovirus major late transcription unit. Nature 287:246–248

Bachenheimer S, Darnell JE (1975) Adenovirus 2 mRNA is transcribed as part of a high molecular weight precursor RNA. Proc Natl Acad Sci USA 72:4445–4449

Baker CC, Ziff E (1980) Biogenesis, structures and sites of encoding of the 5′ termini of adenovirus 2 mRNAs. Cold Spring Harbor Symp Quant Biol 44:415–428

Barrell BG, Air GM, Hutchison CA (1976) Overlapping genes in bacteriophage OX174. Nature 264:34–41

Barrett T, Wolstenholme AJ, Mahy BJ (1979) Transcription and replication of influenza virus RNA. Virology 98:211–225

Beltz GA, Flint SJ (1979) Inhibition of HeLa cell protein synthesis during adenovirus infection: restriction of cellular messenger RNA sequences to the nucleus. J Mol Biol 131:353–373

Benz EW, Wydro RM, Nadal-Ginard B, Dina D (1980) Moloney murine sarcoma proviral DNA is a transcriptional unit. Nature 288:665–669

Beremond MW, Blumenthal T (1979) Overlapping genes in RNA phage: a new protein implicated in lysis. Cell 18:257–266

Berget SM, Sharp PA (1979) Structure of the late adenovirus 2 heterogeneous nuclear RNA. J Mol Biol 129:547–565

Berget SM, Moore C, Sharp PA (1977) Spliced segments at the 5′ terminus of adenovirus late mRNA. Proc Natl Acad Sci USA 74:3171–3175

Berk AJ, Sharp PA (1977) UV mapping of the adenovirus 2 early promoters. Cell 12:45–55

Berk AJ, Sharp PA (1978a) Spliced early mRNAs of simian virus 40. Proc Natl Acad Sci USA 75:1274–1278

Berk AJ, Sharp PA (1978b) Structure of the adenovirus 2 early mRNAs. Cell 14:695–711

Berk AJ, Lee F, Harrison T, Williams J, Sharp PA (1979) Pre-early adenovirus 5 gene product regulates synthesis of early viral messenger RNAs. Cell 17:935–944

van Beveran C, Goddard JG, Berns A, Verma LM (1980) Structure of Moloney leukemia viral DNA: nucleotide sequence of the 5′ long terminal repeat and adjacent cellular sequences. Proc Natl Acad Sci USA 77:3307–3311

Bina-Stein M, Thoren M, Salzman N, Thompson JA (1979) Rapid sequence determination of the late SV40 16S mRNA leader by using inhibitors of reverse transcriptase. Proc Natl Acad Sci USA 76:731–735

Birg F, Favaloro J, Kamen R (1977) Analysis of polyoma virus nuclear RNA by mini-blot hybridization. Proc Natl Acad Sci USA 74:3138–3142

Bishop JM (1978) Retroviruses. Annu Rev Biochem 47:37–88

Blanchard JM, Weber J, Jelinek W, Darnell JE (1979) In vitro RNA:RNA splicing in adenovirus 2 mRNA formation. Proc Natl Acad Sci USA 75:5344–5348

Bratosin S, Horowitz M, Laub O, Aloni Y (1978) Electron microscopic evidence for splicing of SV40 late mRNAs. Cell 13:783–790

Breathnach R, Benoist C, O'Hare K, Gannon F, Chambon P (1978) Ovalbumin gene: evidence for a leader sequence in mRNA and DNA sequences at the exon-intron boundaries. Proc Natl Acad Sci USA 75:4853–4857

Buchman AR, Burnett L, Berg P (1980) The SV40 nucleotide sequence. In: Tooze J (ed) Molecular biology of tumor viruses: DNA tumor viruses. Cold Spring Harbor, NY, pp 799–829

Canaani D, Khana C, Mukamel A, Groner Y (1979) Sequence heterogeneity at the 5′ termini of late SV40 19S and 16S mRNAs. Proc Natl Acad Sci USA 76:3078–3082

Celma ML, Dhar R, Pan J, Weissman SM (1977) Comparison of the nucleotide sequence of the messenger RNA from the major structural protein of SV40 with the DNA sequence encoding the amino acids of the protein. Nucleic Acids Res 4:2549–2559

Chow LT, Broker TR (1978) The spliced structures of adenovirus-2 fiber message and other late mRNAs. Cell 15:497–510

Chow LT, Roberts JM, Lewis JB, Broker TR (1977a) A map of cytoplasmic RNA transcripts from lytic adenovirus type 2 determined by electron microscopy of RNA:DNA hybrids. Cell 11:819–836

Chow LT, Gelinas RE, Broker TR, Roberts RJ (1977b) An amazing sequence arrangement at the 5′ ends of adenovirus 2 messenger RNA. Cell 12:1–8

Chow LT, Broker TR, Lewis JB (1979) Complex splicing patterns of RNAs from the early regions of adenovirus 2. J Mol Biol 134:265–303

Cohen JC, Shank PR, Morris VL, Cardiff R, Varmus HE (1979) Integration of the DNA of mouse mammary tumor virus in virus-infected normal and neoplastic tissue of the mouse. Cell 16:333–345

Cole CN, Landers T, Goff SP, Manteuil-Brutlag S, Berg P (1977) Physical and genetic characterization of deletion mutants of simian virus 40 constructed in vitro. J Virol 24:277–294

Contreras R, Cole C, Berg P, Fiers W (1979) Nucleotide sequence analysis of two SV40 mutants with deletions in the late region of the genome. J Virol 29:789–793

Cordell B, Weiss SR, Varmus HE, Bishop JM (1978) At least 104 nucleotides are transposed from the 5′ terminus of the avian sarcoma virus genome to the 5′ termini of smaller viral mRNAs. Cell 15:79–91

Crawford LV, Cole CN, Smith AE, Paucha E, Tegtmeyer P, Rundell K, Berg P (1978) Organization and expression of early genes of simian virus 40. Proc Natl Acad Sci USA 75:117–121

Derynck R, Content J, DeClerq E, Volckaert G, Tavernier J, Davos R, Fiers W (1980) Isolation and structure of human fibroblast interferon gene. Nature 285:542–547

Dhar R, Subramanian KN, Pan J, Weissman S (1977) Structure of a large segment of the genome of simian virus 40 that does not encode known proteins. Proc Natl Acad Sci USA 74:827–831

Dhar R, McClements WL, Enquist LW, van de Woude GF (1980) Nucleotide sequence of integrated Moloney sarcoma provirus long terminal repeats and their host and viral junctions. Proc Natl Acad Sci USA 77:3937–3941

Diemal B, Louis C, Sekeris CE (1977) The presence of small molecular weight RNAs in nuclear ribonucleoprotein particles carrying hnRNA. FEBS Letters 73:80–84

Dunn AR, Hassell JA (1977) A novel method to map transcripts: evidence for homology between an adenovirus mRNA and discrete multiple regions of the viral genome. Cell 12:23–36

Dunn AR, Mathews MB, Chow LT, Sambrook J, Keller W (1978) A supplementary adenoviral leader sequence and its role in messenger translation. Cell 15:511–526

Early P, Rogers J, Davis M, Calame K, Bond M, Wall R, Hood L (1980) Two mRNAs can be produced from a single immunoglobulin μ gene by alternative RNA processing pathways. Cell 20:313–319

van der Eb AJ, van Ormondt H, Schrier PI, Kupker JH, Jochemsen H, van der Elsen PJ, DeLeys RJ, Maat J, van Beveren CP, Dijkema R, deWaard A (1980) Structure and function of the transforming genes of human adenoviruses and SV40. Cold Spring Harbor Symp Quant Biol 44:383–400

Evans LH, Dresler S, Kabat D (1977) Synthesis and glycosylation of polyprotein precursors to the internal core proteins of Friend murine leukemia virus. J Virol 24:865–874

Evans R, Weber J, Ziff E, Darnell JE (1979) Premature termination during adenovirus transcription. Nature 278:367–370

Evans RM, Fraser N, Ziff E, Weber J, Wilson M, Darnell JE (1977) The initiation sites for RNA transcription in Ad2 DNA. Cell 12:733–739

Fan H (1977) RNA metabolism of murine leukemia virus: size analysis of nuclear, pulse-labelled, virus-specific RNA. Cell 11:297–305

Fan H, Verma IM (1978) Size analysis and relationship of murine leukemia virus specific mRNAs: evidence for transposition of sequences during synthesis and processing of subgenomic mRNA. J Virol 26:468–478

Fiers W, Contreras R, Haegeman G, Rogers R, van der Voorde A, van Heuverswyn H, van Herreweghe J, Volckaert G, Ysebaert M (1978) Complete nucleotide sequence of SV40 DNA. Nature 273:113–120

Flavell AJ, Cowie A, Legon S, Kamen R (1979) Multiple 5' terminal cap structures in late polyoma virus RNA. Cell 16:357–371

Flavell AJ, Cowie A, Arrand J, Kamen R (1980) Localization of three major capped 5' ends of polyoma virus late mRNA within a single tetranucleotide sequence in the viral genome. J Virol 33:902–908

Flint SJ, Sharp PA (1976) Adenovirus transcription V. Quantitation of the viral RNA sequences in adenovirus 2 infected and transformed cells. J Mol Biol 106:749–771

Flint SJ, Beltz GA (1980) Expression of transforming viral genes in semipermissive cells transformed by SV40 or Adenovirus type 2 or type 5. Cold Spring Harbor Symp Quant Biol 44:89–102

Fluck MM, Benjamin T (1979) Comparison of two early gene functions essential for transformation in polyoma virus and SV40. Virology 96:205–228

Ford JP, Hsu MT (1978) Transcription pattern of in vivo labelled late SV40 RNA: equimolar transcription beyond the mRNA 3' terminus. J Virol 28:795–801

Fraser N, Ziff E (1978) RNA structures near poly(A) of adenovirus 2 late messenger RNAs. J Mol Biol 124:27–51

Fraser NW, Seghal PB, Darnell JE (1979) Multiple discrete sites for premature RNA chain termination in adenovirus 2 infection: enhancement by 5, 6-dichloro-1-B-D-ribofuranosyl benzimidazole. Proc Natl Acad Sci USA 76:2571–2575

Friedman T, Esty A, LaPorte P, Deininger P (1979) The nucleotide sequence and genome organization of the polyoma early region: extensive nucleotide and amino acid homology with SV40. Cell 17:715–724

Ghosh PK, Reddy VR, Swinscoe J, Leibowitz P, Weissman SM (1978a) Heterogeneity and 5' terminal structures of the late RNAs of SV40. J Mol Biol 126:813–846

Ghosh PK, Reddy VR, Swinscoe J, Choudary PH, Leibowitz P, Weissman SM (1978b) The 5' terminal leader sequence of late 16S mRNA from cells infected with SV40. J Biol Chem 253: 3643–3647

Goldberg S, Weber J, Darnell JE (1977) The definition of a large viral transcription unit late in adenovirus 2 infection of HeLa cells: mapping by effects of ultraviolet irradiation. Cell 10:617–621

Goldenberg CJ, Raskas HJ (1979) Splicing patterns of nuclear precursors to the mRNA from adenovirus 2 DNA binding protein. Cell 16:131–138

Graham FG, Harrison TJ, Williams JF (1978) Defective transforming capacity of adenovirus type 5 host-range mutants. Virology 86:10–21

Green MR, Roeder RG (1980a) Transcripts of the adeno-associated virus genome: mapping of the major RNAs. J Virol 36:79–92

Green MR, Roeder RG (1980b) Definition of a novel promoter for the major adenovirus-associated virus mRNA. Cell 22:231–242

Green MR, Lebovitz RM, Roeder RG (1979) Expression of the autonomous parvovirus H1 genome: evidence for a single transcriptional unit and multiple spliced polyadenylated transcripts. Cell 17:967–977

Green MR, Straus SE, Roeder RG (1980) Transcripts of the AAV genome: multiple poly-adenylated RNAs including a potential primary transcript. J Virol 355:560–565

Gruss P, Lai CJ, Dhar R, Khoury G (1979) Splicing as a requirement for biogenesis of functional 16S mRNA of SV40. Proc Natl Acad Sci USA 76:4317–4321

Haegerman G, Fiers W (1978) Evidence for 'splicing' of SV40 16S mRNA. Nature 273:70–73

Haegerman G, van Heuverswyn H, Gheysen D, Fiers W (1979) Heterogeneity of the 5' terminus of late mRNA induced by a viable SV40 deletion mutant. J Virol 31:484–493

Halbert DN, Spector DJ, Raskas H (1979) In vitro translation products specified by the transforming region of adenovirus type 2. J Virol 31:621–629

Hamada H, Igarashi T, Muramatsu M (1980) In vitro splicing of SV40 late mRNA in isolated nuclei from CV-1 cells. Nucleic Acids Res 8:587–599

Hamer D, Smith KD, Boyer SH, Leder P (1979) SV40 recombinants carrying rabbit β-globin gene. Cell 17:725–735

Harrison TJ, Graham FG, Williams JF (1977) Host range mutants of adenovirus type 5 defective for growth in human cells. Virology 77:319–329

Harter ML, Lewis JB (1978) Adenovirus type 2 early proteins synthesized in vitro and in vivo: identification in infected cells of the 38,000 to 50,000 molecular weight protein encoded by the left end of the adenovirus type 2 genome. J Virol 26:737–749

Haseltine W, Baltimore D (1976) Size of murine RNA tumor virus-specific nuclear RNA molecules. J Virol 19:331–337

Hay AJ, Lomniczi B, Bellamy AR, Skehel JJ (1977) Transcription of the influenza virus genome. Virology 83:337–355

Hayward WS (1977) Size and genetic content of viral RNAs in avian oncornavirus infected cells. J Virol 24:47–63

Horowitz M, Bratosin S, Aloni Y (1978) Polyoma infected cells contain at least three spliced late RNAs. Nucleic Acids Res 5:4663–4675

Howard EF (1978) Small nuclear RNA molecules in nuclear ribonucleoprotein complexes from mouse erythroleukemia cells. Biochem 17:3228–3236

Hsu MT, Ford J (1977) Sequence arrangements of the 5' ends of SV40 16S and 19S mRNAs. Proc Natl Acad Sci USA 74:4982–4985

Hsu TW, Sabran JL, Mark GE, Guntaka RV, Taylor JM (1978) Analysis of unintegrated avian RNA tumor virus double stranded DNA intermediates. J Virol 28:810–818

Hughes SH, Shank PR, Spector DH, Kung HJ, Bishop JM, Varmus HE, Vogt PK, Brietman ML (1978) Proviruses of avian sarcoma viruses are terminally redundant, coextensive with unintegrated linear DNA and integrated at many sites. Cell 15:1397–1410

Hunter T, Hutchinson MA, Eckhart W (1978) Translation of polyoma virus T antigens in vitro. Proc Natl Acad Sci USA 75:5917–5921

Hutchinson MA, Hunter T, Eckhart W (1978) Characterization of T antigens in polyoma infected and transformed cells. Cell 15:65–77

Inglis SC, Barrett T, Brown CM, Almond JW (1979) The smallest genome RNA segment of influenza virus contains two genes that may overlap. Proc Natl Acad Sci USA 76:3790–3794

Ito Y, Brocklehurst JR, Dulbecco R (1977a) Virus-specific proteins in the plasma membrane of cells lytically-infected or transformed by polyoma virus. Proc Natl Acad Sci USA 74:4666–4670

Ito Y, Spurr N, Dulbecco R (1977b) Characterization of polyoma virus T antigen. Proc Natl Acad Sci USA 74:1259–1263

Ito N, Spurr N, Griffin BE (1980) Middle T antigen as primary inducer of full expression of the phenotype of transformation by polyoma virus. J Virol 35:219–232

Jones N, Shenk T (1979a) Isolation of adenovirus type 5 host-range deletion mutants defective for transformation of rat embryo cells. Cell 17:683–689

Jones N, Shenk T (1979b) An adenovirus type 5 early gene function regulates expression of other early viral genes. Proc Natl Acad Sci USA 77:3665–3669

Kamen R, Favaloro J, Parker J (1980b) Topography of the three late mRNAs of polyoma virus which encode the virion proteins. J Virol 33: (1980) 637–651

Kamen R, Favaloro J, Parker J, Treisman R, Lania La, Fried M, Mellor A (1980a) Comparison of polyoma virus transcription in productively-infected mouse cells and transformed rodent cell lines. Cold Spring Harbor Symp Quant Biol 44:63–75

Kedes LH (1976) Histone messengers and histone genes. Cell 8:321–331

Kelly TJ, Nathans D (1977) The genome of simian virus 40. Adv Virus Res 21:85–173

Khoury G, Gruss P, Dhar R, Lai CJ (1979) Processing and expression of early SV40 mRNA; a role for RNA conformation in splicing. Cell 18:85–92

Khoury G, Alwine J, Goldman N, Gruss P, Jay G (1980) New chimeric splice junction in adenovirus 2 - SV40 hybrid viral mRNA. J Virol 36:143–151

Kitchingman GR, Westphal H (1980) The structure of adenovirus 2 early nuclear and cytoplasmic RNAs. J Mol Biol 137:23–48

Kitchingman GR, Lai SP, Westphal H (1977) Loop structures in hybrids of early RNA and the separated strands of adenovirus DNA. Proc Natl Acad Sci USA 74:4392–4395

Klessig DF (1977) Two adenovirus mRNAs have a common 5' terminal leader sequence encoded at least 10 kb upstream from their main coding region. Cell 12:9–21

Kopchick JJ, Jamjoom GA, Watson KF, Arlinghaus RB (1978) Biosynthesis of reverse transcriptase from Rauscher murine leukemia virus by synthesis and cleavage of a gag-pol read-through viral polyprotein. Proc Natl Acad Sci USA 75:2016–2020

Krzyzek RA, Collett HS, Lau AF, Perdue ML, Leis JP, Faras AJ (1978) Evidence for splicing of avian sarcoma virus 5'-terminal genomic sequences onto viral specific RNA in infected cells. Proc Natl Acad Sci USA 75:1284–1288

Lai CJ, Nathans D (1975) Mapping the genome of SV40. Cold Spring Harbor Symp Quant Biol 39:53–60

Lai CJ, Khoury G (1979) Deletion mutants of SV40 defective in biosynthesis of late viral mRNA. Proc Natl Acad Sci USA 76:71–75

Lai CJ, Dhar R, Khoury G (1978) Mapping the spliced and unspliced late lytic SV40 RNAs. Cell 14:971–982

Lamb RA, Choppin PW (1979) Segment 8 of the influenza virus genome is unique in coding for two polypeptides. Proc Natl Acad Sci USA 76:4908–4912

Lamb RA, Lai CJ (1980) The sequence of interrupted and uninterrupted mRNAs and cloned DNA coding for the two overlapping non-structural proteins of influenza virus. Cell 21:475–485

Lamb RA, Etkind PR, Choppin PW (1978) Evidence for a ninth influenza viral polypeptide. Virology 91:60–78

Lamb RA, Choppin PW, Channock RM, Lai CJ (1980) Mapping of the two overlapping genes for polypeptides NS1 and NS2 on RNA segment 8 of the influenza virus genome. Proc Natl Acad Sci USA 77:1857–1861

Laub O, Bratosin S, Horowitz M, Aloni Y (1979) The initiation of transcription of SV40 DNA at late times after infection. Virology 92:310–321

Laughlin CA, Westphal H, Carter BJ (1979) Spliced adenovirus-associated virus RNA. Proc Natl Acad Sci USA 76:5567–5571

Lavi S, Groner Y (1977) 5'-terminal sequences and coding regions of late SV40 mRNAs are derived from non-contiguous segments of the viral genome. Proc Natl Acad Sci USA 74:5323–5327

Legon S, Flavell AJ, Cowie A, Kamen R (1979) Amplification in the leader sequence of late polyoma virus RNAs. Cell 16:373–388

Lerner MR, Steitz JA (1979) Antibodies to small nuclear RNAs complexed with proteins are produced by patients with systemic lupus erythematosus. Proc Natl Acad Sci USA 76:5495–5499

Lerner MR, Boyle JA, Mount SM, Wolin SL, Steitz JA (1980) Are snRNP's involved in splicing? Nature 283:220–224

Lev Z, Manor H (1977) Amount and distribution of virus-specific sequences in giant RNA molecules isolated from polyoma infected mouse kidney cells. J Virol 21:831–842

Lewis AM, Martin RG (1979) Oncogenicity of SV40 deletion mutants that induce altered 17-kilodaltons of t-proteins. Proc Natl Acad Sci USA 76:4299–4302

Lewis JB, Anderson CW, Atkins JF (1977) Further mapping of late adenovirus genes by cell-free translation of RNA selected by hybridization to specific DNA fragments. Cell 12:37–44

Lewis JB, Atkins JF, Baum PR, Solem R, Gesteland RF, Anderson CW (1976) Location and identification of the genes for adenovirus type 2 early polypeptides. Cell 7:141–151

Linke HW, Hunter T, Walter G (1979) Structural relationship between the 100,000 and 17,000 molecular weight T-antigens of SV40 as deduced by comparison with the SV40-specific proteins coded by the non-defective adenovirus type 2 - SV40 hybrid viruses. J Virol 29:390–394

Lowy DR, Rands E, Chattopadhyay SK, Garon CF, Hager GL (1980) Molecular cloning of infectious integrated murine leukemia virus DNA from infected mouse cells. Proc Natl Acad Sci USA 77:614–618

Maat J, van Ormondt H (1979) The nucleotide sequence of the transforming Hind III-G fragment of adenovirus type 5 DNA. Gene 6:75–90

Manley JL, Sharp PA, Gefter ML (1979a) RNA synthesis in isolated nuclei: in vitro initiation of adenovirus 2 major late mRNA precursor. Proc Natl Acad Sci USA 76:160–164

Manley JL, Sharp PA, Gefter ML (1979b) RNA synthesis in isolated nuclei: identification and comparison of adenovirus 2 transcripts synthesized in vitro and in vivo. J Mol Biol 135:171–197

Manley JL, Fine A, Campo A, Sharp PA, Gefter ML (1980) DNA-dependent transcription of adenovirus genes in a soluble whole-cell extract. Proc Natl Acad Sci USA 77:3855–3859

Manor H, Wu M, Baran N, Davidson N (1979) Electron microscopic mapping of RNA transcribed from the late region of polyoma virus DNA. J Virol 32:293–303

Mark GE, Taylor JM, Broni B, Krug RM (1979) Nuclear accumulation of influenza viral RNA transcripts and the effects of cycloheximide, actinomycin D and α-amanitin. J Virol 29:744–752

Martin RG, Setlow VP, Edwards CAF, Vembu D (1979) The roles of SV40 tumor antigens in transformation of Chinese hamster lung cells. Cell 17:635–643

Mathews MB (1980) Binding of adenovirus VA RNA to mRNA: a possible role in splicing. Nature 285:575–577

May E, Kress M, May P (1978) Characterization of two SV40 early mRNAs and evidence for a nuclear "prespliced" RNA species. Nucleic Acids Res 5:3083–3099

McGrogan M, Raskas HJ (1978) Two regions of the adenovirus 2 genome specify families of late polysomal RNAs containing common sequences. Proc Natl Acad Sci USA 75:625–629

Mellon P, Duesberg PH (1977) Subgenomic cellular Rous sarcoma virus RNAs contain oligonucleotides from the 3′ half and the 5′ terminus of virion RNA. Nature 270:631–634

Mellor A, Smith AE (1978) Characterization of the amino-terminal tryptic peptides of SV40 small t and large T antigens. J Virol 28:992–996

Miller JS, Ricciardi RP, Roberts BE, Paterson BM, Mathews MB (1980) The arrangement of messenger RNAs and protein coding sequences in the major late transcription unit of adenovirus 2. J Mol Biol 142:455–488

Model P, Webster RE, Zinder ND (1979) Characterization of op3, a lysis-defective mutant of bacteriophage fd. Cell 18:235–246

Murphy EC, Kopchick JJ, Watson KF, Arlinghaus RB (1978) Cell-free synthesis of a precursor polyprotein containing both gag and pol gene products by Rauscher murine leukemia virus 35S RNA. Cell 13:356–369

Murry V, Holliday R (1979) Mechanism for RNA splicing of gene transcripts. FEBS Letters 106:5–7

Nagata S, Mantei M, Weissmann C (1980) The structure of one of eight or more distinct chromosomal genes for human interferon. Nature 287:401–408

Nevins JR (1979) Processing of late adenovirus nuclear RNA to mRNA: kinetics of formation of intermediates and demonstration that all events are nuclear. J Mol Biol 130:493–506

Nevins JR, Darnell JE (1978a) Groups of adenovirus type 2 mRNAs derived from a large primary transcript: possible nuclear origin and possible common 3′ ends. J Virol 25:811–823

Nevins JR, Darnell JE (1978b) Steps in the processing of adenovirus 2 mRNA: poly(A) + nuclear sequences are conserved and poly(A) addition precedes splicing. Cell 15:1477–1493

Oppermann H, Bishop JM, Varmus HE, Levintow L (1977) A joint product of the genes gag and pol of avian sarcoma virus: a possible precursor of reverse transcriptase. Cell 12:993–1005

van Ormondt H, Maat J, de Waard A, van der Eb AJ (1978) The nucleotide sequence of the transforming Hpa 1E fragment of adenovirus type 5 DNA. Gene 4:309–328

Parsons JT, Lewis P, Dierks P (1978) Purification of virus-specific RNA from chicken cells infected with avian sarcoma virus: identification of genome length and subgenome length viral RNAs. J Virol 27:227–238

Paterson BM, Marciani DJ, Papas TS (1977) Cell-free synthesis of the precursor polyprotein for avian myeloblastosis virus DNA polymerase. Proc Natl Acad Sci USA 74:4951–4954

Paucha E, Mellor A, Smith R, Smith AE (1977) The cell-free synthesis of Simian virus 40 T-antigens. EMBO-INSERM Colloq 69:189–198

Paucha E, Mellor A, Harvey R, Smith AE, Hewick RM, Waterfield MD (1978) Large and small tumor antigens from SV40 have identical amino terminal mapping at 0.65 units. Proc Natl Acad Sci USA 75:2165–2169

Perricaudet M, Akusjärvi G, Virtonen A, Pettersson U (1979) Structure of two spliced mRNAs from the transforming region of human subgroup C adenoviruses. Nature 281:694–696

Perricaudet M, LeMoullec JM, Tiollais P, Pettersson U (1980a) Structure of two adenovirus type 12 transforming polypeptides and their evolutionary implications. Nature 288:174–176

Perricaudet M, LeMoullec JM, Pettersson U (1980b) Predicted structures of two adenovirus tumor antigens. Proc Natl Acad Sci USA 77:3778–3782

Persson H, Oberg B, Philipson L (1978) Purification and characterization of an early protein, E14k, from adenovirus type 2 infected cells. J Virol 28:119–139

Philipson L, Andersson P, Olshevsky U, Weinberg R, Baltimore D, Gesteland R (1978) Translation of murine leukemia virus and murine sarcoma virus RNAs in nuclease-treated reticulocyte lysates: enhancement of the gag-pol polypeptide with yeast suppressor tRNA. Cell 13:189–199

Piper RW (1979) Polyoma virus transcription early during productive infection of mouse 3T6 cells. J Mol Biol 131:399–407

Porter AG, Smith JC, Emtage JS (1980) Nucleotide sequence of influenza virus RNA segment 8 indicates that coding regions for NS_1 and NS_2 proteins overlap. Proc Natl Acad Sci USA 77: 5074–5078

Prives C, Gilboa E, Revel M, Winocour E (1977) Cell-free translation of SV40 early messenger RNA coding for viral T antigen. Proc Natl Acad Sci USA 74:457–461

Reddy VB, Thimmappaya B, Dhar R, Subramanian KN, Zain BS, Pan J, Ghosh PK (1978) Genome of simian virus 40. Science 200:494–502

Reddy VB, Ghosh PK, Leibowitz P, Piatak M, Weissman SM (1979a) SV40 early mRNAs. I genomic localization of 3′ and 5′ termini and two major splices in mRNA from transformed and lytically infected cells. J Virol 30:279–296

Reddy VB, Ghosh PK, Lebowitz P, Weissman SM (1979b) Gaps and duplicated sequences in the leaders of SV40 16S RNA. Nucleic Acids Res 5:4195–4214

Reed SI, Alwine JC (1977) An analysis by electron microscopy of early SV40 RNA from a tsA mutant. Cell 11:523–531

Ricciardi R, Miller JS, Roberts BE (1979) Purification and mapping of specific mRNAs by hybridization-selection and cell-free translation. Proc Natl Acad Sci USA 76:4927–4931

Rogers J, Wall R (1980) A mechanism of RNA splicing. Proc Natl Acad Sci USA 77:1877–1879

Rogers J, Early P, Carter C, Calane K, Bond M, Hood L, Wall R (1980) Two mRNAs with different 3′ ends encode membrane-bound and secreted forms of immunoglobulin μ chain. Cell 20: 303–312

Rosenthal LJ, Salmon C, Weil R (1976) Isolation and characterization of poly(A)-containing intranuclear polyoma-specific giant RNAs. Nucleic Acids Res 3:1167–1183

Ross S, Flint SJ, Levine AJ (1980) Identification of the adenovirus early proteins and their genomic map positions. Virology 100:419–432

Rothenberg E, Donoghue D, Baltimore D (1978) Analysis of a 5′ leader sequence on murine leukemia virus 21S RNA: heteroduplex mapping with long reverse transcriptase products. Cell 13: 435–451

Sabran JL, Hsu TW, Yeater C, Kaji A, Mason WS, Taylor JM (1979) Analysis of integrated avian RNA tumor virus DNA in transformed chicken, duck and quail fibroblasts. J Virol 29:170–178

Sambrook J, Greene R, Stringer J, Mitchison T, Hu SL, Botchan M (1980) Analysis of the sites of integration of viral DNA sequences in rat cells transformed by adenovirus 2 or SV40. Cold Spring Harbor Symp Quant Biol 44:569–584

Sanger F, Air GM, Barrell BG, Brown NL, Coulson AR, Fiddes JC, Hutchison AC, Slocombe PM, Smith M (1977) The nucleotide sequence of bacteriophage ∅X174 DNA. Nature 265:687–698

Schaffhausen BS, Silver JE, Benjamin TL (1978) Tumor antigens in cells productively-infected by wild-type polyoma virus and mutant N9-18. Proc Natl Acad Sci USA 75:79–83

Schlegel R, Benjamin T (1978) Cellular alterations dependent upon the polyoma virus hr-t function: separation of mitogenic from transforming capacities. Cell 14:587–599

Seghal PB, Fraser NW, Darnell JE (1979) Early Ad2 transcription units: only promoter proximal RNA continues to be made in the presence of DRB. Virology 94:185–191

Seif R (1980) Polyoma middle t antigen: a tumor progression factor. J Virol 35:479–487

Seif R, Martin RG (1979) SV40 Small t antigen is not required for the maintenance of transformation but may act as a promoter (co-carcinogen) during establishment of transformation in resting rat cells. J Virol 32:979–988

Seif I, Khoury G, Dhar R (1979a) BKV splice sequences based on analysis of preferred donor and acceptor sites. Nucleic Acids Res 6:3387–3398

Seif I, Khoury G, Dhar R (1979b) The genome of human papovavirus, BKV. Cell 18:963–977

Shank PB, Hughes SM, Kung H-J, Majors JE, Quintrell N, Guntaka RV, Bishop JM, Varmus HE

(1978) Mapping unintegrated avian sarcoma virus DNA: termini of linear DNA bear 300 nucleotide repeats present once or twice in two species of circular DNA. Cell 15:1383–1395

Shenk TE, Carbon J, Berg P (1976) Construction and analysis of viable deletion mutants of simian virus 40. J Virol 18:664–671

Shimotohno K, Mizutani S, Temin H (1980) Sequence of retrovirus provirus resembles that of bacterial transposable elements. Nature 285:550–554

Silver JE, Schaffhausen BS, Benjamin TL (1978) Tumor antigens induced by non-transforming mutants of polyoma virus. Cell 15:485–496

Simmons DT, Martin MA (1978) Common methionine-containing peptides near the amino-terminal end of primate papovavirus tumor antigens. Proc Natl Acad Sci USA 75:1131–1135

Simmons DT, Chang C, Martin MA (1979) Multiple forms of polyoma virus tumor antigens from infected and transformed cells. J Virol 29:881–887

Singer PA, Singer HH, Williamson AR (1980) Different species of messenger RNA encode receptor and sensory IgM μ chains differing at their carboxy-termini. Nature 285:294–300

Sleigh MJ, Topp WC, Hamich R, Sambrook JF (1978) Mutants of SV40 with an altered small t protein are reduced in their ability to transform cells. Cell 14:79–88

Smart JE, Ito Y (1978) Three species of polyoma virus tumor antigen share common peptides probably near the amino termini of the proteins. Cell 15:1427–1437

Smith AE, Smith R, Paucha E (1978) Extraction and fingerprint analysis of SV40 large and small T antigens. J Virol 28:140–153

Soeda E, Arrand JE, Smolar N, Griffin BE (1979) Polyoma virus DNA I. Sequence from the early region that contains the origin of replication and codes for small, middle and (part of) large T antigens. Cell 17:354–370

Soeda E, Arrand JR, Smolar N, Walsh JE, Griffin B (1980) Coding potential and regulatory signals of the polyoma virus genome. Nature 283:445–453

Spector DJ, McGrogan M, Raskas HJ (1978) Regulation of the appearance of cytoplasmic RNAs from region 1 of the adenovirus 2 genome. J Mol Biol 126:395–414

Spector DJ, Crossland LD, Halbert DN, Raskas HJ (1980) A 28k polypeptide is the translation product of 9S RNA encoded by region 1A of adenovirus 2. Virology 102:218–221

Stark BC, Kile R, Bowman EJ, Altman S (1978) Ribonuclease P: an enzyme with an essential RNA component. Proc Natl Acad Sci USA 75:3717–3721

Streuli M, Nagata S, Weissmann C (1980) At least three human type interferons: structure of 2. Science 209:1343–1347

Subramanian KN (1979) Segments of SV40 DNA spanning most of the leader sequence of the major late mRNA are dispensable. Proc Natl Acad Sci USA 76:2556–2560

Sugisaki H, Sugimoto K, Takanami M, Shiroki H, Saito I, Shimojo H, Sawada Y, Vemizu Y, Uesugi S, Fujinaga K (1980) Structure and gene organization in the transforming Hind III fragment of adenovirus 12. Cell 20:777–786

Sutcliffe JG, Shimmick TM, Verma IM, Lerner RA (1980) Nucleotide sequence of Moloney leukemia virus: 3' end reveals details of replication, analogy to bacterial transposons and an unexpected gene. Proc Natl Acad Sci USA 77:3302–3306

Tal J, Ron D, Tattersall P, Bratosin S, Aloni Y (1979) About 30% of minute virus of mice RNA is spliced out following polyadenylation. Nature 279:649–651

Taylor JM, Ilmensee R, Litwin S, Herring L, Broni B, Krug RM (1977) Use of specific radioactive probes to study transcription and replication of the influenza genome. J Virol 21:530–540

Thimmappaya B, Weissman S (1977) The early region of SV40 DNA may have more than one gene. Cell 11:837–843

Thimmappaya B, Shenk T (1979) Nucleotide sequence analysis of viable deletion mutants lacking segments of the SV40 genome coding for small t antigen. J Virol 30:668–678

Thompson JA, Radonovich MF, Salzman NP (1979) Characterization of the 5'-terminal structures of SV40 early mRNAs. J Virol 31:437–446

Tsai M-J, Ting AC, Nordstrom JL, Zimmer W, O'Malley BW (1980) Processing of high molecular weight ovalbumin and ovomucoid precursor RNAs to messenger RNA. Cell 22:219–230

Villareal LP, White RT, Berg P (1979) Mutational alterations with the SV40 leader segment generate altered 16S and 19S mRNAs. J Virol 29:209–219

Volckaert G, van der Voorder A, Fiers W (1978) Nucleotide sequence of the SV40 small t gene. Proc Natl Acad Sci USA 75:2160–2164

Volckaert G, Feunteun J, Crawford LV, Berg P, Fiers W (1979) Nucleotide sequence deletions within the coding region for small t-antigen of SV40. J Virol 30:674–682

Ward DC, Tattersall P (1978) The replication of mammalian parvoviruses. Cold Spring Harbor, N.Y.

Wasylyk B, Kedinger C, Corden J, Brison O, Chambon P (1980) Specific in vitro initiation of transcription on conalbumin and ovalbumin genes and comparison with adenovirus 2 early and late genes. Nature 285:367–373

Weber J, Jelinek W, Darnell JE (1977) The definition of a large viral transcription unit late in Ad2 infection: mapping of nascent RNA molecules labelled in isolated nuclei. Cell 10:611–616

Weber J, Blanchard JM, Ginsberg H, Darnell JE (1980) Order of polyadenylic acid addition and splicing events in early adenovirus mRNA formation. J Virol 33:286–291

Weil PA, Luse DS, Segall J, Roeder RG (1979) Selective and accurate initiation of transcription at the adenovirus 2 major late promoter in a soluble system dependent on purified RNA polymerase II and DNA. Cell 18:469–484

Weiss SR, Varmus HE, Bishop MJ (1977) The size and genetic composition of virus-specific RNAs in the cytoplasm of cells producing avian sarcoma-leukosis viruses. Cell 12:983–992

Wilson MC, Fraser NW, Darnell JE (1979) Mapping of RNA initiation sites by high doses of UV-irradiation: evidence for three independent promoters within the left-hand 11% of the Ad2 genome. Virology 94:175–184

Wilson MC, Sawicki SG, Salditt-Georgieff M, Darnell JE (1978) Adenovirus type 2 mRNA in transformed cells: map positions and differences in transport time. J Virol 25:97–103

Wold BJ, Klein WH, Hough-Evans BR, Britten RJ, Davidson N (1978) Sea urchin embryo mRNA sequences expressed in the nuclear RNAs of adult tissue. Cell 14:941–950

Wold WSM, Green M (1979) Adenovirus type 2 early polypeptides immunoprecipitated by antisera to five lines of adenovirus-transformed cells. J Virol 30:297–310

van de Woude GF, Oskarrson MK, Enquist LW, Nomura S, Sullivan M, Fischinger PJ (1979) Cloning of integrated Moloney sarcoma proviral DNA sequences in bacteriophage λ. Proc Natl Acad Sci USA 76:4464–4468

Yamamoto T, deCrombrugghe B, Pastan I (1980) Identification of a functional promoter in the long terminal repeat of Rous sarcoma virus. Cell 22:787–798

Yang VW, Flint SJ (1979) Synthesis and processing of adenoviral RNA in isolated nuclei. J Virol 32:394–407

Yang VW, Lerner MR, Steitz JA, Flint SJ (1981) A small, nuclear ribonucleoprotein is required for splicing of adenoviral early RNA sequences. Proc Natl Acad Sci USA 78:1371–1375.

Yoshida K, Fujinaga K (1980) Unique species of mRNA from adenovirus type 7 early region 1 in cells transformed by adenovirus type 7 DNA fragment. J Virol 36:337–352

van Zaane D, Gielkins ALJ, Herselink WG, Bloomers HPJ (1977) Identification of Rauscher murine leukemia virus-specific mRNAs for the synthesis of gag and env gene products. Proc Natl Acad Sci USA 74:1855–1859

Zain BS, Roberts RJ (1979) Sequences from the beginning of the fiber messenger RNA of adenovirus 2. J Mol Biol 131:341–352

Zain S, Sambrook J, Roberts RJ, Keller W, Fried M, Dunn AR (1979) Nucleotide sequence analysis of the leader segments in a cloned copy of adenovirus 2 fiber mRNA. Cell 16:851–861

Zieve G, Penman S (1976) Small RNA species of the HeLa cell: metabolism and subcellular localization. Cell 8:19–31

Ziff EB, Evans RM (1978) Coincidence of the promoter and capped 5′ terminus of RNA from the adenovirus 2 major late transcription unit. Cell 15:1463 –1475

Ziff E, Fraser N (1978) Adenovirus type 2 late mRNAs: structural evidence for 3′ coterminal sequences. J Virol 25:897–906

Mechanism of mRNA Recognition by Eukaryotic Ribosomes During Initiation of Protein Synthesis

Marilyn Kozak*

1   Introduction 81
2   Characteristics of Initiation Regions in Eukaryotic Messenger RNAs 85
3   Possible Mechanisms for Selection of Initiation Sites by Eukaryotic Ribosomes . . . 91
4   Evaluation of the Scanning Mechanism 94
4.1 A Summary of the Evidence 94
4.2 Variations on the Theme 99
4.3 Messages Which Seem to Violate the First-AUG-Rule 100
4.4 How Can the Exceptions Be Explained? 102
5   Questions and Speculations 105
5.1 An Economical Message Might Initiate at the First and the
     Second AUG Codon 105
5.2 Role of 5'-Terminal Methylated Residues 106
5.3 Determinants of Messenger Efficiency 106
5.4 Peculiarities of Viral Messenger RNAs 108
References 110

1 Introduction

There has been considerable speculation about what features in messenger RNA direct ribosomes to the site where peptide-bond formation is to begin. In prokaryotic systems, a substantial body of evidence supports *Shine* and *Dalgarno's* proposal (1974) that base pairing occurs between the pyrimidine-rich 3'-end of 16S ribosomal RNA and a purine-rich sequence located approximately ten nucleotides to the left of the AUG initiator codon (*Steitz* and *Jakes* 1975; *J.J. Dunn* et al. 1978; *Steitz* 1979). This interaction plays a central role in recognition of initiation sites by bacterial ribosomes, although other features in prokaryotic mRNAs also influence the efficiency of ribosome binding (*Lodish* 1970; *Taniguchi* and *Weissmann* 1978; *Borisova* et al. 1979; *Fiil* et al. 1980; *Iserentant* and *Fiers* 1980). The structural similarities between prokaryotic and eukaryotic ribosomes (*Boublik* and *Hellmann* 1978; *Gourse* and *Gerbi* 1980; *Tanaka* et al. 1980) and the obvious parallels in the overall process of peptide-bond formation indicate a high degree of conservation during evolution of the protein synthesis machinery. On the other hand, eukaryotic translational systems display certain peculiarities which argue against the notion that the mechanism of initiation in eukaryotes is more or less an extension of the accepted prokaryotic me-

---

* Department of Biological Sciences, University of Pittsburgh, Pittsburgh, PA 15260, USA

TABLE 1. SEQUENCES OF THE 5'-UNTRANSLATED REGIONS OF EUKARYOTIC CELLULAR MESSENGER RNAs

AUCUCAGGAGCAGGAGCACCGGCAGCGCCGCCUGCAGAGCCGGCAGUACCUCACCAUGGCCAUGGCAGGCGUCUUC	[b]Chicken ovomucoid
m^{7}GpppACAUACAGCUAGAAAGCUGUAUUGCCUUUAGCAGUCAGCUCGAC/AGACAACUCAGAGUUCACCAUGGGCUCCACUCGGUGCAGCA	[b]Chicken ovalbumin
m^{7}GpppAUCACAGACCCAGAGGGACGGUCUGUCACCCCGUCUCCCUCCUCCUCAACACCAGCCUGCCCACACCAAGCUCAUCCUCUGCACC	[b]Chicken conalbumin
m^{7}GpppACACUCUUCUGGUCCCAGUCCGACGACUCAGAGGAACCACCACCAUGGUGCUGUCUCCCGCUGAC	[b]Rabbit α-globin
m^{7}GpppACUUCUCCUGGUCCCACAGACUCAGAGAGAACCCACCAUGGUGCUGUCUCCUGCCGAC	[b]Human α-globin
m^{7}GpppACUUCUGAUUCUGACAGCACUCGAGGAAGAAACCAUGGUGCUCUCGGGGAAGAC	[b]Mouse α-globin
m^{7}GpppACACUUGCUUUUGACACAACUGUGUUCACUAGCAACCUCCCAAAACAGACAGAAUGGUGCAUCUGUCCAGUGAG	[b]Rabbit β-globin
m^{7}GpppACAUUUGCUUCUGACACAACUGUGUUCACUAGCAACCUCAAACAGACACCAUGGUGCACCUGACUCCUGAG	[b]Human β-globin
ACACUUCUUCUGACAUAACAGUGUUCACUAGCAACCUCAAACAGACACCAUGGUGCAUCUGACUCCUGAG	[b]Human δ-globin
m^{7}GpppACACUCGCUUCUGGAAC[G/C]GUCUGAG[A]UAUCAAUAAGCUCCUAGUCCAGACGCCAUGGGCCAUUUCACAGAGGAG	[b]Human γ-globin
AUAUCUGCUUCUGACACAAC[U]GUGUUCACUAGCAACCUCAGACAGACACCAUGGUGCAUCUGACUCCUGAG	[b]Human ε-globin
m^{7}GpppACAUUUGCUUCUGACA[A]CUCACAACCCCAGAAACAGACAUCAUGGUGCACCUGACUGAUGCU	[b]Mouse β-globin (major)
m^{7}GpppACGUUUGCUUCUGA[G]UCUGUGUGUUGGACUUGCAAC[U]CAGAAACAGACAUCAUGGUGCACCUGAUGCU	[b]Mouse β-globin (minor)
ACACUUGCUUCUGACACAACUGUGUUCACUAGCAACCUCAGACAAACAGACACCAUG	[b]Goat β-globin
GCUCAGACCUCCUCCGACGACAGCCACACGCUACCCUCCUCCACCGCCACCAUGGUGCACUGGACUGCUGAG	[b]Chicken β-globin
m^{7}GpppAUCAGUCGGCUUCCAACUCCUCGAGAUGAGAGUCAAAACCUUUGUG	[d]Silkworm fibroin
UUUAUCAGCCUUCUCCAGGUUUACUCAACUUUGAGAAGAAGAUUGUACCUUAAGACGUGUGUAAAUAAGUGUCGCAAAAGACAUG	[b]Bovine preproparathyroid hormone
(A)ACCCUAAGUGACAGCCUACAACCAUAGACCAAGCAG/GUCAUUGUUCCAACAUGGCCCUGUGGAUGCGCCUUC	[b]Rat preproinsulin I
AGCCCUCCAGGACAGGCUGCAUCAGAGGAGGCCAUCAAGCAG/AUCACUGUCCUUCUGCCAUGGCCCUGUGGAUGCGCCUC	[c]Human preproinsulin
AGCCGAUGGAAUAAAAAAUAUUCCUUUCCCUUCUCAGAAG/GCCUCCCCAGCUCAUCAUGGGCUUACUCAGCAUG	[c]Chicken preproinsulin
...AAACCAGCUCAAGGCUGUAUCCUCCGUCCUCCUCAACACCUCAUCACCUCCCUCCUUACUCACAG/UUCUACUCAGCAUGGUCCGC	[b]Anglerfish preproinsulin
ACAGCCUAGGGCUGCGAUUUCCGCCAAACUGGACGGCAAUCCUAGCGUGAAGGCUGGAUUUUAUCCCCGCUGCCCGCCAUUGAACUGC	Mouse dihydrofolate reductase
UAAGGCCCGGAGCGGGCGCGCCGCCUGCAGGCAGGAGGUGACGGGAGGGCGGGCAUCGUCGUGAGAUCGUGCACAUC	[b]Chicken β-tubulin
AUUCGUUUUGGUUAACCCCGACGACCGUAAUCAAGAUGGCUGAG	Histone H1 (S. purpuratus)
AUUCAAGCAGCUCGAACAUUGUUACGUCUGACGUUCUGAAUUACUCGAUUAUCUCAAACCUCAACAAACAUCAUGUCUGGACGCAGGAAAGAGU	[b]Histone H2A "
AUUCACAGUAUCCAAAGAAUAUUUGCUUGACAUACUCGUUUCUCGUCGUUUCUGCGAUCGUUUACGACCCACAAGCGACC	[b]Histone H2B "
AUUCAUCCCGUCACUCGUAUUUGGACAUCGUCAAUUUCCGUUCAACUCAUAUGGCCACGCACCGACC	[b]Histone H3 "
AUUGCCUUAGCGUAAAUAUUCCUACACAGGAACACAAACCAUGUCCGGACGUGGUAAAAG	Histone H4 "
ACUUGUUUGGUUAACUCCGUACGCACGCGGUUACCAAGGUUUACCAAGUUACCCGCGACACUGACACUGCACACUGCCAAGAAA	[d]Histone H1 (P. miliaris) clone h22
AACCAUUCAAGCCAGCGACGCCACUCGUUCGUUCACCUCGUCUCUCAGCGUCGGCAUCCGUUCGCUCCUAGAAUCAUCAUGUCUGGAGAGGUAAAAGU	[b]Histone H2A "
GCACUCACAGUACCAAAAGCAUUGCUCGUGACACUCGCUGGUUCUGCUCCUAGAACAUCAGAAAACUCAUCUCCACCAUG	[b]Histone H2B "

AUUCAUCUCGUCACCCUCGUUUGAAACACUGUCUCCCAAUCACCAAG**AUG**GCACGAACCAAGCAGACG   [b] Histone H3

AAUCGCUCAGCGAAAACGUCCAGUCGCAUCGCACUCGCAUCUCAUCUCCAUA**AUG**UCAGGCCGUGGUAAAGGA   [b] Histone H4   "

UUCUAAACUGCAACCUUUCGAAGCCUUUGCUCUGGCACAACAGGUAGGCGACACGUUGUGUUCAAU**AUG**ACCAACAAGUGUCCUCUC   [c] Human fibroblast interferon

AGAACCUAGAGCCCAAGGUUCAGAGUCACCCAUCUCAGCAGAUACUGCCAGAGUAUCUGCCAUAUCUACA**AUG**GCCCUCGCCCUUUGCUUUA   [c] Human leukocyte interferon type α1

UGAGCCUAAACCUUAGGCUCACCCAUUUCAACCAGUCUCAGCGCAUCUGCCACUCACA**AUG**GCCUUGACCUUUGCUUUA   [c] Human leukocyte interferon

AUUCUCAACGUAAAUCAGAGAUUCCAACCGCAGUGGAAGGCAGCAGCACAUG / AAAUAAAUUAGUGUGUAGAAGAAUCUUGACAUG   [b] Mouse α-amylase (salivary)

m7GpppGACAACUUCAAAGCAAA**AUG**AAGUUCGUUCCUGCUGCUU   [b] Mouse α-amylase (pancreatic)

AUUCAAUUCAAACAAGCAAAGAUGAACAAGCAAAGAUGGACACACAUCGCGGAAGCGUAAGCUGAGCAACAAACAACCAAGCCAGCGAACAAGCCUAAACCUGACAAGCAAAGAUCUGC-   [d] Drosophila 70K heat shock protein

AAUAAAGUGCAAGGUUAAAGGUGAAUCAAUUAAAACCAACCUGAAAUACUGACCAACUCGUAAAUCAACC-

AAGAAGUCAUUAUUGUGAAGACAAGAGAAGACAUCUGAAUACUUCAACAGUCUGAAUUACACACACA**AUG**CCUCGUAUUGGAAUCUUG   [b] Chicken lysozyme

AGUCCCGUGUGUACGACACCUGGCCAACGAU**AUG**AGGUCUUUGCGAAGAUGUUG   [b] Dictyostelium actin clone 5

AUCAUUAUUAAUAAAAUCAUUAAAAUAUAUAUAAAAAA**AUG**GACGGUGAAGAUGGUUCAA   [b]   "   "   "   clone 6

UAAUUCAAAAAAUAAAUCAAAUAAAUAAAUAAUAUAUAAUAA**AUG**GAUGGUGAAGAUGGUUCAA   [b]   "   "   "   clone 8

UCAAUACUAAUUCAAAUCAAAUAUAUAUAUAAAAUCAUUUAAAUAAAUUGACGGUGAAGAUGGUUCAA   [b] Yeast actin

...AUUCUUCCUUCCCUUUCUACUCAAACCCAGAAGAAGAAAAGAGAAAAGGUCAAUCUUUGGUUA^AGAAUAGGAUC-
UUCUACUACAUCAGCUUUUAGAGUUUUCUCACGCCUCUAUCGuCAAAAUUUACUGCUAAUUUCUCUCCCCAAGAUCCAAAAUUUACUGCUAAUUUCUGAUAAAUUCUCAACAACUCAACAAAU**AUG**UCAUACCCAAGGUUUAGAGU/AGGUUGCUGC   [d] Dictyostelium discoidin I

AUCAUUAAAUGAAAAUCUGAAAAUUUCAUUGUUUCCUCCCAAAAUUUUAAAAUUCAACACCAAUUAAAAUCUCACCCAAGGUUUUAGU   [d]   "   "   "

AUCAUUAAAACUGAAAAAUUUAAAAUUAAAAUCUUUUUUAAAAUUCAACACCAAUUAAAAUCAUUUUUAAAAUCAUUUUUAGGU

...CAGUAACCGCCCUGAACACACUCCAGAGAAGGAGCGCCAU**GGA**UAUCUCUCUG/AGGUUGCUGC   [b] Human chorionic gonado-tropin (α subunit)

AUCAUUAAAUGAAAAUCUGAAAAUUUCAUUGUUUCCUCCCAAAAUUUUAAAAUUCAACAGCAGCCAGGUGUCAGCC   [b] Rat prolactin

...AGUGGUUCCUUUAGGACUGUGGGGGAAGUGUGGUCCCAGGUCGUCAACAGCCAGGUGUCAGCC

...GGAUCCGUGGACACGGCCUGAGCUGCUCAGGGCCUACAGGCCUCCCGGACG   [c] Human growth hormone

...GUGGACAGAUCACUGAGUGGCGAUGGCGACGACUCUCAGACU   [c] Rat growth hormone

...AAUAUUCUUUCCUUAUACAUUAGGUCCUUUGUAGCAUAAAUUACUAUACUUCUAUAGACACGCAAAAUACACUAACAUAAUA**AUG**ACAGUUCAAGGCCGGU   [b] Yeast iso-1-cytochrome c

...UUUUUAAACACCCAAGGAACCUUAGAAGACGAAUUAAUACACAUAAUAAUAAAAA**AUG**GUUAGAGUUGCUAUUAAC   [b] Yeast glyceraldehyde-3-phosphate dehydrogenase

AUCAUUCUCAGCCUUUGAUUUUCCUCAUCAUAUCAAACAAACAAAGAGUAAACA**AUG**AAACACAAAGAGCAUCCUU   [c] Silkmoth chorion gene 401a   *B-family*

AUCAUUAUUGAGUUUCCCUCAUUAAUAUCAUCAUACAGUCAAAA**AUG**CAGCCAAAGCACUUUCUC   [c] Silkmoth chorion gene 10a

GUCAUUCUGAAUUUAAUAUUCAUCAUCAGUGCAAACA**AUG**UCAACCUUCCGCUUUCUA   [c] Silkmoth chorion gene 18b   *A-family*

AUCAUUCUAGAUUCAGCAUUCAGCAUUCUGGAUCAUA**AUG**UCUACUCGUUGGAUCAUUCUUUCGUUUCUUG   [c] Silkmoth chorion gene 292a

[a] The AUG initiator codon is shown in boldface. Although all of the messenger RNAs listed in this table are believed to be capped, I have shown the m^7G cap only on those messages for which the 5'-proximal sequence was determined directly. Many of the sequences listed in the table were deduced indirectly by analysis of cDNA. Because the cDNA copy may stop short of the 5'-end of the message, it is sometimes difficult to pinpoint the precise start site of transcription. I have written three dots at the 5'-end of sequences which are known to be incomplete. For the remaining messages, the available evidence suggests that the sequence listed includes all or nearly all of the 5'-untranslated segment. Due to errors in copying by reverse transcriptase (*Richards* et al. 1979), there may be minor discrepancies in the sequence immediately adjacent to the 5'-terminus of some messages. In cases where the start site of transcription is staggered, asterisks indicate alternative sites of capping. Methylation of cap-adjacent nucleotides varies from one messenger species to another, and is not shown. Splice sites are indicated by a diagonal slash. Sequences derived solely from analysis of genomic DNA are not included in the table unless there is supplementary evidence identifying the (approximate) start site for transcription, and demonstrating colinearity of the 5'-noncoding region of the message with the gene. I have also omitted a few messages for which sequence information is available, but in which the functional initiator codon has not been identified unambiguously. Five criteria (indicated by italicized superscript letters) were used to identify functional initiator codons: (a) The AUG codon was protected against nuclease digestion by 80S ribosomes, under conditions of initiation. (b) The nucleotide sequence following the putative initiator codon corresponds to the known N-terminal amino acid sequence of the *nascent* protein. (In some cases, amino acid and nucleotide sequence data were derived from two different organisms. Although the correspondence is not always perfect in such cases, it is adequate to identify the site of initiation.) (c) The initiator codon was identified based on the known N-terminal amino acid sequence of the *mature* protein, and the expectation that the nascent form of the protein carries an additional hydrophobic "signal peptide" at the amino terminus. (d) The AUG in question is followed by an open reading frame (i.e., free of terminator codons) of sufficient length to encode a protein of the expected size. This criterion, although weak, seems acceptable in cases where the molecular weight of the protein is known and the next AUG triplet in the message is a considerable distance downstream from the first. (e) Data obtained by analyzing N-terminal tryptic peptides synthesized in vitro are consistent with initiation occurring at the indicated site. The sequences shown in the table are from the following references: *Chicken ovomucoid* − *Catterall* et al. 1980. *Chicken ovalbumin* − *Kuebbing* and *Liarakos* 1978; *McReynolds* et al. 1978. *Chicken conalbumin* − *Cochet* et al. 1979. *Rabbit α-globin* − *Baralle* 1977b; *Heindell* et al. 1978. *Human α-globin* − *Baralle* 1977c; *Chang* et al. 1977; *Wilson* et al. 1980. *Mouse α-globin* − *Baralle* and *Brownlee* 1978; *Pavlakis* et al. 1980. *Rabbit β-globin* − *Baralle* 1977a; *Efstratiadis* et al. 1977; *Lockard* and *RajBhandary* 1976. *Human β-globin* − *Baralle* 1977c; *Chang* et al. 1977. *Human δ-globin* − *Spritz* et al. 1980. *Human γ-globin* − *Chang* et al. 1978; *Slightom* et al. 1980. *Human ε-globin* − *Baralle* et al. 1980. The 5'-terminus shown for the δ- and ε-globin mRNAs is the most likely cap site, based on homology with other β-like globin genes. *Mouse β-globin* (major) − *Baralle* and *Brownlee* 1978; *Konkel* et al. 1979; *Pavlakis* et al. 1980. *Mouse β-globin* (minor) − *Baralle* and *Brownlee* 1978; *Konkel* et al. 1979. *Goat β-globin* − *Haynes* et al. 1980. *Chicken β-globin* − *Richards* et al. 1979. *Silkworm fibroin* − *Tsujimoto* and *Suzuki* 1979. *Bovine pre-proparathyroid hormone* − In the cDNA sequence reported by *Kronenberg* et al. (1979a), the region corresponding to the 5'-terminal ∼ 50 nucleotides of the message apparently became inverted during cloning. The correct sequence as shown above was recently determined by C.A. Weaver, D.F. Gordon and B. Kemper (personal communication). *Rat preproinsulin I* − *Cordell* et al. 1979; *Lomedico* et al. 1979. *Human preproinsulin* − *Bell* et al. 1980. *Chicken preproinsulin* − *Perler* et al. 1980. In the case of human and chicken preproinsulin mRNAs, the 5'-terminus and the end points of the intervening sequence were tentatively located by comparison with the rat sequence. *Anglerfish preproinsulin* − *Hobart* et al. 1980. *Mouse dihydrofolate reductase* − *Nunberg* et al. 1980. Contrary to an earlier report, the 5'-noncoding region of the mouse dihydrofolate reductase message does not appear to be spliced (*C. Simonsen* and *R. Schimke*, personal communication). *Chicken β-tubulin* − *Valenzuela* et al. 1981. *Strongylocentrotus purpuratus histone messages* − *Sures* et al. 1978, 1980. *Psammechinus miliaris histone messages* (clone h22) − *Schaffner* et al. 1978; *Busslinger* et al. 1980; *Hentschel* et al. 1980. *Human fibroblast interferon* − *Houghton* et al. 1980; *Derynck* et al. 1980. *Human leukocyte interferon* (type α1) − *Mantei* et al. 1980; *Nagata* et al. 1980. *Human leukocyte interferon* − *Goeddel* et al. 1980. *Mouse α-amylase messages* − *Hagenbüchle* et al. 1980. *Drosophila 70K heat shock protein* − *Török* and *Karch* 1980. 5'-noncoding sequences have been determined for two additional copies of

the 70K heat-shock genes (*Ingolia* et al. 1980). One of these (BH1) differs in 18 positions from the sequence shown above. The differences include single base changes, insertions consisting of one to three nucleotides, and two deletions consisting of three and nine nucleotides, respectively. The other copy of the 70K gene, designated G13, differs in only four positions from that shown above. AUG triplets are absent from the 5'-untranslated region of all three *Drosophila* messages encoding 70K heat-shock proteins. *Chicken lysozyme* − *Jung* et al. 1980. *Dictyostelium actin messages* − *Firtel* et al. 1979 and unpublished data from *R. Firtel*. *Yeast actin* − *Ng* and *Abelson* 1980. The sequence reported by *Gallwitz* and *Sures* (1980) is identical to that shown except for a 3 bp deletion (UCA underlined). *Dictyostelium discoidin* − *Rowekamp* et al. 1980 and unpublished data from *R. Firtel. Human chorionic gonadotropin* (α subunit) − *Fiddes* and *Goodman* 1979. *Rat prolactin* − *Cooke* et al. 1980. *Human growth hormone* − *Martial* et al. 1979. *Rat growth hormone* − *Seeburg* et al. 1977. *Yeast iso-1-cytochrome c* − *Smith* et al. 1979. The length shown for the 5'-noncoding region of this message is the best estimate that can be made from available evidence (*Boss* et al. 1980). *Yeast glyceraldehyde-3-phosphate dehydrogenase* − *Holland* and *Holland* 1979. *Silkmoth chorion genes* − *Jones* and *Kafatos* 1980

chanism. For example, the monocistronic character of eukaryotic messenger RNAs and the facilitating effect of the 5'-terminal m^{7}G cap are features, not observed in prokaryotes, which must be assimilated into any model for translational initiation in eukaryotes. Although extrapolation from prokaryotes to eukaryotes seems ill-advised, there is every reason to believe that, within the eukaryotic kingdom, messenger RNAs ranging in origin from yeast cells to mice to plant and animal viruses are all initiated via fundamentally the same mechanism.

2 Characteristics of Initiation Regions in Eukaryotic Messenger RNAs

Definition of the "ribosome binding site" in a eukaryotic message is not straightforward. The region of the message *protected* against nuclease by a 40S ribosomal subunit (with associated initiation factors) can extend up to 65 nucleotides (*Kozak* and *Shatkin* 1978b). This is considerably bigger than the 25–30 nucleotide fragment protected by an 80S ribosome. It is not clear whether the "extra" sequences protected by the 40S ribosomal subunit are important for the initiation process. Neither 80S-protected nor 40S-protected mRNA fragments can *rebind* efficiently to ribosomes unless the fragment retains the m^{7}G cap (*Kozak* and *Shatkin* 1978a). Thus, the 5'-terminal cap – which is not protected by the ribosome if the cap-to-AUG distance is greater than about 50 nucleotides – nevertheless must be considered part of the initiation region. There are many other experiments, of course, which implicate the m^{7}G cap in translational initiation (*Shatkin* 1976; *Filipowicz* 1978). The current working hypothesis, for which evidence is presented in Section 4, is that a 40S ribosomal subunit binds initially at or near the (capped) 5'-end of a message and subsequently migrates along the RNA chain, stopping when it encounters the first AUG codon. If this mechanism is correct, it seems reasonable to define the "initiation region" as the entire sequence extending from the 5'-terminus up to the AUG initiator codon. This definition is obviously too broad, since portions of the 5'-noncoding region have been deleted from some messages without impairing translation (*Villarreal* et al. 1979; *Sangar* et al. 1980). Nevertheless, this seems at the moment to be the most practical definition.

Tables 1 and 2 show the sequences of the initiation regions from a large number of cellular and viral messages. The length of the 5'-noncoding region varies tremendously

TABLE 2.   SEQUENCES OF THE 5'-UNTRANSLATED REGIONS OF PLANT AND ANIMAL VIRUS MESSENGER RNAs

ppAGUAAAGACAGGAAACUUUACUGACUAAC**AUG**GCAAACAACAGAACAAC	[a,b]Satellite tobacco necrosis genome
m[7]GpppAAUAGCAAUCAGCCCAAC**AUG**GAAUCCACAAAGAACUC	[b]Turnip yellow mosaic: coat protein
m[7]GpppGUAUUUUUCAACAACAUUACAACCACAACAACAAACAACACAUUACAAUUAC**AUG**GCAUACAACACAGACAGCU	[a]Tobacco mosaic virus genome
m[7]GpppGUUUUAAAUA**AUG**UCUUACAAGUAUCACUACU	[b]Tobacco mosaic: coat protein
m[7]GpppGUAUUUAAUA**AUG**UCGACAUUCAGGAACUGGU	[b]Brome mosaic RNA-4: coat protein
m[7]GpppGUAAAAAUACCAACUAAAUUCGUUCGGCGAACAUCGGUUUUUCAGUAGUAGGAUCAUCUAAUUCUAUUUUACCAACAUCGUAAUAGUUUCUCCC	[d]Brome mosaic RNA-3
m[7]GpppGUUUUAUUUUAAUUUCUAAUAGGUCUUCAAUAGUUUCCCC	[a,b]Alfalfa mosaic RNA-4: coat protein
m[7]GpppGUUUUCACUUACACACGCUUGGUGCAAGAUGAGAUUAAUCAACUCAAUUCAAUUAUUACAGUGUAAUUCGUACU-	[a]Alfalfa mosaic RNA-3
UUUCGUAAGUAGGUUUCUGUAAAAGCGUUUCUGUUUAAAUUUGGCCUAACGAAUUCGUACUCUCGUGAUGAAGUGUGU-	[a]Reovirus σ1 protein
UAGCCAUUACCUAUCCGUAAUAGAUGCGUAAUUCGUAAUUCGUAAUUCAUUCCAUUCGUAUUUCGUGAGUGAGUUGUAGUGAUUACAGGAGAAUACAAAACAAAU	[a]Reovirus σ2 protein (s46)
m[7]GpppGCUAUUGGUCGG**AUG**GAUG GCUCGGCCUGCGUCCUA	[a]Reovirus σNS protein (s45)
m[7]GpppGCUAUUCGCUGGUCAGUU**AUG**UAUG GCUUCCUCACUCAGAG	[a]Reovirus σ3 protein (s54)
m[7]GpppGCUAUUUUG(CCUCUCC,C)AGACGUUGUCGACCGGUACUCUGCAAAGAUG GGGAACG(CU,CUUC)CU	[a]Reovirus µ1 protein (m52)
m[7]GpppGCUAAAGUGACCGUUGUCACUGCAAGAUG GGGAACG(CU,CUUC)CU	[a]Reovirus µNS protein (m44)
m[7]GpppGCUAAUCGCGGUCAGG**AUG**GAAGCG GAAUUCCAAGG	[a]Reovirus µ2 protein (m36)
m[7]GpppGCUAAUUCGGUUAAUUCGGAUAAUUCUCACAAAAGUU	[a]Reovirus large message
m[7]GpppAACAGCAAUC**AUG**GAAGUCCACGAUUUUGAG	[a]Vesicular stomatitis (Indiana) NS
m[7]GpppAACAGAUAUCACGAUCUAAGUGUAUACCCAAUCCAUCAUC**AUG**GUUCCUUAAAGAAGAUU	[a] " " " " L protein
m[7]GpppAACAGAUCGAUCGAUCUGUAUUCCUUGCACUACUUA**AUG**GUGCUUUUGUACUUA	[a] " " " " M protein
m[7]GpppAACAGAAUAAUCAAA**AUG**GCUCCUACAGUCAAGAGA	[a] " " " " G protein
m[7]GpppAACAGAGAUAAUCAAA**AUG**GCUCCUACAGUUAAGAGA	[a] " " " " N protein
m[7]GpppACUCUUCCGCAUCGUGUCUGCGGCCAGCUGUUGGG;/CUCGCGGUUGAGGACAAACUCUCGGCGUCUUUCCAGUA-	[a] " " " " (New Jersey) N protein
CUCUUGGAUCGGAAACCGUCGGCCUCCGAAC/GGUACUCCGCCACCGAGGACCUGCAUCGACCGGAUCG-	[b]Adenovirus 2 hexon protein
GAAAACCUCUCGAGAAAGCGUCUAACCAGUCACAGUCGCA/AGAGGAGCUGCAGGAGUCCGCAUCGACCGGAUCG-	
m[7]GpppACUCUUCCGCAUCGUGUCUGCGGCCAGCUGUUGGG;/CUCGCGGUUGAGGACAAACUCUCGGCGUCUUUCCAGUA-	[b]Adenovirus 2 fiber protein
CUCUUGGAUCGGAAACCGUCGGCCUCCGAAC/GUACUCCGCCACCGAGGACCUGCAUCGACCGGAUCG-	
GAAAACCUCUCGAGAAAGGCGUCUAACCAGUCACACAGUCCGCA/AGAUG AAACGCGGCCAGACCGGCUCU	[b]Adenovirus 2 late polypeptide IX
m[7]GpppAUCUGUUUUGCAGCGCCUCCGACCCGGACUGAAAAG**AUG**AGCAUAUAUCUGCCAC	Adenovirus 5 early region E1a
ACUCUUGAGUGCCAGCGAGUAGGACAAACUCUCCGCCACCGGACUGAAAAGAGACAUAUUAUCUGCCAC	

```
...GAGUUUCUCGCCAGCUCAUUUUCACGGCGCCAUUAAUGAGAACUGAAAUGACUCCC
                                  ACAUCUGACCUCAUGGAGGCUUGGGAGGUGUUUG

m7GpppGCCUCUGAGCUAUCCAGAAGUAGUGAGGAGGCUUUUGAGGCCUCCGUUAAGGUUCGUAGGUCAUGGACUGAA-

m7GpppAUUUCAGGCCAUGGUGCUGCGCCGGCUGUCACGCGUCCGUUAAGGUUCGUAGGUCAUGGACUGAA-
AGUAAAAAACAGCUCACGCCUUUUUGUGUUGUUUAGAGCUUUUGUCAAUUUUGUGAAGGGAGAUACU-
GUUGACGGGAAACGCAAAAACCAGAAAGGUUAACUG/GCCUGUACGGAAGUGUUACUUCUGCUCUAAAAGCUUAUGAAGAUGGCCCCAACAAAA

m7GpppAUUCCACAGCUGGUUCUUUCCGCCUCAGAA/GAGCUUUUGCUGCAAUUUUGUGAAGGGAGAUACU-
GUUGACGGGAAACGCAAAAACCAGAAAGGUUAACUG/GCCUGUACGGAAGUGUUACUUCUGCUCUAAAAGCUUAUGAAGAUGGCCCCAACAAAA

m7GpppAUUCCACAGCUGGUUCUUUCCC-
GCCUCAGAAGGUACCUUACCAAGGUCCUCUUUCCAGAGGUUAUUUCAGGUUAUUUCAGCCAUGGUGCUGCGCCGCCUCCGGUUAAG/GUCCAUGGGUGCUGCUUUAACACUG
     m7GpppAUUUCAGGCCAUGCCAUGGUGCUGCUUCGCUCGGCUGCCGGCGGUCUCCAGCCUCCGGUUAAG/GUCCAUGGGUGCUGCUUUAACACUG

m7GpppGACAUUUUCUAUUUUUAAG[AGUCGGGAGGAGAAAAUUACUGUUGGAGGCCCUUCCGCCACUUCUGAAGCUGAUCAA]n/GGC-
                          UGUACGGUGAUAUCACCUACCUAUUGGGCAACAGUCAUAGAGGAAGAUGGCCCCAAAAGAAAAGC

m7GpppGACAUUUUCUAUUUUUAAG[AGUCGGGAGGAGAAAAUUACUGUUGGAGGCCCUUCCGCCACUUCUGAAGCUGAUCAA]n,GUAAGUGAAUUUUCAAAUGGAGGCCGCCACUGACUAUU

m7GpppGACAUUUUCUAUUUUUAAG[AGUCGGGAGGAGAAAAUUACUGUUGGAGGCCCUUCCGCCACUUCUGAAGCUGAUCAA]n/GAA-
                    UACAGCGGUACCUACACACAGGAAGAGGUCCUACUGUAAAAUAGAAAAUAUGGCGUUGAUACCAUGGCGG

          ACCGGAGGGAGCAA/AGCAAAAGCAGGGUGACAAAGACAUAAUGAAUUCCAACACUGUGUCA
          AGUGUUCGC/

          AUCCUUUUGCAA/GCAAAAGCAGGUAGAUAUUUAAAGAUGAGUCUUCUAACCGAGGU
          CUGGUUGCGG//

          GUUCAUCAUCCCU//GCAAAAGCAGGUAGAUAUUUAAAGAUGAGUCUUCUAACCGAGGU

m7GpppGCCAUUUGACCAUUCACCACAUUGGUGUGCACCUGGGUUGAUGGUGGGAUGGCGGACCUCGGACCUACGAC-
ACCUGCAUGAAGCAGCAGGUCUCCAACUCCCGACGUGAUUUGGUGGGAAGUGGUGGGUCGGCCCCACGACGGC-
GUGGCCAUCCUGGUCUCCAUCCUGCUGCUCGUCGCUUUCGGAGGGCGAGGGGGCUCGCGCUU-
AGGGAGCAGCAAGCUGAGUACCGUCGUCGGAGGAUGAUGCAGUGGGGACGGGAGCCCUGGGCGAUCAAGCAGCAUGGAAGCCGCGCGAUCACAUUAAGGUG

ACACCGAGCGACCCUGCAGCCCCAUCGCCGUCAAGCAGCGUCCGCAGAUCCUUGGUGGUGGGAAACUCCC-
GCACCUUCUGGCCCAGCCCCUUGUAGAAGCGCGUAGAGGCGCGUAUGUGCCUUCGUACCCCGGCCAU
```

[d] Adenovirus 12 early region Ela
[b] Adenovirus 5 early region Elb
[b] SV40 early mRNAs (T and t antigens)
[e] SV40 major late 16S mRNA (encoding VP1)
SV40 minor 16S mRNA
[d] The two most abundant species of } SV40 late 19S mRNA, encoding VP2
[b] Polyoma virus late 16S mRNA (encoding VP1)
[b] Polyoma late 19S (encoding VP2)
[b] Polyoma late 18S (encoding VP3)
[d] Human influenza (A) hemagglutinin (subtype H3)
[d] Human influenza (A) NS proteins
[b] Fowl plague virus matrix protein
[b] Rous sarcoma virus genome RNA (encoding the gag polyprotein)
[d] Herpes thymidine kinase

[a] All of the messages listed are believed to be capped, with the exception of satellite tobacco necrosis virus genome RNA. Criteria used in assembling this table are described in the footnote to Table 1. Sequence data are taken from the following references: *Satellite tobacco necrosis virus genome* − *Leung* et al. 1979; *Browning* et al. 1980. *Turnip yellow mosaic virus coat protein* − *Guilley* and *Briand* 1978. *Tobacco mosaic virus genome* − *Jonard* et al. 1978; *Richards* et al. 1978. *Tobacco mosaic virus coat protein* − *Guilley* et al. 1979. *Brome mosaic virus coat protein* (RNA-4) − *Dasgupta* et al. 1975. *Brome mosaic virus RNA-3* − *Ahlquist* et al. 1979. *Alfalfa mosaic virus coat protein* (RNA-4) − *Koper-Zwarthoff* et al. 1977. The nucleotide in position 26 of RNA-4 varies among different strains of alfalfa mosaic virus; A, G, and U have been found in that position (*Swinkels* and *Bol* 1980). *Alfalfa mosaic virus RNA-3* − *L. Pinck,* personal communication. *Koper-Zwarthoff* et al. (1980) have analyzed the first 101 nucleotides of RNA-3 from a different strain of AMV. Their sequence, which differs considerably from that shown, suggests that the 5′-untranslated region may contain a nonfunctional AUG codon at position 78 to 80. Additional data are needed, however, to confirm the sequence. The 5′-proximal sequence of the message encoding *reovirus* protein σl was determined by *Li* et al. (1980). The 80S ribosome-protected portion of that message has been partially sequenced (*M. Kozak,* unpublished data) and the data support the identification of the 5′-proximal AUG as the initiator codon. Sequences for messages encoding other small (σ) and medium-sized (μ) reovirus proteins are from *Kozak* (1977) and *Darzynkiewicz* and *Shatkin* (1980). The 5′-proximal ribosome-protected sequence of one of the large reovirus messages was determined by *M. Kozak* (unpublished). *Vesicular stomatitis virus* messages: Indiana strain − *Rose* 1978, 1980; New Jersey strain − *Rowlands* 1979. *Adenovirus 2 hexon protein* − *Akusjärvi* and *Pettersson* 1979. *Adenovirus 2 fiber protein* − *Zain* et al. 1979. *Adenovirus 2 late polypeptide IX* − *Aleström* et al. 1980. *Adenovirus 5 early region E₁a* − *Perricaudet* et al. 1979; *Van Ormondt* et al. 1980. *Adenovirus 12 early region E₁a* − *Perricaudet* et al. 1980. *Adenovirus 5 early region E₁b* − *Van Ormondt* et al. 1980; *Anderson* and *Lewis* 1980. *SV40 early mRNAs* − *Reddy* et al. 1978b, 1979; *Haegeman* and *Fiers* 1980. *SV40 major late 16S mRNA* − *Ghosh* et al. 1978a. The minor species of SV40 16S mRNA listed in the table is band 9 described by *Reddy* et al. (1978a). *SV40 late 19S mRNA* − the sequences shown are those of the abundant messenger species 11 and 16 described by *Ghosh* et al. (1978b). There is extensive heterogeneity in the 5′-portion of SV40 late mRNAs, and only a few of the structures are given in the table. The sequences shown for *polyoma virus late mRNAs* were determined by *Arrand* et al. (1980). The 5′-ends of the messages were mapped by *Flavell* et al. (1980), and the splicing sites were determined by *Kamen* et al. (1980) and *Treisman* (1980). Multiple species of polyoma virus mRNAs are derived by repetition of the 57 nucleotide sequence enclosed in brackets (*Legon* et al. 1979; *Zuckermann* et al. 1980; *Treisman* 1980). Human *influenza virus (type A) hemagglutinin* − *Dhar* et al. 1980; *MinJou* et al. 1980. Human *influenza virus (type A) NS protein* − *Dhar* et al. 1980; *Lamb* and *Lai* 1980. Fowl Plague *influenza virus matrix protein* − *Caton* and *Robertson* 1980; *Robertson* 1979. The 5′-noncoding region of influenza virus mRNAs is derived by transferring the 5′-terminal 10 to 15 nucleotides from a cellular message to the nascent viral transcript (*Krug* et al. 1979). A variety of cellular messages can serve as donor, thus generating heterogeneous 5′-termini in the viral mRNA population. *Rous sarcoma virus genome* − *Haseltine* et al. 1977; *Shine* et al. 1977; *R. Swanstrom* and *J.M. Bishop,* personal communication. *Herpes simplex thymidine kinase* − *McKnight* 1980

− from 10 to more than 300 nucleotides. The extremely short and extremely long 5′-noncoding sequences are found predominantly on viral messages. Leader regions of cellular messages are somewhat more uniform; most fall within the range of 40–80 nucleotides, as shown in Figure 1. It is interesting that all of the drosophila heat-shock messages fall outside this range: the 5′-noncoding sequence varies from 111 to 253 nucleotides in five heat-shock genes that have been characterized (*Ingolia* et al. 1980; *Ingolia* and *Craig* 1981). The difference between viral and cellular messages might be related to the higher translational efficiency observed with many viral messages, although (as explained in Section 5.3) there is no simple correlation between translational efficiency and length of the 5′-noncoding region. The 5′-untranslated regions of eukaryotic messages also show enormous variation in composition. For example, the A + U content varies from 32% in chick-

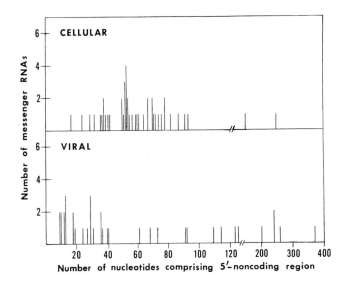

Fig. 1. Length of the 5′-noncoding portion of eukaryotic messenger RNAs. The number of nucleotides between the 5′-terminus and the AUG initiator codon is shown for cellular (upper panel) and viral messages (lower panel). The data represent only those messages in Tables 1 and 2 for which the entire 5′-noncoding sequence is known. The message for the drosophila 70K heat-shock protein is included (*Ingolia* et al. 1980), but other heat-shock messages are not shown in this figure or in Table 1 because identification of the functional initiator codon is still tentative

en ovomucoid mRNA (*Catterall* et al. 1980) to 77% in the 5′-untranslated region of tobacco mosaic virus genome RNA (*Richards* et al. 1978) and more than 90% in the actin messages of slime molds (*Firtel* et al. 1979). In most of the messages listed in Tables 1 and 2, the G content of the 5′-noncoding region is lower than the 25% that would be expected on a random basis.

In contrast with the variability in length and overall composition of 5′-untranslated segments, the sequences flanking the AUG initiator codon show rather striking uniformity. Table 3 (part A) shows that in 85% of eukaryotic messages the nucleotide immediately following the initiator codon is a purine − most often guanosine. On the 5′-side of the AUG codon, 95% of eukaryotic messages have a purine (most often adenosine) in position −3; and, in 56% of the messages examined, cytidine occurs in position −4. Thus, CAxxAUG$_A^G$ might be considered a consensus sequence for eukaryotic initiation sites. As a control of sorts, I surveyed the sequences surrounding AUG triplets which are not involved in translation; part B of Table 3 shows a much more random distribution of nucleotides flanking AUG triplets in the introns of eukaryotic genes. Interestingly, sequences flanking the initiator codon in prokaryotic messages (Table 3, part C) are similar to eukaryotic initiation sites in that adenosine frequently occurs in position −3, and either adenosine or guanosine in position +4. While it is tempting to attribute functional significance to the conserved sequences flanking eukaryotic initiator codons, presence of a purine in positions −3 and +4 cannot be an absolute requirement because a few messages deviate from the pattern. Comparison of the 5′-proximal sequence of the N message in two strains of vesicular stomatitis virus reveals only three differences, one of which involves

Table 3. Analysis of Sequences Flanking AUG Codons[a]

	Position −4	Position −3	Position −2	Position −1	Position +4	Position +5	Position +6
A. Sequences Flanking the Initiator AUG in Eukaryotic Messages							
U	11%	1%	24%	12%	11%	14%	42%
A	22%	83%	35%	25%	22%	27%	15%
C	56%	4%	33%	49%	4%	43%	15%
G	11%	12%	8%	14%	63%	16%	28%
B. Sequences Flanking AUG Triplets Which Occur in Introns of Eukaryotic Genes							
U	26%	31%	25%	33%	32%	24%	26%
A	30%	35%	33%	28%	28%	33%	36%
C	25%	17%	19%	22%	20%	21%	24%
G	19%	17%	23%	17%	20%	22%	14%
C. Sequences Flanking the Initiator Codon in Prokaryotic Messages							
U	19%	17%	36%	30%	14%	16%	34%
A	49%	60%	29%	32%	42%	28%	46%
C	18%	18%	24%	28%	11%	41%	11%
G	14%	5%	11%	10%	33%	15%	9%

[a] The AUG codon is numbered +1 to +3, and numbering continues (+4 etc.) into the coding portion of the message. Nucleotides in the 5′-noncoding region of the message are assigned negative numbers beginning with the residue immediately preceding the AUG triplet. In addition to the sequences listed in Tables 1 and 2, the following messenger RNAs were also included in part A: Semliki Forest virus capsid protein (*Garoff* et al. 1980), hepatitis B virus surface antigen (*Valenzuela* et al. 1979), Rous sarcoma virus *src* protein (*Czernilofsky* et al. 1980), polyoma virus early mRNAs (*Friedmann* et al. 1978), the 16K protein from adenovirus 2, early region 3 (*Hérissé* et al. 1980), rainbow trout protamine (*Jenkins* 1979), chicken α-globin (*Richards* and *Wells* 1980). *Xenopus* β-globin (*Williams* et al. 1980), bovine ACTH-β-LPH precursor protein (*Nakanishi* et al. 1980), yeast iso-2-cytochrome c (*Montgomery* et al. 1980), yeast his 4 gene (*Farabaugh* and *Fink* 1980), and four mouse immunoglobulin genes (*Bernard* et al. 1978; *Seidman* et al. 1979; *Early* et al. 1980; *Sakano* et al. 1980). The initiation site for SV40 VP3 was included (*Reddy* et al. 1978b) but VP1 was omitted since it is not known whether translation in vivo begins at position 239 or 245. A total of 106 messages is represented in part A. The intervening sequences surveyed in part B are from the chick ovalbumin gene (*Robertson* et al. 1979), silkworm fibroin (*Tsujimoto* and *Suzuki* 1979), rat preproinsulin (*Lomedico* et al. 1979), mouse α-globin (*Nishioka* and *Leder* 1979), mouse β-globin (*Konkel* et al. 1978), rabbit β-globin (*Van Ooyen* et al. 1979), and two mouse immunoglobulin genes (*Bernard* et al. 1978; *Early* et al. 1980). For part C, the seventy-two prokaryotic initiation sites listed by *Atkins* (1979) and by *Post* and *Nomura* (1980) were used

the residue immediately following the initiator codon: AUGG is changed to AUGU (*Rowlands* 1979).

Because prokaryotic ribosome binding sites nearly always contain a terminator codon − either UAA or UGA − closely preceding the initiator codon, *Atkins* (1979) has speculated that terminator codons and release factors might be involved in the initiation process in prokaryotes. Inspection of the 5′-untranslated sequences of eukaryotic messages reveals that the frequency of nonsense codons (UAA, UGA or UAG) is approximately as expected on a random basis: one terminator in any frame per seven codons. The terminator codons occur at varying distances from the AUG triplet, and there is no reason to suspect their involvement in the initiation process in eukaryotes.

The most striking characteristic of eukaryotic initiation regions is absence of AUG triplets from the 5'-noncoding portion of the mRNA. In 90 out of the 95 messages listed in Tables 1 and 2, the AUG codon located closest to the 5'-end is the one used to initiate translation. The few exceptions to this rule are discussed in Section 4.3. Splicing has been detected within the 5'-noncoding region of many viral and a few cellular messages – including those of ovalbumin (*Catterall* et al. 1978), bovine ACTH-β-LPH precursor protein (*Nakanishi* et al. 1980), mouse α-amylase (*Young* et al. 1981) and preproinsulin (*Lomedico* et al. 1979; *Bell* et al. 1980; *Perler* et al. 1980). It is curious that, in each of the preproinsulin genes, the rather short intron that interrupts the 5'-untranslated segment contains one or more AUG triplets. Thus one might argue that the intervening sequence, although quite short, must nevertheless be removed – if absence of AUG codons upstream from the initiation site is important for mRNA function, as proposed below.

Although GUG triplets occur in the 5'-proximal portion of many eukaryotic messages, there is no evidence that GUG can function as an initiator codon in eukaryotes. In the presence of low concentration (2 mM) magnesium chloride, only synthetic polymers that contained AUG were translated in an ascites cell-free system; GUG-containing polymers worked only when the magnesium concentration was increased to 5 mM (*Brown* and *Smith* 1970). The conclusion that GUG cannot normally initiate translation is supported by genetic studies in yeast (*Stewart* et al. 1971). Direct analysis of nucleotide sequences (Tables 1, 2) has so far revealed not a single eukaryotic message in which GUG initiates translation. This contrasts with prokaryotes, where GUG does function as the initiator codon, albeit infrequently (*Atkins* 1979). In rare instances bacterial ribosomes can even initiate at AUA (*Belin* et al. 1979) or UUG codons (*Files* et al. 1975). There are a number of structural differences between prokaryotic and eukaryotic initiator Met-tRNA species which may account for the greater flexibility in bacteria. One possibility is that the hypermodified residue N^6-(threoninocarbonyl)adenosine adjacent to the anticodon in eukaryotic (but not prokaryotic) initiator Met-tRNA restricts the ability of the eukaryotic species to mispair with GUG or other codons (*Ofengand* 1977; *Sherman* et al. 1980a). Whatever the reason, AUG seems to be the only functional initiator codon in eukaryotes.

3 Possible Mechanisms for Selection of Initiation Sites by Eukaryotic Ribosomes

Various mechanisms have been proposed to explain how eukaryotic ribosomes might recognize the unique initiator codon in a message.

The "scanning model" postulates an entry site for 40S ribosomal subunits which is distinct from the AUG-containing site. The hypothesis is that a 40S subunit (with associated initiation factors and Met-tRNA) binds initially at the 5'-end of the message and subsequently migrates toward the interior of the mRNA, stopping when it encounters the first AUG codon. According to this mechanism, the initiator codon is defined simply by its position: the AUG closest to the 5'-terminus is the one used to initiate protein synthesis. Evidence supporting this idea has been reviewed previously (*Kozak* 1978, 1980e); an updated summary of the evidence is presented in the following section.

Whereas the scanning mechanism postulates sequential interactions, an alternative possibility is that the ribosome interacts simultaneously with the 5'-terminus and the

AUG triplet. Since the distance between the m^7G cap and the initiator AUG codon varies among eukaryotic messages from 10 to more than 300 nucleotides, the two-site recognition mechanism requires that secondary/tertiary folding within the 5'-region of the message brings the cap and the AUG close together. Were this true, denaturing the message should impair ribosome binding; but this does not appear to happen. On the contrary, denaturation seems to enhance the efficiency of initiation (*Payvar* and *Schimke* 1979; *Kozak* 1980a). The two-site recognition model is also contradicted by the finding that, after removal of the m^7G cap from reovirus mRNA, wheat germ ribosomes continued to bind exclusively (albeit with lower efficiency) at the authentic initiator codon (*Kozak* and *Shatkin* 1978a). Many spurious internal "initiation sites" were activated by cleaving the message, however (*Kozak* 1980b). This runs contrary to the notion that the 5'-terminus and the AUG codon must be properly oriented in order for ribosomes to bind, since the chance occurrence of such an elaborate recognition signal should be low.

A third hypothesis is that the 40S ribosomal subunit enters at the 5'-end of a message and subsequently repositions itself at the AUG-containing site, *without traversing the entire 5'-noncoding sequence.* Since there is no evidence for initiation at multiple sites, even when the 5'-segment of a message contains several nearby AUGs, the mechanism by which the ribosome is transferred from the 5'-terminus must be precise. The "bind-and-jump" model requires an additional signal to tell the ribosome *which* AUG triplet to aim for. The recognition feature could be a hairpin loop preceding the AUG codon, as occurs in rat preproinsulin mRNA (*Lomedico* et al. 1979), chick ovalbumin mRNA (*Schroeder* et al. 1979), and the message encoding the T antigen of SV40 and BK virus (*Yang* and *Wu* 1979). But hairpin loops are not found in a comparable position in many other eukaryotic messages. The sequence CUUPyUG, common to globin mRNAs (*Baralle* and *Brownlee* 1978), is not present in the leader region of most of the other messages listed in Tables 1 and 2. Many eukaryotic initiation sites have the form $CAxxAUG^G_A$, as mentioned above; but this sequence is not universal nor is it unique to initiator AUGs.

The most popular suggestion is that recognition of the initiator AUG might be mediated by base pairing between the 3'-end of 18S ribosomal RNA and a complementary sequence located to the left (*Hagenbüchle* et al. 1978; *Azad* and *Deacon* 1980) or right of the AUG triplet (*Both* 1979; *Tsujimoto* and *Suzuki* 1979). Some eukaryotic messages do have a sequence complementary to the purine-rich tract 3'-UAGGAAGGCGU-5' which is present near the 3'-end of 18S rRNA, but occurrence of the required sequence within the 5'-proximal region of eukaryotic mRNAs does not appear to be statistically significant (*DeWachter* 1979). Noting the absence of a common sequence upstream of the AUG triplet, *Baralle* and *Brownlee* (1978) proposed that a base-pairing mechanism might operate in eukaryotes similar to that which occurs in prokaryotes, except that it is the AUG codon itself that pairs with ribosomal RNA. Such an interaction would not help to explain how ribosomes distinguish the *unique* initiator AUG from all others, however. In recent studies, a psoralen derivative was used to crosslink apposed regions of mRNA and ribosomal RNA within 40S and 80S initiation complexes (*Nakashima* et al. 1980). The results suggest that the 3'-terminus of 18S rRNA is positioned near the 5'-end of reovirus and a number of other viral mRNAs. But further experiments are needed to verify this interpretation. The same type of crosslinked complex could be formed with capped poly(U), which has little potential to base pair with the 3'-end of 18S rRNA. Thus, although these experiments demonstrate that messenger RNA and 18S rRNA are closely apposed in initiation complexes, additional work is needed to determine if the two RNA components are actually base paired, precisely which portions of each RNA are involved, and whether the interaction has functional significance. Although the 5'-noncoding sequences of many eukaryotic messages reveal little potential for base pairing with the 3'-end of 18S ribosomal RNA, there are some striking exceptions. The leader regions of adenovirus early and late mRNAs (*Baker* et al. 1979; *Ziff* and *Evans* 1978), polyoma virus late 16S mRNA (*Legon* 1979; *Soeda* et al. 1980), ovalbumin (*Kuebbing* and *Liarakos* 1978), interferon (*Houghton* et al. 1980), and a few other messages show an impressive 6–9 nucleotide complementarity with the purine-rich segment near the 3'-end of 18S rRNA. The problem is that the putative "Shine/Dalgarno sequence" in these messages occurs a considerable distance upstream from the AUG codon. Thus, if that sequence in eukaryotic mRNAs has functional significance, it seems more likely that interaction with rRNA might enhance the efficiency of translation – perhaps by stabilizing a "preinitiation complex" – than that it would help to identify the correct initiator codon.

If an additional signal (apart from the 5'-terminus and the AUG codon) is needed to identify the initiation site, it cannot be very elaborate in view of the large number of adventitious sites that become active upon fragmentation of a message (*Kozak* 1980b). Moreover, genetic studies with yeast iso-1-cytochrome c mutants have provided strong evidence that selection of the initiator AUG is not dictated by the flanking nucleotide sequences (*Sherman* et al. 1980b). Although these experiments do not rule out a "bind-and-jump" mechanism, it becomes difficult to imagine what feature(s) might serve to identify a particular AUG triplet as the target.

A fourth possibility is that the functional initiator codon is chosen by default: it might be the only AUG *not* sequestered by the secondary/tertiary structure of the message. This "conformational model" predicts that the functional AUG should always be located in an exposed region. There are several examples of eukaryotic messages, however, in which the initiator codon is likely to be involved in a stable base-paired structure (*Ahlquist* et al. 1979; *Schroeder* et al. 1979; *Tsujimoto* and *Suzuki* 1979; *Soeda* et al. 1980; *Pavlakis* et al. 1980). On the other hand, a preliminary analysis of the secondary structure of globin mRNA suggests that several *internal* (noninitiator) AUG codons are highly *exposed* (*Pavlakis* et al. 1980). The conformational model predicts that denaturation of a message should activate new initiation sites. Contrary to this prediction, recent studies showed that 80S initiation complexes continue to form predominantly, if not exclusively, at the 5'-proximal AUG in unfolded reovirus mRNA (*Kozak* 1980a, d). [The story is a little more complicated if one incubates denatured mRNA with 40S subunits in the absence of 60S subunits. Under those conditions, many "extra" 40S subunits bound to unfolded reovirus mRNA (*Kozak* 1980a). This appeared to be due to excessive *migration* of 40S subunits, however, rather than direct binding of ribosomes to spurious sites in the denatured template. Even when the template was extensively unfolded, 40S ribosomes were able to enter only at the 5'-terminus of reovirus mRNA.]

Although alternative mechanisms have not been rigorously disproven, the available evidence seems most consistent with the scanning model. The following section outlines the evidence in more detail.

4 Evaluation of the Scanning Mechanism

4.1 A Summary of the Evidence

Various types of experiments, carried out in many different laboratories, have provided evidence consistent with the scanning model.

1. The mechanism rationalizes the facilitating effect of the m⁷G cap, which is at the putative entry site for 40S ribosomes. The importance of the methylated cap was shown by comparing the translational activity of capped and uncapped forms of a given message (*Both* et al. 1975; *Lockard* and *Lane* 1978; *Muthukrishnan* et al. 1978), and by demonstrating that in vitro translation of capped mRNAs is inhibited by addition of cap analogues (*Hickey* et al. 1976) or anti-cap antibodies (*Munns* et al. 1979). An overwhelming body of evidence documenting the importance of the cap has been presented in previous reviews (*Shatkin* 1976; *Filipowicz* 1978; *Banerjee* 1980) and need not be repeated here. It is noteworthy that the m⁷G cap enhances translation even in messages in which the initiator codon is hundreds of nucleotides downstream from the 5′-terminus (*Beemon* and *Hunter* 1977; *Kamen* et al. 1978). In attempting to deduce how the cap exerts its effect, one point that must be remembered is that ribosomes initiate at the *same* 5′-proximal AUG codon irrespective of the presence or absence of the terminal m⁷G (*Shih* et al. 1976; *Kozak* and *Shatkin* 1978a). Thus, although a methylated cap greatly increases the efficiency of initiation, the cap does not function as a recognition signal telling the ribosome *where* to bind. It seems to be the 5′-end of an RNA molecule as such, not the m⁷G cap, that comprises the primary recognition site for ribosome attachment. It follows that one need not postulate different initiation mechanisms for capped versus uncapped messages.

2. Ribosome binding is prevented by circularization of the message (*Kozak* 1979a). Linear forms of various (uncapped) synthetic polymers were shown to bind to wheat germ and reticulocyte ribosomes in vitro, but the same polymers failed to bind after they were circularized by RNA ligase. These observations have been repeated recently using a 5′-terminal fragment from tobacco mosaic virus RNA (*Konarska* et al. 1981). Loss of activity upon circularization of the template suggests that, even without the m⁷G cap, the 5′-terminus of a message plays an essential role in ribosome attachment.

3. Fragmentation of a message allows ribosomes to bind to sequences derived from the interior of the RNA molecule. Binding of ribosomes to spurious internal sites has been observed upon fragmentation of a variety of messages including cowpea mosaic virus (*Pelham* 1979a), foot-and-mouth disease virus mRNA (*Sangar* et al. 1980), ovalbumin mRNA (*Schroeder* et al. 1979), reovirus mRNA (*Kozak* 1980b), adenovirus mRNA (*Lawrence* 1980), Rous sarcoma virus RNA (*Beemon* and *Hunter* 1978), Moloney murine sarcoma virus RNA (*Papkoff* et al. 1980), and polyoma virus cRNA (*Legon* 1979). Fragments derived from the interior of reovirus mRNA bound more efficiently after mild denaturation, which may make the uncapped ends more accessible. Internal sites are *not* accessible to ribosomes in *intact* reovirus mRNA, even after extensive denaturation (*Kozak* 1980a, d). The multiplicity of "initiation sites" that are activated as a consequence of cleavage implies that the sequence requirements for ribosome binding are not very elaborate. Thus, these experiments with fragmented mRNA suggest that presence of an exposed 5′-end on an RNA molecule is necessary *and may be sufficient* to permit ribosome attachment.

4. The scanning model predicts that 40S ribosomal subunits should be able to attach

to RNA molecules which lack an AUG codon. This has, indeed, been observed with a 29-nucleotide fragment derived from the 5′-end of brome mosaic virus RNA-3 (*Ahlquist* et al. 1979) and with a variety of synthetic ribopolymers such as $m^7GpppG^mC(U)_n$, $m^7GpppG^mC(A,C)_n$ and $m^7GpppG^mC(U,C)_n$ (*Both* et al. 1976). On the other hand, *not every RNA fragment forms stable complexes* with 40S ribosomes. Negative results might be expected if the RNA molecule has a great deal of secondary structure (such that it lacks a *free* 5′-terminus) or if the template is very short, in which case the 40S ribosome might bind and immediately run off.

5. The model predicts that when ribosomes are incubated in vitro with a heterogeneous set of RNA fragments, 40S subunits should interact with (and protect from nuclease digestion) a greater variety of sequences than 80S ribosomes. That is, a 40S ribosome should be able to attach to almost any RNA fragment, whereas a 60S subunit should join only if the sequence includes an AUG codon. Consistent with this prediction, two-dimensional fingerprints of protected mRNA fragments recovered from 40S initiation complexes were far more complex than fingerprints of 80S-protected fragments (*Legon* et al. 1977; *Legon* 1979). (In view of the somewhat contradictory results described in the following paragraph, systematic studies are needed – using RNA templates of known sequence – to confirm that an AUG codon is needed for 60S joining.)

6. Messages with a long 5′-noncoding region permit more than one ribosome to bind in the presence of an inhibitor of elongation, such as sparsomycin. Binding of several ribosomes to the long 5′-leader segment of tobacco mosaic virus genome RNA (*Filipowicz* and *Haenni* 1979), brome mosaic virus (BMV) RNA-3 (*Ahlquist* et al. 1979), and polyoma virus late mRNAs (*Legon* 1979) is consistent with the notion that there is an entry site for ribosomes upstream from the AUG codon. (The long 5′-noncoding region in BMV RNA-3 actually permitted binding of a second *80S* ribosome – an interesting result *not* predicted by the scanning model. It is not known, however, if the 80S complex that forms upstream from the AUG codon is a functional intermediate or an abortive complex.)

7. A key postulate of the scanning mechanism is that 40S subunits must be able to migrate. This was first demonstrated by analyzing initiation complexes formed with reovirus mRNA and wheat germ ribosomes, in the presence of the antibiotic edeine (*Kozak* and *Shatkin* 1978b). Edeine seems to impair the ability of ribosomes to recognize the AUG codon, perhaps because the drug perturbs the binding of Met-tRNA. The result is that the first-bound 40S subunit *bypasses* the 5′-proximal AUG and advances into the interior of the message, making room for additional ribosomes to enter at the 5′-end. Thus, we found that edeine promoted formation of rapidly sedimenting complexes in which *each reovirus mRNA molecule was associated with several 40S subunits*. (Reovirus messenger RNAs are monocistronic and the 5′-noncoding region is quite short. Thus, the normal initiation complex, in the absence of edeine, consists of a single 40S subunit centered at the 5′-proximal AUG codon.) Control experiments indicated that edeine did not permit "extra" 40S ribosomes to attach *directly* to internal sites in reovirus messenger RNA. For example, when the mRNA was preincubated with wheat germ ribosomes in the presence of sparsomycin, allowing an 80S ribosome to bind at the normal initiation site and thus block the 5′-end of the message, subsequent incubation with edeine did not permit additional 40S subunits to bind. If 40S ribosomes can enter only at the 5′-end of the message, as this experiment suggests, and yet become distributed throughout the length of the RNA chain, then 40S subunits must migrate extensively after binding. This phenomenon is not induced by edeine; migration occurs in the absence of antibiotics if

the magnesium concentration is lowered (*Kozak* 1979b) or if denatured mRNA is used as template (*Kozak* 1980a). The ability of 40S subunits to migrate has been shown more directly by attaching a ^{32}P-labeled poly(A) tail to the 3′-end of brome mosaic virus RNA-4. When this template was incubated in the presence of edeine for 2 minutes (just long enough to allow one or two 40S ribosomes to attach near the 5′-end) and an inhibitor of initiation was then added, during the ensuing 3–6 minutes the prebound 40S subunits *advanced far enough to protect the ^{32}P-labeled segment against hydrolysis by nuclease.* Migration of 40S subunits under these conditions required ATP hydrolysis (*Kozak* 1980c).

The experiments just described demonstrate the ability of 40S ribosomes to migrate *beyond* the AUG codon when the initiation process is perturbed; but does migration occur *within* the 5′-untranslated region, as the scanning model requires? When initiation complexes were formed in the absence of ATP, a 40S subunit appeared to be trapped upstream from the AUG codon (*Kozak* 1980c). This result supports a two-step initiation mechanism in which entry of a 40S ribosome at the 5′-terminus of a message is followed by (ATP-dependent) migration.

8. Examination of the 5′-proximal nucleotide sequences of over 90 eukaryotic messages has revealed that, in most cases, translation begins at the AUG codon closest to the 5′-terminus. The data are summarized in Tables 1 and 2, and the few exceptions are discussed in the following section. Absence of AUG triplets from the 5′-untranslated region of most eukaryotic messenger RNAs − including a number of messages in which the 5′-noncoding segment is hundreds of nucleotides long − provides striking support for the scanning mechanism. A further prediction of the model is that, if a new AUG triplet were introduced upstream from the natural initiator codon, the adventitious AUG should supplant the natural AUG codon. To test this prediction, sodium bisulfite was used to convert an A*C*G sequence (fortuitously located in the 5′-noncoding region of two reovirus messages) to AUG. Subsequent sequence analysis of the ribosome-protected mRNA fragments recovered from sparsomycin-blocked 80S initiation complexes revealed that most of the ribosomes were indeed situated at the "unnatural" 5′-proximal AUG created by the bisulfite treatment (*Kozak* 1980d).

In an elegant genetic analysis of yeast iso-1-cytochrome c mutants, *Sherman* and colleagues showed that when the normal initiator codon was inactivated by mutation, introduction of a new AUG codon almost anywhere within a 37-nucleotide region restored translation (*Sherman* et al. 1980b). The N-terminal region of the yeast iso-1-cytochrome c gene has the sequence

AA<u>A</u> <u>UUA</u> <u>AUA</u> *AUG* ACU GAA <u>UUC</u> <u>AAG</u> GCC GGU UCU GCU <u>AAG</u>.

The AUG shown in italics is the initiator codon in the wild-type gene, and the underlined sequences indicate positions where an AUG initiator codon has been introduced in various revertants. The data provide strong evidence for a mechanism in which ribosomes initiate at the 5′-proximal AUG codon *irrespective of the flanking sequences.* [Comparison of the N-terminal amino acid sequences of wild-type yeast iso-1- and iso-2-cytochrome c (*Montgomery* et al. 1980) suggests, amusingly, that Nature may have mimicked Sherman's experiment in relocating the AUG initiator codon in one of those genes.]

9. The scanning model rationalizes the monocistronic character of eukaryotic messages (*Jacobson* and *Baltimore* 1968; *Petersen* and *McLaughlin* 1973). Even in yeast, where there are coordinately regulated genes for various biochemical pathways − superficially reminiscent of bacterial operons − the messenger RNAs have been shown to be monocistronic (*Hopper* and *Rowe* 1978). There are numerous examples of viral messages which

I. THE PRIMARY TRANSCRIPTS ARE MONOCISTRONIC mRNAs.

    (a) The genome is segmented, with each   (b) The viral genes are linked, but
        segment encoding one protein.   internal promoters permit each
                                         gene to be transcribed separately.

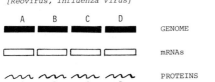   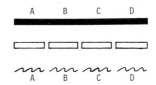

II. THE POLYCISTRONIC PRIMARY TRANSCRIPT IS TRANSLATED INTO A "POLYPROTEIN," WHICH IS
    CLEAVED TO GENERATE THE MATURE VIRAL PROTEINS.

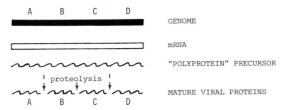

III. THE POLYCISTRONIC PRIMARY TRANSCRIPT DIRECTS TRANSLATION OF ONLY THE 5'-PROXIMAL GENE
     PRODUCT. GENERATION OF SUBGENOMIC mRNAs IS REQUIRED TO TRANSLATE THE REMAINING CISTRONS.

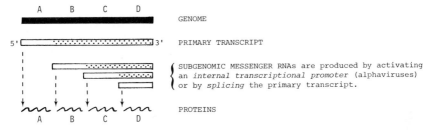

Fig. 2. An outline of strategies adopted by animal viruses to cope with the inability of eukaryotic ribosomes to initiate within the interior of a polycistronic transcript. For simplicity, each virus is diagrammed as if it encodes four proteins, designated A through D. Viruses belonging to Group Ia have fragmented genomes, with each segment encoding one protein. Segmentation of the genome guarantees that the messenger RNAs will be monocistronic. Alternatively, monocistronic messages can be produced if a polycistronic genome contains separate transcriptional promoters at the beginning of each gene, as shown for Group Ib. Whereas the primary transcripts are monocistronic in Group I viruses, the primary transcript is polycistronic in Groups II and III. When confronted with a polycistronic transcript, eukaryotic ribosomes generally initiate only at the 5'-proximal AUG, from which point peptide-bond formation continues until the first in-phase nonsense codon is encountered. In a formal sense, Group II viruses have solved the problem of how to express downstream cistrons by eliminating nonsense codons at the intercistronic junctions. Thus, the polycistronic picornavirus message, which is identical to the genome, is translated end-to-end − or nearly so − yielding a polyprotein which is subsequently clipped by proteases to generate the mature viral proteins. The picornavirus genome is "polycistronic" only if one counts the number of functional proteins it encodes; from the point of view of a ribosome, the genome is a single long cistron.

are structurally polycistronic; that is, the transcript encodes two or more polypeptides. In nearly every instance, however, translation is limited to the 5'-proximal cistron (*Smith* 1977). Figure 2 illustrates the diverse strategies adopted by animal viruses to cope with the problem that eukaryotic ribosomes cannot initiate within the interior of an RNA chain.

This peculiar restriction on initiation seems to reflect not the structure of eukaryotic messages but the properties of the eukaryotic translational machinery. Thus, even with a polycistronic mRNA from bacteriophage lambda, only the first cistron was translated in a wheat germ cell-free extract (*Rosenberg* and *Paterson* 1979). In the case of the polycistronic genomic message of RNA phages, it seems clear that authentic phage polypeptides – including coat protein (located in the center of the genome), replicase (located near the 3'-end), and lysis peptide (overlapping the coat and replicase cistrons) – can be synthesized in eukaryotic cell-free extracts (*Davies* and *Kaesberg* 1973; *Morrison* and *Lodish* 1973; *Atkins* et al. 1979). However, recent studies in which R17 RNA was incubated with

---

In the case of Group III viruses, a ribosome enters at the 5'-end of the primary transcript and proceeds *until it is halted by a nonsense triplet at the end of coding region A;* cistrons B, C, and D (stippled) are not translated. The strategy usually employed to activate the "silent" cistrons involves generating smaller transcripts from which upstream AUG codons have been eliminated. In the case of alphaviruses (group A arboviruses), the requisite subgenomic message is produced by initiating transcription at an internal site in the genome (*Brzeski* and *Kennedy* 1978; *Sawicki* et al. 1978). This contrasts with papovaviruses, adenoviruses, and retroviruses, which generate smaller messages by splicing the primary transcript. Group III viruses characteristically produce families of overlapping mRNAs which share a common 3'-terminus but have staggered 5'-termini. Depending upon where the 5'-termini of the smaller messages map, coding regions A through D may be partially overlapping, as in adenovirus and papovavirus late mRNAs, or non-overlapping, as in retroviruses and alphaviruses. I have attempted to depict only the most general features in the diagram. Detailed descriptions of the transcriptional/translational strategy of particular viruses are given in the following references. Expression of the *reovirus* genome – *Shatkin* and *Both*, 1976; *McCrae* and *Joklik* 1978. Organization of the *influenza virus* genome – *Inglis* et al. 1977. [An "extra" influenza virus message, generated by splicing one of the primary transcripts, has recently been described by *Lamb* and *Lai* (1980) and *Inglis* et al. (1980).] *Testa* et al. (1980) present evidence for a model in which *vesicular stomatitis virus* mRNAs are transcribed from multiple promoters. An alternative mechanism involving a polycistronic transcript has been proposed for VSV (*Herman* et al. 1980), but there is no evidence that the large transcript serves as a precursor to mRNA. *Vaccinia virus* probably transcribes each gene independently, at least during the early phase, since the effect of ultraviolet irradiation on synthesis of each message appears to be proportional to the size of the encoded protein (*Pelham* 1977; *Bossart* et al. 1978). The interpretation that each message is independently initiated is supported by the diversity of sequences found at the 5'-termini of in vitro transcripts (*Keith* et al. 1980) and by direct mapping of some early vaccinia mRNAs (*Wittek* et al. 1980). Under some circumstances, however, high-molecular-weight transcripts are synthesized by vaccinia cores (*Paoletti* 1977). Thus, classification of poxviruses in Group I must be considered tentative. The general scheme shown for *picornaviruses* is based on studies by *Jacobson* and *Baltimore* (1968), *Jacobson* et al. (1970) and *Villa-Komaroff* et al. (1975). Studies by *Knauert* and *Ehrenfeld* (1979) suggest a slightly more complicated picture for poliovirus, which is mentioned in the text. Expression of *polyoma virus* late genes – *Siddell* and *Smith* 1978; *Hunter* and *Gibson* 1978; *Kamen* et al. 1980. *SV40* late genes – *Lebowitz* and *Weissman* 1979. *Adenovirus* late genes – *J.S. Miller* et al. 1980. *Alphavirus* translation – *Cancedda* et al. 1975; *Glanville* et al. 1976. The role of subgenomic mRNAs in translation of *retrovirus* proteins has been described by *Pawson* et al. (1977) and *Weiss* et al. (1977). Proteolytic cleavage of high-molecular-weight precursors is also involved in generating the mature proteins of retroviruses and alphaviruses, which therefore share certain features of Group II viruses. In the case of *parvoviruses* (*Laughlin* et al. 1979) and *coronaviruses* (*Stern* and *Kennedy* 1980a, b) the structure of the mRNAs follows the pattern of Group III viruses. The coding potential of the various subgenomic messages has not yet been confirmed, however

wheat germ ribosomes suggested that cleavage of the phage RNA was a prerequisite for initiation at the internal cistrons (*Kozak* 1980b).

10. A final prediction of the scanning model, in contrast with the other mechanisms described in Section 3, is that initiation should be relatively insensitive to major perturbations in the 5'-proximal region of the message. Translation was remarkably unaffected by *deletion* of 5'-noncoding sequences in SV40 mRNA (*Haegeman* et al. 1979; *Subramanian* 1979; *Villarreal* et al. 1979), polyoma virus early mRNA (*Bendig* and *Folk* 1979), foot-and-mouth disease virus RNA (*Sangar* et al. 1980), and rabbit β-globin mRNA (*Kronenberg* et al. 1979b). Although each of these shortened messages clearly directed synthesis of normal polypeptide(s), in most cases the efficiency of translation of the altered message could not be determined. In the case of one deletion mutant affecting polyoma virus early mRNA, translational efficiency appeared to be reduced (*Bendig* et al. 1980). Translation was not prevented by *insertion* of 180 nucleotides upstream from the initiator codon in adenovirus fiber mRNA (*A.R. Dunn* et al. 1978). In studies with bisulfite-modified reovirus mRNA, extensive *alteration* of the primary sequence flanking the AUG codon did not impair ribosome binding (*Kozak* 1980d). Given the ability of eukaryotic ribosomes to tolerate such drastic changes in messenger RNA structure, it is not surprising that the 5'-untranslated regions of some closely related messages display considerable evolutionary divergence. Examples include the actin genes in slime molds (*Firtel* et al. 1979), the genes for yeast iso-1- and iso-2-cytochrome c (*Montgomery* et al. 1980), silkmoth chorion genes belonging to the same multigene family (*Jones* and *Kafatos* 1980), two genes encoding histone H2B in yeast (*Wallis* et al. 1980), isocoding histone messages in sea urchins (clones h19 and h22, *Busslinger* et al. 1980), and the late mRNAs of SV40 vs those of polyoma virus (*Arrand* et al. 1980). Comparison of the 5'-noncoding regions of ten mammalian β-like globin genes reveals only a short common sequence (CUUPyPyG) near the cap; substitutions occur in almost every other position upstream of the initiator codon (*Efstratiadis* et al. 1980). All of this variation suggests that ribosomes do not recognize, or at least do not require, a precise sequence in the 5'-untranslated portion of messenger RNA. Finally, as noted above, irreversible *denaturation* of reovirus mRNA did not diminish its capacity to interact with ribosomes (*Kozak* 1980a). Thus, one is led to postulate a mechanism for initiation in eukaryotes in which neither the primary nor the secondary structure of the message plays an obligatory role in directing ribosome binding.

4.2 Variations on the Theme

A number of variations on the scanning model have been suggested. One possibility is that the 40S ribosomal subunit bypasses AUG codons which are sequestered in base-paired structures, and that translation begins at the first *exposed* AUG. This mechanism was suggested to account for failure to initiate at the first AUG triplet in SV40 late mRNAs (*Ghosh* et al. 1978a, b; *Lebowitz* and *Weissman* 1979; *Piatak* et al. 1979) The idea seems to be contradicted, however, by several other messages in which the functional AUG codon apparently is located in a stable base-paired region of the RNA (*Ahlquist* et al. 1979; *Schroeder* et al. 1979; *Tsujimoto* and *Suzuki* 1979; *Soeda* et al. 1980; *Pavlakis* et al. 1980). This is, admittedly, a weak rebuttal since the available information about the native secondary structure of messenger RNAs is meager. On the other hand, experiments with reovirus mRNAs suggest that the best way to induce a 40S ribosome to bypass an AUG triplet is not to sequester it, but to abolish the secondary structure of the region (*Kozak* 1980a).

A nother proposed variation on the scanning mechanism is that a 60S subunit might couple with the 40S subunit at or near the 5'-terminal entry site, and it is the 80S ribosome which then scans the 5'-proximal region of the message in search of the first AUG. This idea is compatible with the observed binding of a second 80S ribosome (rather than just a 40S subunit) within the long 5'-noncoding region that precedes the AUG initiator codon in brome mosaic virus RNA-3 (*Ahlquist* et al. 1979). It has not been shown, however, (and indeed it seems unlikely) that an 80S complex which assembles upstreams of the AUG codon can subsequently migrate, in the presence of sparsomycin. On the other hand, 40S subunits are capable of migrating after attaching at the 5'-end of a message (*Kozak* and *Shatkin* 1978b; *Kozak* 1980c). Analysis of the 40S ribosome-protected regions of vesicular stomatitis virus (*Rose* 1978), polyoma virus (*Legon* 1979), satellite tobacco necrosis virus (*Browning* et al. 1980), and reovirus mRNAs (*Kozak* 1977) revealed that, with each of these messages, stable *40S initiation complexes were positioned at the AUG initiator codon*. Thus, 40S ribosomal subunits, in the absence of 60S subunits, are capable of both migrating and recognizing the AUG "stop signal".

4.3 Messages Which Seem to Violate the First-AUG-Rule

Two experimental approaches have revealed apparent exceptions to the rule that initiation of translation is confined to the first AUG triplet in a message. One approach involves analysis of the products of in vitro protein synthesis. There are a number of reports in which a single messenger RNA species directs synthesis of two or more proteins (one of which usually predominates) which appear to be independently initiated. This has been shown most convincingly with the genome RNA of poliovirus (*Celma* and *Ehrenfeld* 1975; *Knauert* and *Ehrenfeld* 1979), and a possible explanation for the poliovirus phenomenon is mentioned in the following section. Initiation at a second site within the interior of the message has also been claimed for tobacco necrosis virus (*Salvato* and *Fraenkel-Conrat* 1977), Southern bean mosaic virus (*Salerno-Rife* et al. 1980), carnation mottle virus (*Salomon* et al. 1978), alfalfa mosaic virus RNA-3 (*Pinck* et al. 1979), and cowpea mosaic virus genome RNA (*Pelham* 1979b). In most of these cases, with the notable exception of poliovirus, the possibility that a second initiation site was activated by cleavage of the message must be considered. *Lawrence* (1980) has emphasized the ease with which messenger RNA undergoes cleavage, generating translatable fragments, during incubation in reticulocyte cell-free extracts. Wheat germ extracts are also contaminated with ribonucleases, although the nuclease activity can be minimized by incubating at low temperatures. Formation of *disomes* in the absence of protein chain elongation would seem to constitute good evidence that ribosomes can indeed bind to a second, internal site in certain messenger RNAs (*Neeleman* and *Van Vloten-Doting* 1979; *Pelham* 1979b; *Pinck* et al. 1979). This criterion is meaningless, however, if the message contains a long 5'-noncoding region which may allow a queue of ribosomes to bind upstream of the *single* initiator codon (*Ahlquist* et al. 1979; *Filipowicz* and *Haenni* 1979). In view of these technical difficulties, there is not a single well-documented demonstration of a eukaryotic message in which ribosomes can initiate at both the 5'-proximal and a second internal cistron.

I have omitted from the above discussion some very preliminary reports in which the possibility of internal initiation is raised (*Dolja* et al. 1979; *Somogyi* and *Dobos* 1980), as well as a few reports in which early experiments suggesting internal initiation have been contradicted by more recent data. One of these concerns the 14S mRNA for calf lens α-crystallin, which appeared from early experiments to be a bicistronic message (*Chen* and *Spector* 1977). More recent data indicate, however, that each polypeptide is translated from a different species of mRNA (*Cohen* et al. 1978). Similarly, the 13S mRNA from maize that directs synthesis of two zein components (*Larkins* et al. 1976) has been shown to consist of two separable mRNAs (*Wienand* and *Feix* 1978). In the case of tobacco rattle virus, although *Fritsch* et al. (1977) reported that RNA-2 directs synthesis of both coat protein and a 31,000 dalton polypeptide, more recent data suggest that each protein is translated from a separate mRNA species (*Pelham* 1979c; *Bisaro* and *Siegel* 1980). Conflicting results have been obtained with the 42S RNA genome of Sindbis and Semliki Forest virus, which encodes both structural and nonstructural proteins. *Van Steeg* et al. (1979) detected initiation at both sites in their in vitro studies. This might be attributed to cleavage of the message, however, since only the 5'-proximal nonstructural proteins were initiated on 42S RNA in several other studies (*Glanville* et al. 1976; *Bonatti* et al. 1980). Early reports that flavivirus 42S RNA directs synthesis of several independently initiated proteins (*Westaway* 1977) must also be reevaluated in the light of recent evidence for a single initiation site in the flavivirus genome (*Wengler* et al. 1979a).

The second approach which has unequivocally revealed exceptions to the first-AUG-rule involves determination of nucleotide sequences. In two messages – *chicken preproinsulin* (*Perler* et al. 1980) and *Semliki Forest virus genome RNA* (*Wengler* et al. 1979b) – nonfunctional AUG codons occur very close to the cap. [Semliki Forest virus RNA is not included in Table 2 because the sequence around the functional initiator codon is not known. The conclusion that translation does not begin at the 5'-proximal AUG is based on the presence of an in-phase terminator codon a short distance downstream, and on the failure of 40S ribosomes to protect the m^{7}G cap on the related Sindbis virus genome (*Cancedda* and *Shatkin* 1979).] Since ribosomes might be expected to have a "blind spot" between the cap-binding site and the AUG-recognition site, AUG codons occurring within the first few residues adjacent to the cap might not be recognized. Brome mosaic virus RNA-4 is probably the best available yardstick; in that message the functional AUG occurs in position 10–12. In other messages in which the 5'-penultimate and subpenultimate nucleotides are methylated, or in which the nucleotide composition of the cap-adjacent region differs from BMV, the point at which the ribosome begins "scanning" might be shifted by a couple of residues. In any event, messages in which a nonfunctional AUG codon occurs very close to the cap do not necessarily contradict the scanning model.

Other messages in which the first AUG (which occurs at a considerable distance from the cap) is not the functional initiator codon pose more of a problem. Translation begins at the second AUG in *mouse α-amylase mRNA* derived from salivary glands or liver tissue (*Hagenbüchle* et al. 1980, 1981) and in a *Dictyostelium* message designated M4 (*A. Kimmel* and *R. Firtel*, personal communication). (In the case of the M4 message, the functional initiator codon was tentatively identified based on the presence of a long open reading frame. Since a protein encoded by M4 mRNA has not been demonstrated, however, I have not included it in Table 1. It is possible, although not likely, that that message directs synthesis of only the short peptide resulting from initiation at the first AUG.) Comparison of the nucleotide sequence of the *Rous sarcoma virus* 38S genome (*R. Swanstrom* and *J.M. Bishop*, personal communication) with the known N-terminal amino acid sequence of the *gag* polyprotein precursor (*Palmiter* et al. 1978) reveals that translation of *gag* begins at the fourth AUG codon – 372 nucleotides from the 5′-end of the message. Sequences derived from the 5′-portion of the RSV genome are known to be transposed to the 5′-end of the subgenomic mRNAs encoding the *env* and *src* proteins (*Mellon* and *Duesberg* 1977; *Cordell* et al. 1978; *Krzyzek* et al. 1978); the transposed segment is about 360 nucleotides long (*J.M. Bishop*, personal communication). Thus, at least three AUG triplets, each followed closely by an in-phase terminator codon, occur upstream from the functional initiator codon in the RSV *env* and *src* messages, too. There are hints that the 5′-untranslated region of *src* mRNA is several hundred nucleotides long, and contains even more than three AUG codons (*Czernilofsky* et al. 1980; *Quintrell* et al. 1980). *SV40 late messenger RNAs* provide another violation of the rule that ribosomes initiate exclusively at the 5′-proximal AUG. The third AUG triplet in 16S mRNA serves as the initiator codon for capsid protein VP1, and the second AUG in 19S mRNA is the initiator codon for capsid protein VP2, as shown in Table 2. [It is possible that the same species of SV40 19S mRNA directs synthesis of both VP2 and VP3, since only trace amounts of a smaller message – lacking the AUG initiator codon for VP2 – have been detected in infected cells (*Ghosh* et al. 1978b; *Piatak* et al. 1979). On the other hand, *Hunter* (1979) showed that the template for SV40 VP2 migrates in acrylamide gels marginally more slowly than the template for VP3. Thus, SV40 is probably like the polyoma virus system, in which *Siddell* and *Smith* (1978) have demonstrated separate messages for VP2 and VP3.]

In summary, there are at least nine eukaryotic messenger RNAs in which translation does not begin at (or is not limited to) the first AUG triplet: chicken preproinsulin mRNA, the 42S genome of Semliki Forest virus, mouse α-amylase mRNA from salivary glands or liver, the M4 message from *Dictyostelium,* three mRNAs from Rous sarcoma virus, and the late 16S and 19S messages of SV40.

4.4 How Can the Exceptions Be Explained?

How do ribosomes select the correct internal AUG codon in these exceptional messenger RNAs? In our present state of ignorance, we cannot even be sure how to phrase the question. Is it that ribosomes initiate at an internal AUG triplet *instead of* the 5′-proximal AUG codon? Or is it that ribosomes are *not limited to* the first AUG triplet in these messages? There are hints that the latter alternative might operate with Rous sarcoma virus and SV40 mRNAs. When 80S initiation complexes were formed in vitro with Rous sarcoma virus genome RNA and the ribosome-protected regions of the RNA were subsequently analyzed (*Darlix* et al. 1979), sequences flanking the *first* AUG triplet were efficiently protected against nuclease – even though the *gag* coding region begins some 300 nucleotides downstream. In the case of SV40 late 16S mRNA, analysis of the long leader sequence preceding the VP1 coding region reveals a curious situation: the first AUG codon (position 11–13 in the major form of 16S mRNA shown in Table 2) is followed by a long open reading frame, extending for 183 nucleotides and terminating just before the splice junction (*Celma* et al. 1977). Since a protein corresponding to that sequence had never been detected, *Sherman Weissman* dubbed the region an "agnogene". However, *Gilbert Jay* et al. (1981) recently made the exciting discovery that the 62 amino acid "agnoprotein" is synthesized in large amounts in virus-infected cells. It seems most likely, although not yet demonstrated directly, that the leader portion of 16S mRNA is the template for synthesis of the agnoprotein. Assuming this to be true, the unusual thing about SV40 16S mRNA (and perhaps RSV 38S mRNA, as well) is *not* that the 5′-proximal AUG is ignored, but that another downstream AUG triplet is also functional. One can envision a number of mechanisms by which this might happen.

1. Ribosomes might bind *independently* at the 5′-proximal AUG and at the internal AUG codon preceding the VP1 sequence in 16S mRNA. This would necessitate a signal identifying that AUG as the target. The signal directing ribosomes to bind internally cannot reside in the first 195 nucleotides of 16S mRNA, since that portion of the leader has been deleted (or replaced by other sequences) without impairing the ability to translate VP1 (*Subramanian* 1979). On the other hand, substitution of the VP1 coding sequence (and five nucleotides preceding the AUG triplet) by the coding and most of the 5′-noncoding sequence of rabbit β-globin mRNA did not prevent ribosomes from finding the correct internal initiator codon in 16S mRNA − in this case, that of β-globin (*Mulligan* et al. 1979). This implies that the putative signal for internal binding does not reside in the sequences immediately flanking the VP1 initiator codon. Perhaps the strongest argument against independent binding at the VP1 start site in 16S mRNA is that ribosomes fail to translate the VP1 cistron when it occurs near the 3′-end of 19S mRNA.

2. An intriguing possibility is that, upon completing translation of the agnoprotein, a ribosome might remain associated with the template and subsequently *reinitiate* at the start site of the VP1 protein. Although this mechanism is possible with the 16S message, the explanation cannot be extrapolated to the late 19S message which directs synthesis of VP2. As shown in Figure 3, AUG_{253} (the initiator codon for the agnoprotein) is present near the 5′-end of both 16S and late 19S mRNA. Since ribosomes are known to initiate at AUG_{253} in the 16S message, it seems likely that they do so in the 19S message as well. In the case of 16S mRNA, a ribosome initiating at position 253 will terminate at position 439 − upstream of the AUG initiator codon for VP1. In the case of 19S mRNA, however, a ribosome initiating at position 253 would not encounter an in-phase terminator codon until position 527 − which is beyond the initiator codon for VP2. Thus, the idea that a ribosome terminates one protein and reinitiates at the next available AUG triplet is not very likely; one would have to postulate that the ribosome can move forward *or backward* in search of an AUG codon.

3. An alternative mechanism is that after a 40S ribosomal subunit attaches at the 5′-end of the message and begins to migrate it may stop at the first AUG triplet *or it may migrate beyond* − advancing to the second, third or fourth AUG codon before the 60S subunit joins and translation begins. In other words, the scanning mechanism operates, but in a somewhat relaxed manner. This sort of "exaggerated migration" has been demonstrated in vitro with denatured reovirus mRNA (*Kozak* 1980a), although there is no experimental justification for extrapolating those results to native SV40 RNA. The relaxed scanning mechanism predicts that initiation should occur at the second AUG triplet in SV40 16S mRNA − as well as at the first and third AUG codons, which are now known to be functional. A ribosome initiating at the second AUG (position 303 in the genome) would encounter a nonsense codon after incorporating just two amino acids, however; this makes it difficult to test the prediction. A relaxed scanning mechanism would ex-

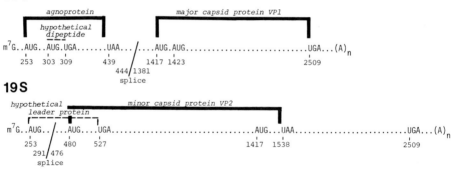

Fig. 3. Arrangement of initiator and terminator codons in the late messenger RNAs of Simian Virus 40. To facilitate comparison of the two messages, the numbers used in this figure to identify triplets and splice sites refer to their position in the DNA genome (*Reddy* et al. 1978b). AUG_{253} in this figure corresponds to the AUG codon in position 11–13 of the major late 16S mRNA sequence shown in Table 2. SV40 late mRNAs are heterogeneous, and I have shown only one form of each message. The diagram is not drawn to scale. The 16S mRNA species is the presumed template for both the agnoprotein (initiating at AUG_{253}) and the major capsid protein VP1. The dipeptide that would result from initiation at AUG_{303} has not been demonstrated. It is not known whether translation of VP1 normally begins at AUG_{1417} or AUG_{1423}. The nucleotide sequence following AUG_{1423} corresponds to the N-terminal amino acid sequence of the mature VP1 protein (*Van de Voorde* et al. 1976; *Kempe* et al. 1979) and the flanking nucleotides (AAG · AUG · GCC) resemble the "consensus sequence" for eukaryotic initiation sites. On the other hand, AUG_{1417} was identified as the functional initiator codon for translation of VP1 in vitro (*A. Mellor, R. Hewick* and *A. Smith*, personal communication). For simplicity, I shall consider AUG_{1417} to be the site of initiation of VP1. The only product known to be translated from 19S mRNA is VP2, initiating at AUG_{480}. Although the hypothetical leader peptide encoded by 19S mRNA (AUG_{253}–UGA_{527}) has not yet been detected, it seems reasonable to expect that region to be translated inasmuch as the 5'-proximal sequences (including AUG_{253}) are identical in the 16S and 19S transcripts. Note that the sequence encoding the C-terminal portion of the hypothetical 19S leader peptide overlaps the sequence encoding the N-terminal portion of VP2. This is in contrast with the 16S mRNA, in which a ribosome translating the agnogene would terminate upstream from the initiator codon for VP1

plain why the initiator codon for SV40 VP1 is accessible to ribosomes in 16S mRNA but not in 19S mRNA, and why translation of the Rous sarcoma virus *env* and *src* proteins requires production of subgenomic messages. In other words, *even in those unusual messages in which ribosomes initiate at an AUG codon which is not first in line, the requirement for a nearby 5'-terminus persists.*

An assumption underlying the foregoing discussion is that the predominant species of SV40 16S and 19S mRNAs are the functional messages for VP1 and VP2, respectively. But SV40 late mRNAs are known to be heterogeneous (*Ghosh* et al. 1978b; *Reddy* et al. 1978a). The transcripts diagrammed in Figure 3 represent only the most abundant form of each message. It is possible that VP1 is translated from a minor species of 16S mRNA, such as that reproduced in Table 2, in which the upstream AUG codons are absent; rare forms of SV40 19S mRNA have also been identified in which the 5'-leader sequence lacks AUG codons (*Ghosh* et al. 1978b). This explanation seems less likely in the case of Rous sarcoma virus messages, since the majority of intracellular viral mRNA molecules contain the same 5'-terminal sequence as the genome (*Cordell* et al. 1978). On the other hand, there is evidence for a small population of RSV transcripts containing altered lead-er sequences (*Stoltzfus* and *Kuhnert* 1979). I did not discuss picornaviruses in the fore-going section because the available data are not sufficient to pinpoint the functional ini-tiator codon. There are hints, however, that translation might not begin at the first AUG triplet in foot-and-mouth disease virus (FMDV) mRNA. In one strain of FMDV, the first AUG codon occurs 33-35 nucleotides from the 5'-end of the genome (*Harris* 1980). A large fragment derived from the 3'-end of virion RNA (and thus lacking AUG_{33-35}) appears to direct synthesis of the same polypeptides as full-length FMDV RNA (*Sangar* et al. 1980). Thus, one must conclude either that AUG_{33-35} is bypassed by ribosomes when full-length virion RNA is used as the template, or that full-length RNA is cleaved during incubation in the extract, prior to being translated. One cannot decide whether a ribosome is breaking the rules (i.e., bypassing the 5'-proximal AUG codon) unless one knows which form of RNA the ribosome sees.

5 Questions and Speculations

5.1 An Economical Message Might Initiate at the First and the Second AUG Codon

One consequence of the scanning mechanism is that the second AUG triplet in a mes-sage might be viewed as a potential "secondary ribosome binding site". If a small percent-age of 40S subunits were to bypass the normal initiation site and stop instead at the sec-ond AUG, two polypeptides might be synthesized from a single message. *Rose*(1980) has presented evidence for low-level binding of ribosomes at the second AUG during in vitro translation of one of the vesicular stomatitis virus messages, although there is no evidence that this occurs in vivo. The interesting phenomenon that *Knauert* and *Ehren-feld* have described (1979) in which ribosomes initiate at either or both of two sites in poliovirus mRNA – synthesizing two quite unrelated polypeptides – might have its ex-planation in the ability of ribosomes to sometimes bypass the first, and initiate at the se-cond AUG. Knowledge of the 5'-proximal sequence of poliovirus mRNA should help to unravel this phenomenon.

From a different perspective, it would seem that one way to ensure exclusive and effi-cient translation of the "correct" polypeptide might be to place a second AUG very close to, and in the same reading frame as, the first. This sort of redundancy is noticeable in a number of eukaryotic messages, including those of chicken ovomucoid (*Catterall* et al. 1980), bovine preproparathyroid hormone (*Kronenberg* et al. 1979a), rat preproinsulin (*Cordell* et al. 1979; *Lomedico* et al. 1979), bovine growth hormone (*W.L. Miller* et al. 1980), SV40 VP1 (*Ghosh* et al. 1978a), adenovirus 2 hexon protein (*Akusjärvi* and *Pettersson* 1979), and the 16K protein encoded by adenovirus 2 early region 3 (*Hérissé* et al. 1980; *Persson* et al. 1980). Obviously, it is more likely that the second AUG in each of these mes-sages reflects a need for methionine in the corresponding position of the polypeptide, than that the second AUG enhances the fidelity of initiation. But the possibility exists. In the case of an immunoglobulin light chain mRNA which has the sequence AUGxx-xAUG, initiation at both AUGs has been demonstrated in vitro (*Zemell* et al. 1978), con-sistent with the notion that a second in-phase initiator codon can serve as a back up to the first. On the other hand, adenovirus type 2 hexon protein, synthesized in vitro, has a unique amino-terminal sequence (*Anderson* and *Lewis* 1980). If AUG triplets 5 and 6 (just downstream from the normal initiator codon) function as alternate initiation sites in Ad2 hexon mRNA, they do so with very low efficiency. The fact that the initiator codon is *not* reiterated, either in tandem or at two nearby sites, in *most* eukaryotic messages suggests that a single AUG triplet generally functions quite efficiently to stop migration of the 40S subunit and to initiate peptide-bond formation.

5.2 Role of 5′-Terminal Methylated Residues

The mechanism by which the methylated cap promotes initiation remains obscure, although there are some intriguing hints. Denaturation of mRNA obviates the requirement for m^7G (*Kozak* 1980a). This raises the possibility that the cap might mediate unfolding of the 5′-terminus of native messenger RNA, thereby facilitating ribosome entry. The observation that messenger RNAs are less dependent on the m^7G cap at low ionic strength (*Weber* et al. 1977, 1978; *Herson* et al. 1979), which increases the conformational flexibility of mRNA, might be taken as support for this hypothesis. The facilitating effect of the cap must be due, at least in part, to interaction with one or more cap-binding proteins. A likely candidate for this role has been identified by *Sonenberg* et al. (1978, 1980).

The significance of methylation of the 5′-penultimate and subpenultimate nucleotides also remains to be explained. The extent of methylation of these residues varies from one cellular message to another (*Lockard* 1978; *Pavlakis* et al. 1980), and some viral messages lack 2′-O-methylated residues adjacent to the cap (*Colonno* and *Stone* 1976; *Hefti* et al. 1976; *Cleaves* and *Dubin* 1979). In vivo experiments using inhibitors of methylation have shown that 2′-O-methylation of the penultimate nucleotide is not absolutely required for translation (*Dimock* and *Stoltzfus* 1979; *Kaehler* et al. 1979). Although 2′-O-methylation of the cap-adjacent residue was reported to enhance binding of synthetic polymers to ribosomes in certain cell-free extracts (*Muthukrishnan* et al. 1976), the effect has not been observed consistently (*Keith* et al. 1978). Since 2′-O-methylation causes the 5′-terminus of the RNA molecule to have a more extended structure (*Kim* and *Sarma* 1978), its role may be to augment the m^7G cap in making the 5′-end of the RNA chain more accessible to ribosomes.

5.3 Determinants of Messenger Efficiency

The scanning mechanism may explain how ribosomes select the correct site for initiation of protein synthesis, but the model does not address the question of what makes one message more efficient than another. The fact that messenger RNAs do show marked differences in translational efficiency indicates that one or more steps in the initiation process are subject to modulation. The existence of messenger-discriminatory initiation factors (*Golini* et al. 1976; *Gette* and *Heywood* 1979) is part of the answer – but what features in messenger RNAs underlie their differential response to initiation factors? Although I emphasized above that drastic alteration of the 5′-untranslated segment of a message does not impair the fidelity of initiation, one might expect (even though experimental evidence is lacking) that the 5′-noncoding portion of a message would modulate translational efficiency. Thus, the very interesting observation that the leader sequence on mouse α-amylase mRNA varies, depending on the tissue of origin, might provide a basis for regulating expression of that enzyme (*Hagenbüchle* et al. 1981).

If one considers the entire spectrum of messenger RNAs listed in Tables 1 and 2, it is evident that translational efficiency is not simply related to length of the 5'-noncoding region (*Herson* et al. 1979). On the other hand, in a number of studies in which a small set of related viral messages were compared, there was an inverse relationship between translational efficiency and length of the 5'-noncoding segment. Examples include brome mosaic virus mRNAs (*Shih* and *Kaesberg* 1976; *Chroboczek* et al. 1980), vesicular stomatitis virus mRNAs (*Lodish* and *Froshauer* 1977), turnip yellow mosaic virus RNAs (*Benicourt* and *Haenni* 1978), and the adenovirus message for polypeptide IX *versus* other late adenovirus messages (*Cherney* and *Wilhelm* 1979). But other studies contradict the simple conclusion that the most efficient messages are those in which the AUG initiator codon is closest to the cap. For example, β-globin mRNA – which has a somewhat longer 5'-noncoding region than α-globin mRNA – is more efficiently translated both in vitro and in vivo (*Lodish* 1971). Among the four small reovirus messages, the species (s1) with the *shortest* 5'-untranslated segment seems to be translated *least* efficiently (*Levin* and *Samuel* 1980). SV40 infected cells provide another example. Under conditions of hypertonic stress (which presumably discriminate against less efficient messages) translation of the late viral 16S mRNA, which has an extraordinarily long 5'-leader segment, seems to be more resistant than bulk host mRNA (*England* et al. 1975; *Wolgemuth* et al. 1980). Thus, *if* a long leader tends to reduce translational efficiency, there must be ways to circumvent the effect of length. It may be that conformational folding within a long leader region, rather than length per se, lowers translational efficiency.

A negative effect of secondary structure has been postulated to explain the difference in efficiency between α- and β-globin mRNAs (*Baralle* 1977b). *Pavlakis* et al. (1980) showed that the AUG initiator codon in β-globin mRNA is more accessible to nucleases (and hence more exposed) than in α-globin mRNA. Studies with base-substituted reovirus mRNAs also suggested an inverse correlation between translational efficiency and the amount of secondary structure in a message (*Kozak* 1980a). Obviously, much additional work is needed to define which specific regions of the message are important in this regard. Efficient initiation might require exposure of the 5'-terminus, the AUG codon, or the entire sequence in between the 5'-terminus and the initiator codon. Enhanced translation following treatment of messenger RNA with methylmercury hydroxide (*Payvar* and *Schimke* 1979) is consistent with the notion that secondary/tertiary structure has a negative effect on ribosome binding.

Although I have argued above that eukaryotic ribosomes tolerate extensive sequence variation in the 5'-noncoding region of mRNA, the nucleotides immediately flanking the AUG initiator codon are not random. It seems more than coincidental that most eukaryotic initiation sites (see Table 3) have the sequence AUG*G* – complementary to 3'-UAC*C*-5' in the anticodon loop of eukaryotic Met-tRNA$_i$. [Yeast cells are an exception: the anticodon loop in yeast Met-tRNA$_i$ has the sequence 3'-UACU-5'. The complementary sequence AUGA occurs in only one of the six yeast messages for which sequence information is currently available.] The most common initiation sequence in prokaryotic messenger RNAs is AUG*A*, complementary to 3'-UAC*U*-5' in the anticodon loop of prokaryotic Met-tRNA$_f$. In the case of one prokaryotic message, there is evidence that the A residue flanking the initiator codon enhances translation (*Taniguchi* and *Weissmann* 1978). In view of the great number of spurious "initiation sites" that can be activated by fragmentation of reovirus mRNA (*Kozak* 1980b) or by mutational relocation of the AUG codon in the yeast cytochrome c gene (*Sherman* et al. 1980b), presence of a particular set of flanking sequences cannot be an absolute requirement for initiation in eukaryotes. *Sherman* et al. (1980b) have noted, on the other hand, that the efficiency of translation in certain cytochrome c revertants is influenced by the sequence preceding the AUG triplet. It might be that interaction of Met-tRNA with the initiator codon is facilitated by particular flanking nucleotides, in somewhat the same way as the sequences neighboring terminator codons have been shown to modulate the efficiency of binding of suppressor tRNAs (*Akaboshi* et al. 1976; *Colby* et al. 1976; *Feinstein* and *Altman* 1978).

Finally, one must consider the possibility that distant regions of the message might influence initiation events. *Deletion* of 3'-noncoding sequences from rabbit β-globin mRNA apparently did not impair its ability to be translated in vitro (*Kronenberg* et al. 1979b). High molecular weight nuclear RNA from polyoma virus-infected cells was a competent template for synthesis of capsid protein VP2 in vitro, suggesting that *extra sequences* at the 3'-end of a message do not interfere with translation of the 5'-proximal cistron (*Kamen* et al. 1978). Similarly, *Setzer* et al. (1980) discerned no functional difference among multiple forms of mouse dihydrofolate reductase mRNA in which the 3'-untranslated region varied from 80 to over 900 nucleotides. On the other hand, the 3'-noncoding region does seem to influence the in vivo stability of some messages. When the normally untranslated 3'-region of α-globin mRNA is translated (as in production of Hb Constant Spring), the stability of α-globin mRNA is drastically reduced (*Weatherall* and *Clegg* 1979). Although the poly(A) segment commonly found on eukaryotic messages is not an absolute requirement for in vitro translation (*Soreq* et al. 1974), in long term experiments presence of a 3'-terminal poly(A) tract was shown to enhance reinitiation (*Soreq* et al. 1974; *Doel* and *Carey* 1976). Whether the poly(A) tail merely stabilizes mRNA against degradation by nucleases or directly promotes reinitiation of translation remains to be determined.

5.4 Peculiarities of Viral Messenger RNAs

Viral messages have been observed to differ from host mRNAs in their sensitivity to interferon (*Metz* 1975; *Yakobson* et al. 1977), high salt (*England* et al. 1975; *Nuss* et al. 1975; *Carrasco* and *Smith* 1976; *Cherney* and *Wilhelm* 1979; *Garry* et al. 1979a, b), and certain antibiotics (*Warrington* and *Wratten* 1977; *Ramabhadran* and *Thach* 1980). The implied difference in the structure of (most) viral versus (most) cellular messages often makes it possible for viruses to usurp the translational machinery of the host cell. In the case of picornaviruses, it has been known for some time that the viral mRNA is uncapped (*Hewlett* et al. 1976; *Nomoto* et al. 1976). Thus, the observation that poliovirus inhibits translation of capped, cellular messages by inactivating a cap-binding protein (*Trachsel* et al. 1980) came as no surprise – although the experimental proof was not obtained easily! A more subtle mechanism of host shut off is required for viruses whose messenger RNAs, like those of the host cell, rely on the m^{7}G cap. With some strains of vesicular stomatitis virus (*Lodish* and *Porter* 1980), reovirus (*Zweerink* and *Joklik* 1970), adenovirus (*Anderson* et al. 1973), influenza virus (*Skehel* 1972), alphaviruses (*Atkins* 1976; *Lachmi* and *Kääriäinen* 1977), and frog virus 3 (*Elliott* et al. 1980), inhibition of host protein synthesis occurs only late in the infection, and the most likely cause of the inhibition is competition by the vast excess of viral mRNA. But other mechanisms also operate with some of these viruses. *Stanners* et al. (1977) and *Davis* and *Wertz* (1980) have described some interesting mutants of vesicular stomatitis virus in which the level of protein synthesis is modulated by factors other than the quantity of functional viral mRNA. Adenovirus produces a striking inhibition of host mRNA transport (*Beltz* and *Flint* 1979) which undoubtedly contributes to viral takeover of the cellular machinery. *Skup* and *Millward* (1980a, b) have suggested that, during the late stages of reovirus infection, the translational machinery might be altered in a way that allows uncapped mRNA to be translated efficiently. During the course of infection by many cytolytic viruses the plasma membrane becomes leaky, and *Carrasco* (1978) has speculated that the resulting increase in intracellular Na^+ might be responsible for the preferential translation of viral mRNA. This mechanism is supported by studies carried out with Sindbis virus-infected chick cells (*Garry* et al. 1979a, b). Neither ionic changes nor competition by viral mRNA can explain the dramatic shut off of host protein synthesis that occurs during the *early* stages of infection by herpes simplex virus (*Fenwick* and *Walker* 1978) or vaccinia virus (*Person* and *Beaud* 1978). Changes in the translational machinery have been demonstrated following infection by vaccinia virus (*Sagot* and *Beaud* 1979; *Schrom* and *Bablanian* 1979; *Beaud* and *Dru* 1980; *Person* et al. 1980), but there are as yet no clues as to how the altered components discriminate between viral and cellular mRNAs.

An intriguing question about RNA viruses concerns the mechanism(s) by which ribosomes are excluded from the population of viral "plus strands" which must participate in other functions − such as replication and assembly of progeny virions. Noncovalent circularization of the RNA genome may accomplish this objective for Sindbis virus (*Frey* et al. 1979). The genomic RNA of retroviruses tends to form dimers in which the 5'-terminal portions of two RNA molecules are joined noncovalently (*Bender* and *Davidson* 1976). In the case of picornaviruses (*Lee* et al. 1977; *Sangar* et al. 1977; *Hruby* and *Roberts* 1978), calicivirus (*Schaffer* et al. 1980), cowpea mosaic virus (*Daubert* et al. 1978; *Stanley* et al. 1978), tobacco ringspot virus (*Mayo* et al. 1979), and Southern bean mosaic virus RNA (*Ghosh* et al. 1979), a protein is covalently bound to the 5'-terminus of the RNA genome. This might be another ploy to free the RNA of ribosomes so that it may be replicated and packaged into virions. Although our current understanding of the translation initiation mechanism predicts that the 5'-linked protein should effectively prevent ribosome binding, direct proof of this has been difficult to obtain due to the ubiquity in cell-free extracts of an enzyme that cleaves the protein/RNA linkage (*Ambros* et al. 1978). This activity seems to be lower in reticulocyte lysates than in other cell-free extracts, and *Golini* et al. (1980) have exploited this finding to show that poliovirus RNA with covalently-linked protein *can* bind to reticulocyte ribosomes. This interesting and unexpected result will be easier to evaluate when the exact RNA sequence selected by ribosomes (in the presence and absence of 5'-terminal protein) has been identified. Since in vitro translation of protein-linked RNA is at variance with the earlier observation that all of the poliovirus mRNA extracted from polysomes in vivo has a free 5'-terminus (*Nomoto* et al. 1977), additional studies are needed to clarify the situation. On the other hand, it is clear that the 5'-linked protein is not *required* for translation, since prior treatment with protease did not impair in vitro translation of mengovirus RNA (*Perez-Bercoff* and *Gander* 1978), foot-and-mouth disease virus RNA (*Sangar* et al. 1980) or cowpea mosaic virus RNA (*Stanley* et al. 1978).

Acknowledgments/Notes. I am grateful to many colleagues who sent preprints, and who permitted me to cite their unpublished data. The ubiquitous occurrence of an adenylic acid residue three nucleotides upstream from the AUG initiator codon was first pointed out to me by Dr. David Baltimore. Work from my laboratory was supported by a research grant and a Career Development Award from the National Institute of Allergy and Infectious Diseases.

The literature search for this review extends through December, 1980. Portions of the text were adapted from an earlier review which was published in *Protein Biosynthesis in Eukaryotes* (edited by R. *Perez-Bercoff*) Plenum Publishing Co., New York, 1981.

References

Ahlquist P, Dasgupta R, Shih DS, Zimmern D, Kaesberg P (1979) Two-step binding of eukaryotic ribosomes to brome mosaic virus RNA3. Nature 281:277–282

Akaboshi E, Inouye M, Tsugita A (1976) Effect of neighboring nucleotide sequences on suppression efficiency in amber mutants of T4 phage lysozyme. Molec Gen Genet 149:1–4

Akusjärvi G, Pettersson U (1979) Sequence analysis of adenovirus DNA: complete nucleotide sequence of the spliced 5' noncoding region of adenovirus 2 hexon messenger RNA. Cell 16:841–850.

Aleström P, Akusjärvi G, Perricaudet M, Mathews MB, Klessig DF, Pettersson U (1980) The gene for polypeptide IX of adenovirus type 2 and its unspliced messenger RNA. Cell 19: 671–681

Ambros V, Pettersson RF, Baltimore D (1978) An enzymatic activity in uninfected cells that cleaves the linkage between poliovirion RNA and the 5' terminal protein. Cell 15:1439–1446

Anderson CW, Lewis JB (1980) Amino-terminal sequence of adenovirus type 2 proteins: hexon, fiber, component IX, and early protein 1B–15K. Virology 104:27–41

Anderson CW, Baum PR, Gesteland RF (1973) Processing of adenovirus 2 induced proteins. J Virol 12:241–252

Arrand JR, Soeda E, Walsh JE, Smolar N, Griffin BE (1980) Polyoma virus DNA: sequence from the late region that specifies the leader sequence for late mRNA and codes for VP2, VP3, and the N-terminus of VP1. J Virol 33:606–618

Atkins GJ (1976) The effect of infection with Sindbis virus and its temperature-sensitive mutants on cellular protein and DNA synthesis. Virology 71:593–597

Atkins JF (1979) Is UAA or UGA part of the recognition signal for ribosomal initiation? Nucleic Acids Res 7:1035–1041

Atkins JF, Steitz JA, Anderson CW, Model P (1979) Binding of mammalian ribosomes to MS2 phage RNA reveals an overlapping gene encoding a lysis function. Cell 18:247–256

Azad AA, Deacon NJ (1980) The 3'-terminal primary structure of five eukaryotic 18S rRNAs determined by the direct chemical method of sequencing. The highly conserved sequences include an invariant region complementary to eukaryotic 5S rRNA. Nucleic Acids Res 8:4365–4376

Baker CC, Herisse J, Courtois G, Galibert F, Ziff E (1979) Messenger RNA for the Ad2 DNA binding protein: DNA sequences encoding the first leader and heterogeneity at the mRNA 5' end. Cell 18:569–580

Banerjee AK (1980) 5'-Terminal cap structure in eucaryotic messenger ribonucleic acids. Microbiol Reviews 44:175–205

Baralle FE (1977a) Complete nucleotide sequence of the 5' noncoding region of rabbit β-globin mRNA. Cell 10:549–558

Baralle FE (1977b) Structure-function relationship of 5' noncoding sequence of rabbit α- and β-globin mRNA. Nature 267:279–281

Baralle FE (1977c) Complete nucleotide sequence of the 5' noncoding region of human α- and β-globin mRNA. Cell 12:1085–1095

Baralle FE, Brownlee GG (1978) AUG is the only recognisable signal sequence in the 5' noncoding regions of eukaryotic mRNA. Nature 274:84–87

Baralle FE, Shoulders CC, Proudfoot NJ (1980) The primary structure of the human ε-globin gene. Cell 21:621–626

Beaud G, Dru A (1980) Protein synthesis in vaccinia virus-infected cells in the presence of amino acid analogs: a translational control mechanism. Virology 100:10–21

Beemon K, Hunter T (1977) In vitro translation yields a possible Rous sarcoma virus *src* gene product. Proc Natl Acad Sci USA 74:3302–3306

Beemon K, Hunter T (1978) Characterization of Rous sarcoma virus *src* gene products synthesized in vitro. J Virol 28:551–566

Belin D, Hedgpeth J, Selzer GB, Epstein RH (1979) Temperature-sensitive mutation in the initiation codon of the rIIB gene of bacteriophage T4. Proc Natl Acad Sci USA 76:700–704

Bell GI, Pictet RL, Rutter WJ, Cordell B, Tischer E, Goodman HM (1980) Sequence of the human insulin gene. Nature 284:26–32

Beltz GA, Flint SJ (1979) Inhibition of HeLa cell protein synthesis during adenovirus infection. J Mol Biol 131:353–373

Bender W, Davidson N (1976) Mapping of poly(A) sequences in the electron microscope reveals unusual structure of type C oncornavirus RNA molecules. Cell 7:595–607

Bendig MM, Folk WR (1979) Deletion mutants of polyoma virus defining a nonessential region between the origin of replication and the initiation codon for early proteins. J Virol 32:530–535

Bendig MM, Thomas T, Folk WR (1980) Regulatory mutants of polyoma virus defective in DNA replication and the synthesis of early proteins. Cell 20:401–409

Benicourt C, Haenni A-L (1978) Differential translation of turnip yellow mosaic virus mRNAs in vitro. Biochem Biophys Res Commun 84:831–839

Bernard O, Hozumi N, Tonegawa S (1978) Sequences of mouse immunoglobulin light chain genes before and after somatic changes. Cell 15:1133–1144

Bisaro DM, Siegel A (1980) A new viral RNA species in tobacco rattle virus-infected tissue. Virology 107:194–201

Bonatti S, Sonenberg N, Shatkin AJ, Cancedda R (1980) Restricted initiation of protein synthesis on the potentially polycistronic Sindbis virus 42S RNA. J Biol Chem 255:11473–11477

Borisova GP, Volkova TM, Berzin V, Rosenthal G, Gren EJ (1979) The regulatory region of MS2 phage RNA replicase cistron. IV. Functional activity of specific MS2 RNA fragments in formation of the 70S initiation complex of protein biosynthesis. Nucleic Acids Res 6:1761–1774

Boss JM, Darrow MD, Zitomer RS (1980) Characterization of yeast iso-1-cytochrome c mRNA. J Biol Chem 255:8623–8628

Bossart W, Nuss DL, Paoletti E (1978) Effect of UV irradiation on the expression of vaccinia virus gene products synthesized in a cell-free system coupling transcription and translation. J Virol 26:673–680

Both GW (1979) A possible involvement of coding sequences in mRNA-ribosome interaction in eukaryotes. FEBS Letters 101:220–224

Both GW, Banerjee AK, Shatkin AJ (1975) Methylation-dependent translation of viral messenger RNAs in vitro. Proc Natl Acad Sci USA 72:1189–1193

Both GW, Furuichi Y, Muthukrishnan S, Shatkin AJ (1976) Effect of 5'-terminal structure and base composition on polyribonucleotide binding to ribosomes. J Mol Biol 104:637–658

Boublik M, Hellmann W (1978) Comparison of *Artemia salina* and *Escherichia coli* ribosome structure by electron microscopy. Proc Natl Acad Sci USA 75:2829–2833

Brown JC, Smith AE (1970) Initiator codons in eukaryotes. Nature 226:610–612

Browning KS, Leung DW, Clark JM (1980) Protection of satellite tobacco necrosis virus ribonucleic acid by wheat germ 40S and 80S ribosomes. Biochemistry 19:2276–2283

Brzeski H, Kennedy SIT (1978) Synthesis of alphavirus-specified RNA. J Virol 25:630–640

Busslinger M, Portmann R, Irminger JC, Birnstiel ML (1980) Ubiquitous and gene-specific regulatory 5' sequences in a sea urchin histone DNA clone coding for histone protein variants. Nucleic Acids Res 8:957–977

Cancedda R, Shatkin AJ (1979) Ribosome-protected fragments from Sindbis 42S and 26S RNAs. Eur J Biochem 94:41–50

Cancedda R, Villa-Komaroff L, Lodish HF, Schlesinger M (1975) Initiation sites for translation of Sindbis virus 42S and 26S messenger RNAs. Cell 6:215–222

Carrasco L (1978) Membrane leakiness after viral infection and a new approach to the development of antiviral agents. Nature 272:694–699

Carrasco L, Smith AE (1976) Sodium ions and the shut-off of host cell protein synthesis by picornaviruses. Nature 264:807–809

Caton AJ, Robertson JS (1980) Structure of the host-derived sequences present at the 5' ends of influenza virus mRNA. Nucleic Acids Res 8:2591–2603

Catterall JF, O'Malley BW, Robertson MA, Staden R, Tanaka Y, Brownlee GG (1978) Nucleotide sequence homology at 12 intron-exon junctions in the chick ovalbumin gene. Nature 257:510–513

Catterall JF, Stein JP, Kristo P, Means AR, O'Malley BW (1980) Primary sequence of ovomucoid messenger RNA as determined from cloned complementary DNA. J Cell Biol 87:480–487

Celma ML, Ehrenfeld E (1975) Translation of poliovirus RNA in vitro: detection of two different initiation sites. J Mol Biol 98:761–780

Celma ML, Dhar R, Pan J, Weissman SM (1977) Comparison of the nucleotide sequence of the messenger RNA for the major structural protein of SV40 with the DNA sequence encoding the amino acids of the protein. Nucleic Acids Res 4:2549–2559

Chang JC,Temple GF, Poon R, Neumann KH, Wai Kan Y (1977) The nucleotide sequences of the untranslated 5' regions of human α- and β-globin mRNAs. Proc Natl Acad Sci USA 74: 5145–5149

Chang JC, Poon R, Neumann KH, Wai Kan Y (1978) The nucleotide sequence of the 5' untranslated region of human γ-globin mRNA. Nucleic Acids Res 5:3515–3522

Chen JH, Spector A (1977) The bicistronic nature of lens α-crystallin 14S mRNA. Proc Natl Acad Sci USA 74:5448–5452

Cherney CS, Wilhelm JM (1979) Differential translation in normal and adenovirus type 5 infected human cells and cell-free systems. J Virol 30:533–542

Chroboczek J, Puchkova L, Zagorski W (1980) Regulation of brome mosaic virus gene expression by restriction of initiation of protein synthesis. J Virol 34:330–335

Cleaves GR, Dubin DT (1979) Methylation status of intracellular dengue type 2 40S RNA. Virology 96:159–165

Cochet M, Gannon F, Hen R, Maroteaux L, Perrin F, Chambon P (1979) Organization and sequence studies of the 17–piece chicken conalbumin gene. Nature 282:567–574

Cohen LH, Westerhuis LW, de Jong WW, Bloemendal H (1978) Rat α-crystallin a chain with an insertion of 22 residues. Eur J Biochem 89:259–266

Colby DS, Schedl P, Guthrie C (1976) A functional requirement for modification of the wobble nucleotide in the anticodon of a T4 suppressor tRNA. Cell 9:449–463

Colonno RJ, Stone HO (1976) Newcastle disease virus mRNA lacks 2'-O-methylated nucleotides. Nature 261:611–614

Cooke NE, Coit D, Weiner RI, Baxter JD, Martial JA (1980) Structure of cloned DNA complementary to rat prolactin messenger RNA. J Biol Chem 255:6502–6510

Cordell B, Weiss SR, Varmus HE, Bishop JM (1978) At least 104 nucleotides are transposed from the 5' terminus of the avian sarcoma virus genome to the 5' termini of smaller viral mRNAs. Cell 15:79–91

Cordell B, Bell G, Tischer E, DeNoto FM, Ullrich A, Pictet R, Rutter WJ, Goodman HM (1979) Isolation and characterization of a cloned rat insulin gene. Cell 18:533–543

Czernilofsky AP, Levinson AD, Varmus HE, Bishop JM, Tischer E, Goodman HM (1980) Nucleotide sequence of an avian sarcoma virus oncogene (src) and proposed amino acid sequence for gene product. Nature 287:198–203

Darlix J-L, Spahr P-F, Bromley PA, Jaton J-C (1979) In vitro, the major ribosome binding site on Rous sarcoma virus RNA does not contain the nucleotide sequence coding for the N-terminal amino acids of the gag gene product. J Virol 29:597–611

Darzynkiewicz E, Shatkin AJ (1980) Assignment of reovirus mRNA ribosome binding sites to virion genome segments by nucleotide sequence analyses. Nucleic Acids Res 8:337–350

Dasgupta R, Shih DS, Saris C, Kaesberg P (1975) Nucleotide sequence of a viral RNA fragment that binds to eukaryotic ribosomes. Nature 256:624–628

Daubert SD, Bruening G, Najarian RC (1978) Protein bound to the genome RNAs of cowpea mosaic virus. Eur J Biochem 92:45–51

Davies JW, Kaesberg P (1973) Translation of virus mRNA: synthesis of bacteriophage Qβ proteins in a cell-free extract from wheat embryo. J Virol 12:1434–1441

Davis NL, Wertz GW (1980) A VSV mutant synthesizes a large excess of functional mRNA but produces less viral protein than its wild-type parent. Virology 103:21–36

Derynck R, Content J, DeClercq E, Volckaert G, Tavanier J, Devos R, Fiers W (1980) Isolation and structure of a human fibroblast interferon gene. Nature 285:542–547

De Wachter R (1979) Do eukaryotic mRNA 5′ noncoding sequences base-pair with the 18S ribosomal RNA 3′ terminus? Nucleic Acids Res 7:2045–2054

Dhar R, Chanock RM, Lai C-J (1980) Nonviral oligonucleotides at the 5′ terminus of cytoplasmic influenza viral mRNA deduced from cloned complete genomic sequences. Cell 21: 495–500

Dimock K, Stoltzfus CM (1979) Processing and function of undermethylated chicken embryo fibroblast mRNA. J Biol Chem 254:5591–5594

Doel MT, Carey NH (1976) The translational capacity of deadenylated ovalbumin messenger RNA. Cell 8:51–58

Dolja VV, Sokolova NA, Tjulkina LG, Atabekov JG (1979) A study of barley stripe mosaic virus. (BSMV) genome. Molec Gen Genet 175:93–97

Dunn AR, Mathews MB, Chow LT, Sambrook J, Keller W (1978) A supplementary adenoviral leader sequence and its role in messenger translation. Cell 15:511–526

Dunn JJ, Buzash-Pollert E, Studier FW (1978) Mutations of bacteriophage T7 that affect initiation of synthesis of the gene 0.3 protein. Proc Natl Acad Sci USA 75:2741–2745

Early P, Huang H, Davis M, Calame K, Hood L (1980) An immunoglobulin heavy chain variable region gene is generated from three segments of DNA: V_H, D and J_H. Cell 19:981–992

Efstratiadis A, Posakony JW, Maniatis T, Lawn RM, O'Connell C, Spritz RA, DeRiel JK, Forget BG, Weissman SM, Slightom JL, Blechl AE, Smithies O, Baralle FE, Shoulders CC, Proudfoot NJ (1980) The structure and evolution of the human β-globin gene family. Cell 21:653–668

Efstratiadis, A., Kafatos, FC, Maniatis, T. (1977). The primary structure of rabbit β-globin mRNA as determined from cloned DNA. Cell 10, 571–585

Elliott RM, Bravo R, Kelly DC (1980) Frog virus 3 replication: analysis of structural and nonstructural polypeptides in infected BHK cells by acidic and basic two-dimensional gel electrophoresis. J Virol 33:18–27

England JM, Howett MK, Tan KB (1975) Effect of hypertonic conditions on protein synthesis in cells productively infected with simian virus 40. J Virol 16:1101–1107

Farabaugh PJ, Fink GR (1980) Insertion of the eukaryotic transposable element Ty1 creates a 5-base pair duplication. Nature 286:352–356

Feinstein SI, Altman S (1978) Context effects on nonsense codon suppression in Escherichia coli. Genetics 88:201–219

Fenwick ML, Walker MJ (1978) Suppression of the synthesis of cellular macromolecules by herpes simplex virus. J Gen Virol 41:37–51

Fiddes JC, Goodman HM (1979) Isolation, cloning and sequence analysis of the cDNA for the α-subunit of human chorionic gonadotropin. Nature 281:351–356

Fiil NP, Friesen JD, Downing WL, Dennis PP (1980) Post-transcriptional regulatory mutants in a ribosomal protein-RNA polymerase operon of E. coli. Cell 19:837–844

Files JG, Weber K, Coulondre C, Miller JH (1975) Identification of the UUG codon as a translational initiation codon in vivo. J Mol Biol 95:327–330

Filipowicz W (1978) Functions of the 5′-terminal m^7G cap in eukaryotic mRNA. FEBS Letters 96:1–11

Filipowicz W, Haenni A-L (1979) Binding of ribosomes to 5′-terminal leader sequences of eukaryotic messenger RNAs. Proc Natl Acad Sci USA 76:3111–3115

Firtel RA, Timm R, Kimmel AR, McKeown M (1979) Unusual nucleotide sequences at the 5′ end of actin genes in Dictyostelium discoideum. Proc Natl Acad Sci USA 76:6206–6210

Flavell AJ, Cowie A, Arrand JR, Kamen R (1980) Localization of three major capped 5′ ends of polyoma virus late mRNA's within a single tetranucleotide sequence in the viral genome. J Virol 33:902–908

Frey TK, Gard DL, Strauss JH (1979) Biophysical studies on circle formation by Sindbis virus 49S RNA. J Mol Biol 132:1–18

Friedmann T, LaPorte P, Esty A (1978) Nucleotide sequence studies of polyoma DNA. J Biol Chem 253:6561–6567

Fritsch C, Mayo MA, Hirth L (1977) Further studies on the translation products of tobacco rattle virus RNA in vitro. Virology 77:722-732

Gallwitz D, Sures I (1980) Structure of a split yeast gene: complete nucleotide sequence of the actin gene in Saccharomyces cerevisiae. Proc Natl Acad Sci USA 77:2546-2550

Garoff H, Frischauf A-M, Simons K, Lehrach H, Delius H (1980) The capsid protein of Semliki Forest virus has clusters of basic amino acids and prolines in its amino-terminal region. Proc Natl Acad Sci USA 77:6376-6380

Garry R, Bishop J, Parker S, Westbrook K, Lewis G, Waite M (1979a) Na^+ and K^+ concentrations and the regulation of protein synthesis in Sindbis virus-infected chick cells. Virology 96:108-120

Garry R, Westbrook K, Waite M (1979b) Differential effects of ouabain on host- and Sindbis virus-specified protein synthesis. Virology 99:179-182

Gette WR, Heywood SM (1979) Translation of myosin heavy chain messenger ribonucleic acid in an eukaryotic initiation factor 3- and messenger-dependent muscle cell-free system. J Biol Chem 254:9879-9885

Ghosh A, Dasgupta R, Salerno-Rife T, Rutgers T, Kaesberg P (1979) Southern bean mosaic viral RNA has a 5'-linked protein but lacks 3' terminal poly(A). Nucleic Acids Res 7:2137-2146

Ghosh PK, Reddy VB, Swinscoe J, Choudary PV, Lebowitz P, Weissman SM (1978a) The 5'-terminal leader sequence of late 16S mRNA from cells infected with simian virus 40. J Biol Chem 253:3643-3647

Ghosh PK, Reddy VB, Swinscoe J, Lebowitz P, Weissman SM (1978b) Heterogeneity and 5'-terminal structures of the late RNAs of simian virus 40. J Mol Biol 126:813-846

Glanville N, Ranki M, Morser J, Kääriäinen L, Smith AE (1976) Initiation of translation directed by 42S and 26S RNAs from Semliki Forest virus in vitro. Proc Natl Acad Sci USA 73:3059-3063

Goeddel D, Yelverton E, Ullrich A, Heyneker H, Miozzari G, Holmes W, Seeburg P, Dull T, May L, Stebbing N, Crea R, Maeda S, McCandliss R, Sloma A, Tabor J, Gross M, Familletti P, Pestka S (1980). Human leukocyte interferon produced by *E. coli* is biologically active. Nature 287:411-416

Golini F, Thach SS, Birge CH, Safer B, Merrick WC, Thach RE (1976) Competition between cellular and viral mRNAs in vitro is regulated by a messenger discriminatory initiation factor. Proc Natl Acad Sci USA 73:3040-3044

Golini F, Semler BL, Dorner AJ, Wimmer E (1980) Protein-linked RNA of poliovirus is competent to form an initiation complex of translation in vitro. Nature 287:600-603

Gourse RL, Gerbi SA (1980). Fine structure of ribosomal RNA. III. Location of evolutionarily conserved regions within ribosomal DNA. J Mol Biol 140:321-339

Guilley H, Briand JP (1978) Nucleotide sequence of turnip yellow mosaic virus coat protein mRNA. Cell 15:113-122

Guilley H, Jonard G, Kukla B, Richards KE (1979) Sequence of 1000 nucleotides at the 3' end of tobacco mosaic virus RNA. Nucleic Acids Res 6:1287-1308

Haegeman G, Fiers W (1980) Characterization of the 5'-terminal cap structures of early simian virus 40 mRNA. J Virol 35:955-961

Haegeman G, Iserentant D, Gheysen D, Fiers W (1979) Characterization of the major altered leader sequence of late mRNA induced by SV40 deletion mutant dl-1811. Nucleic Acids Res 7:1799-1814

Hagenbüchle O, Santer M, Steitz JA, Mans RJ (1978) Conservation of the primary structure at the 3' end of 18S rRNA from eucaryotic cells. Cell 13:551-563

Hagenbüchle O, Bovey R, Young RA (1980). Tissue-specific expression of mouse α-amylase genes: nucleotide sequence of isoenzyme mRNAs from pancreas and salivary gland. Cell 21:179-187

Hagenbüchle O, Tosi M, Schibler U, Bovey R, Wellauer PK, Young RA (1981) Mouse liver and salivary gland α-amylase mRNAs differ only in 5'-nontranslated sequences. Nature 289:643-646

Harris TJR (1980) Comparison of the nucleotide sequence at the 5' end of RNAs from nine aphthoviruses, including representatives of the seven serotypes. J Virol 36:659-664

Haseltine WA, Maxam AM, Gilbert W (1977) Rous sarcoma virus genome is terminally redundant: the 5' sequence. Proc Natl Acad Sci USA 74:989-993

Haynes JR, Rosteck P, Lingrel JB (1980) Unusual sequence homology at the 5' ends of the developmentally regulated β^A, β^C and γ globin genes of the goat. Proc Natl Acad Sci USA 77: 7127–7131

Hefti E, Bishop DHL, Dubin DT, Stollar V (1976) 5'-Nucleotide sequence of Sindbis viral RNA. J Virol 17:149–159

Heindell HC, Liu A, Paddock GV, Studnicka GM, Salser WA (1978) The primary sequence of rabbit α-globin mRNA. Cell 15:43–54

Hentschel C, Irminger J-C, Bucher P, Birnstiel ML (1980) Sea urchin histone mRNA termini are located in gene regions downstream from putative regulatory sequences. Nature 285:147–151

Hérissé J, Courtois G, Galibert F (1980) Nucleotide sequence of the EcoR1 D fragment of adenovirus 2 genome. Nucleic Acids Res 8:2173–2192

Herman RC, Schubert M, Keene JD, Lazzarini RA (1980) Polycistronic vesicular stomatitis virus RNA transcripts. Proc Natl Acad Sci USA 77:4662–4665

Herson D, Schmidt A, Seal S, Marcus A, van Vloten-Doting L (1979) Competitive mRNA translation in an in vitro system from wheat germ. J Biol Chem 254:8245–8249

Hewlett MJ, Rose JK, Baltimore D (1976) 5'-Terminal structure of poliovirus polyribosomal RNA is pUp. Proc Natl Acad Sci USA 73:327–330

Hickey ED, Weber LA, Baglioni C (1976) Inhibition of initiation of protein synthesis by 7-methylguanosine-5'-monophosphate. Proc Natl Acad Sci USA 73:19–23

Hobart PM, Shen L-P, Crawford R, Pictet RL, Rutter WJ (1980) Comparison of the nucleic acid sequence of anglerfish and mammalian insulin mRNA's from cloned cDNA's. Science 210: 1360–1363

Holland JP, Holland MJ (1979) The primary structure of a glyceraldehyde-3-phosphate dehydrogenase gene from *Saccharomyces cerevisiae*. J Biol Chem 254:9839–9845

Hopper JE, Rowe LB (1978) Molecular expression and regulation of the galactose pathway genes in *Saccharomyces cerevisiae*. J Biol Chem 253:7566–7569

Houghton M, Stewart AG, Doel SM, Emtage JS, Eaton MAW, Smith JC, Patel TP, Lewis HM, Porter AG, Birch JR, Cartwright T, Carey NH (1980) The amino-terminal sequence of human fibroblast interferon as deduced from reverse transcripts obtained using synthetic oligonucleotide primers. Nucleic Acids Res 8:1913–1930

Hruby DE, Roberts WK (1978) Encephalomyocarditis virus RNA. III. Presence of a genome-associated protein. J Virol 25:413–415

Hunter T (1979) Functional characterization of the early and late mRNAs of simian virus 40. Virology 95:511–522

Hunter T, Gibson W (1978) Characterization of the mRNA's for the polyoma virus capsid proteins VP1, VP2, and VP3. J Virol 28:240–253

Inglis SC, McGeoch DJ, Mahy BWJ (1977) Polypeptides specified by the influenza virus genome. 2. Assignment of protein coding functions to individual genome segments by in vitro translation. Virology 78:522–536

Inglis SC, Gething M-J, Brown CM (1980) Relationship between the messenger RNAs transcribed from two overlapping genes of influenza virus. Nucleic Acids Res 8:3575–3589

Ingolia TD, Craig EA (1981) Primary sequence of the 5'-flanking regions of the Drosophila heat shock genes in chromosome subdivision 67B. Nucleic Acids Res 9:1627–1642

Ingolia TD, Craig EA, McCarthy BJ (1980) Sequence of three copies of the gene for the major Drosophila heat shock induced protein and their flanking regions. Cell 21:669–679

Iserentant D, Fiers W (1980) Secondary structure of mRNA and efficiency of translation initiation. Gene 9:1–12

Jacobson MF, Baltimore D (1968) Polypeptide cleavages in the formation of poliovirus proteins. Proc Natl Acad Sci USA 61:77–84

Jacobson MF, Asso J, Baltimore D (1970) Further evidence on the formation of poliovirus proteins. J Mol Biol 49:657–669

Jay G, Nomura S, Anderson CW, Khoury G (1981) Identification of the SV40 agnogene product: a DNA binding protein. Nature 291:346–349

Jenkins JR (1979) Sequence divergence of rainbow trout protamine mRNAs; comparison of coding and non-coding nucleotide sequences in three protamine cDNA plasmids. Nature 279: 809–811

Jonard G, Richards K, Mohier E, Gerlinger P (1978) Nucleotide sequence at the 5' extremity of tobacco-mosaic-virus RNA. 2. The coding region (nucleotides 69–236). Eur J Biochem 84: 521–531

Jones CW, Kafatos FC (1980) Structure, organization and evolution of developmentally regulated chorion genes in a silkmoth. Cell 22:855–867

Jung A, Sippel AE, Grez M, Schütz G (1980) Exons encode functional and structural units of chicken lysozyme. Proc Natl Acad Sci USA 77:5759–5763

Kaehler M, Coward J, Rottman F (1979) Cytoplasmic location of undermethylated messenger RNA in Novikoff cells. Nucleic Acids Res 6:1161–1175

Kamen RI, Wheeler T, Smith AE (1978) Polyoma virus high molecular weight nuclear RNA codes for capsid protein VP2 in vitro. Virology 89:461–474

Kamen R, Favaloro J, Parker J (1980) Topography of the three late mRNA's of polyoma virus which encode the virion proteins. J Virol 33:637–651

Keith JM, Muthukrishnan S, Moss B (1978) Effect of methylation of the N^6 position of the penultimate adenosine of capped mRNA on ribosome binding. J Biol Chem 253:5039–5041

Keith JM, Gershowitz A, Moss B (1980) Dinucleotide sequences at the 5' ends of vaccinia virus mRNA's synthesized in vitro. J Virol 36:601–605

Kempe TD, Beattie WG, Weissman S, Konigsberg W (1979) Correlation of the protein and nucleic acid sequences for the major structural protein of simian virus 40. J Biol Chem 254: 7561–7569

Kim CH, Sarma RH (1978) Spatial configuration of the bizarre 5' terminus of mammalian mRNA. J Am Chem Society 100:1571–1590

Knauert F, Ehrenfeld E (1979) Translation of poliovirus RNA in vitro: studies on n-formylmethionine-labeled polypeptides initiated in cell-free extracts prepared from poliovirus infected HeLa cells. Virology 93:537–546

Konarska M, Filipowicz W, Domdey H, Gross HJ (1981) Binding of ribosomes to linear and circular forms of the 5'-terminal leader fragment of tobacco mosaic virus RNA. Eur J Biochem 114:221–227

Konkel DA, Tilghman SM, Leder P (1978) The sequence of the chromosomal mouse β-globin major gene: homologies in capping, splicing and poly(A) sites. Cell 15:1125–1132

Konkel DA, Maizel JV, Leder P (1979) The evolution and sequence comparison of two recently diverged mouse chromosomal β-globin genes. Cell 18:865–873

Koper-Zwarthoff EC, Lockard RE, Alzner-deWeerd B, RajBhandary UL, Bol JF (1977) Nucleotide sequence of 5'-terminus of alfalfa mosaic virus RNA 4 leading into coat protein cistron. Proc Natl Acad Sci USA 74:5504–5508

Koper-Zwarthoff EC, Brederode FT, Veeneman G, van Boom JH, Bol JF (1980) Nucleotide sequences at the 5'-termini of the alfalfa mosaic virus RNAs and the intercistronic junction in RNA 3. Nucleic Acids Res 8:5635–5647

Kozak M (1977) Nucleotide sequences of 5'-terminal ribosome-protected initiation regions from two reovirus messages. Nature 269:390–394

Kozak M (1978) How do eucaryotic ribosomes select initiation regions in messenger RNA? Cell 15:1109–1123

Kozak M (1979a) Inability of circular mRNA to attach to eukaryotic ribosomes. Nature 280:82–85

Kozak M (1979b) Migration of 40S ribosomal subunits on messenger RNA when initiation is perturbed by lowering magnesium or adding drugs. J Biol Chem 254:4731–4738

Kozak M (1980a) Influence of mRNA secondary structure on binding and migration of 40S ribosomal subunits. Cell 19:79–90

Kozak M (1980b) Binding of wheat germ ribosomes to fragmented viral mRNA. J Virol 35:748–756

Kozak M (1980c) Role of ATP in binding and migration of 40 S ribosomal subunits. Cell 22:459–467

Kozak M (1980d) Binding of wheat germ ribosomes to bisulfite-modified reovirus messenger RNA: evidence for a scanning mechanism. J Mol Biol 144:291–304

Kozak M (1980e). Evaluation of the "scanning model" for initiation of protein synthesis in eucaryotes. Cell 22:7–8

Kozak M, Shatkin AJ (1978a) Identification of features in 5' terminal fragments from reovirus mRNA which are important for ribosome binding. Cell 13:201–212

Kozak M, Shatkin AJ (1978b) Migration of 40S ribosomal subunits on messenger RNA in the presence of edeine. J Biol Chem 253:6568–6577

Kronenberg HM, McDevitt BE, Majzoub JA, Nathans J, Sharp PA, Potts JT, Rich A (1979a) Cloning and nucleotide sequence of DNA coding for bovine preproparathyroid hormone. Proc Natl Acad Sci USA 76:4981–4985

Kronenberg HM, Roberts BE, Efstratiadis A (1979b) The 3' noncoding region of β-globin mRNA is not essential for in vitro translation. Nucleic Acids Res 6:153–166

Krug RM, Broni BA, Bouloy M (1979) Are the 5' ends of influenza viral mRNAs synthesized in vivo donated by host mRNAs? Cell 18:329–334

Krzyzek RA, Collett MS, Lau AF, Perdue ML, Leis JP, Faras AJ (1978) Evidence for splicing of avian sarcoma virus 5'-terminal genomic sequences onto viral-specific RNA in infected cells. Proc Natl Acad Sci USA 75:1284–1288

Kuebbing D, Liarakos CD (1978) Nucleotide sequence at the 5' end of ovalbumin messenger RNA from chicken. Nucleic Acids Res 5:2253–2266

Lachmi B, Kääriäinen L (1977) Control of protein synthesis in Semliki Forest virus-infected cells. J Virol 22:142–149

Lamb RA, Lai C-J (1980) Sequence of interrupted and uninterrupted mRNAs and cloned DNA coding for the two overlapping nonstructural proteins of influenza virus. Cell 21:475–485

Larkins BA, Jones RA, Tsai CY (1976) Isolation and in vitro translation of zein messenger ribonucleic acid. Biochemistry 15:5506–5511

Laughlin CA, Westphal H, Carter BJ (1979) Spliced adenovirus-associated virus RNA. Proc Natl Acad Sci USA 76:5567–5571

Lawrence CB (1980) Activation of an internal site for protein synthesis during in vitro translation. Nucleic Acids Res 8:1307–1317

Lebowitz P, Weissman SM (1979) Organization and transcription of the simian virus 40 genome. Curr Top Microbiol Immunol 87:43–172

Lee YF, Nomoto A, Detjen BM, Wimmer E (1977) A protein covalently linked to poliovirus genome RNA. Proc Natl Acad Sci USA 74:59–63

Legon S (1979) The binding of ribosomes to polyoma virus RNA. Possible role of the leader region in initiation site recognition. J Mol Biol 134:219–240

Legon S, Model P, Robertson HD (1977) Interaction of rabbit reticulocyte ribosomes with bacteriophage fl mRNA and of Escherichia coli ribosomes with rabbit globin mRNA. Proc Natl Acad Sci USA 74:2692–2696

Legon S, Flavell AJ, Cowie A, Kamen R (1979) Amplification in the leader sequence of late polyoma virus mRNAs. Cell 16:373–388

Leung DW, Browning KS, Heckman JE, RajBhandary UL, Clark JM (1979) Nucleotide sequence of the 5' terminus of satellite tobacco necrosis virus ribonucleic acid. Biochemistry 18:1361–1366

Levin KH, Samuel CE (1980) Biosynthesis of reovirus-specified polypeptides. Purification and characterization of the small-sized class mRNAs of reovirus type 3: coding assignments and translational efficiencies. Virology 106:1–13

Li J, Keene J, Scheible P, Joklik WK (1980) Nature of the 3'-terminal sequences of the plus and minus strands of the S1 gene of reovirus serotypes 1, 2 and 3. Virology 105:41–51

Lockard RE (1978) Different cap 1 : cap 2 ratios in rabbit α and β globin mRNA. Nature 275:153–154

Lockard RE, Lane C (1978) Requirement for 7-methylguanosine in translation of globin mRNA in vivo. Nucleic Acids Res 5:3237–3247

Lockard RE, RajBhandary UL (1976) Nucleotide sequences at the 5' termini of rabbit α and β globin mRNA. Cell 9:747–760

Lodish HF (1970) Secondary structure of bacteriophage f2 ribonucleic acid and the initiation of in vitro protein biosynthesis. J Mol Biol 50:689–702

Lodish HF (1971) Alpha and beta globin messenger ribonucleic acid: different amounts and rates of initiation of translation. J Biol Chem 246:7131–7138

Lodish HF, Froshauer S (1977) Rates of initiation of protein synthesis by two purified species of vesicular stomatitis virus messenger RNA. J Biol Chem 252:8804–8811

Lodish HF, Porter M (1980) Translational control of protein synthesis after infection by vesicular stomatitis virus. J Virol 36:719–733

Lomedico P, Rosenthal N, Efstratiadis A, Gilbert W, Kolodner R, Tizard R (1979) The structure and evolution of the two nonallelic rat preproinsulin genes. Cell 18:545–558

Mantei N, Schwarzstein M, Streuli M, Panem S, Nagata S, Weissmann C (1980) The nucleotide sequence of a cloned human leukocyte interferon cDNA. Gene 10:1–10

Martial JA, Hallewell RA, Baxter JD, Goodman HM (1979) Human growth hormone: complementary DNA cloning and expression in bacteria. Science 205:602–607

Mayo MA, Barker H, Harrison BD (1979) Evidence for a protein covalently linked to tobacco ringspot virus RNA. J Gen Virol 43:735–740

McCrae MA, Joklik WK (1978) The nature of the polypeptide encoded by each of the 10 double-stranded RNA segments of reovirus type 3. Virology 89:578–593

McKnight SL (1980) The nucleotide sequence and transcript map of the herpes simplex virus thymidine kinase gene. Nucleic Acids Res 8:5949–5964

McReynolds L, O'Malley BW, Nisbet AD, Fothergill JE, Givol D, Fields S, Robertson M, Brownlee GG (1978) Sequence of chicken ovalbumin mRNA. Nature 273:723–728

Mellon P, Duesberg PH (1977) Subgenomic, cellular Rous sarcoma virus RNAs contain oligonucleotides from the 3′ half and the 5′ terminus of virion RNA. Nature 270:631–634

Metz DH (1975) The mechanism of action of interferon. Cell 6:429–439

Miller JS, Ricciardi RP, Roberts BE, Paterson BM, Mathews MB (1980) Arrangement of messenger RNAs and protein coding sequences in the major late transcription unit of adenovirus 2. J Mol Biol 142:455–488

Miller WL, Martial JA, Baxter JD (1980) Molecular cloning of DNA complementary to bovine growth hormone mRNA. J Biol Chem 255:7521–7524

MinJou W, Verhoeyen M, Devos R, Saman E, Fang R, Huylebroeck D, Fiers W, Threlfall G, Barber C, Carey N, Emtage S (1980) Complete structure of the hemagglutinin gene from the human influenza A/Victoria/3/75 (H3N2) strain as determined from cloned DNA. Cell 19:683–696

Montgomery DL, Leung DW, Smith M, Shalit P, Faye G, Hall BD (1980) Isolation and sequence of the gene for iso-2-cytochrome c in *Saccharomyces cerevisiae*. Proc Natl Acad Sci USA 77:541–545

Morrison TG, Lodish HF (1973) Translation of bacteriophage Qβ RNA by cytoplasmic extracts of mammalian cells. Proc Natl Acad Sci USA 70:315–319

Mulligan RC, Howard BH, Berg P (1979) Synthesis of rabbit β-globin in cultured monkey kidney cells following infection with a SV40 β-globin recombinant genome. Nature 277:108–114

Munns TW, Morrow CS, Hunsley JR, Oberst RJ, Liszewski MK (1979) Antibody-nucleic acid complexes. Inhibition of translation of silkmoth chorion messenger ribonucleic acid with antibodies specific for 7-methylguanosine. Biochemistry 18:3804–3810

Muthukrishnan S, Morgan M, Banerjee AK, Shatkin AJ (1976) Influence of 5′-terminal m⁷G and 2′-O-methylated residues on messenger ribonucleic acid binding to ribosomes. Biochemistry 15:5761–5768

Muthukrishnan S, Moss B, Cooper JA, Maxwell ES (1978) Influence of 5′-terminal cap structure on the initiation of translation of vaccinia virus mRNA. J Biol Chem 253:1710–1715

Nagata S, Mantei N, Weissmann C (1980) The structure of one of the eight or more distinct chromosomal genes for human interferon-α. Nature 287:401–408

Nakanishi S, Teranishi Y, Noda M, Notake M, Watanabe Y, Kakidani H, Jingami H, Numa S (1980) The protein-coding sequence of the bovine ACTH-β-LPH precursor gene is split near the signal peptide region. Nature 287:752–755

Nakashima K, Darzynkiewicz E, Shatkin AJ (1980) Proximity of mRNA 5′-region and 18S rRNA in eukaryotic initiation complexes. Nature 286:226–230

Neeleman L, van Vloten-Doting L (1979) Determination of the number of ribosomal binding sites on the RNAs of eukaryotic viruses. Methods in Enzymology 60:410–417

Ng R, Abelson J (1980) Isolation and sequence of the gene for actin in *Saccharomyces cerevisiae*. Proc Natl Acad Sci USA 77:3912–3916

Nishioka Y, Leder P (1979) The complete sequence of a chromosomal mouse α-globin gene reveals elements conserved throughout vertebrate evolution. Cell 18:875–882

Nomoto A, Lee YF, Wimmer E (1976) The 5′ end of poliovirus mRNA is not capped with m⁷G (5′)ppp(5′)Np. Proc Natl Acad Sci USA 73:375–380

Nomoto A, Kitamura N, Golini F, Wimmer E (1977) The 5′-terminal structures of poliovirion

RNA and poliovirus mRNA differ only in the genome linked protein VPg. Proc Natl Acad Sci USA 74:5345–5349

Nunberg JH, Kaufman RJ, Chang A, Cohen S, Schimke RT (1980) Structure and genomic organization of the mouse dihydrofolate reductase gene. Cell 19:355–364

Nuss DL, Oppermann H, Koch G (1975) Selective blockage of initiation of host protein synthesis in RNA-virus-infected cells. Proc Natl Acad Sci USA 72:1258–1262

Ofengand J (1977) tRNA and aminoacyl-tRNA synthetases. In: Weissbach H, Pestka S (eds) Molecular mechanisms of protein biosynthesis. New York, Academic Press, pp 7–79

Palmiter RD, Gagnon J, Vogt VM, Ripley S, Eisenman RN (1978) The NH_2-terminal sequence of the avian oncornavirus *gag* precursor polyprotein ($Pr76^{gag}$). Virology 91:423–433

Paoletti E (1977) In vitro synthesis of a high molecular weight virion-associated RNA by vaccinia. J Biol Chem 252:866–871

Papkoff J, Hunter T, Beemon K (1980) In vitro translation of virion RNA from Moloney murine sarcoma virus. Virology 101:91–103

Pavlakis GN, Lockard RE, Vamvakopoulos N, Rieser L, RajBhandary UL, Vournakis JN (1980) Secondary structure of mouse and rabbit α- and β-globin mRNAs: differential accessibility of α and β initiator AUG codons towards nucleases. Cell 19:91–102

Pawson T, Harvey R, Smith AE (1977) The size of Rous sarcoma virus mRNAs active in cell-free translation. Nature 268:416–420

Payvar F, Schimke RT (1979) Methylmercury hydroxide enhancement of translation and transcription of ovalbumin and conalbumin mRNA's. J Biol Chem 254:7636–7642

Pelham HRB (1977) Use of coupled transcription and translation to study mRNA production by vaccinia cores. Nature 269:532–534

Pelham HRB (1979a) Translation of fragmented viral RNA in vitro: initiation at multiple sites. FEBS Letters 100:195–199

Pelham HRB (1979b) Synthesis and proteolytic processing of cowpea mosaic virus proteins in reticulocyte lysates. Virology 96:463–477

Pelham HRB (1979c) Translation of tobacco rattle virus RNAs in vitro: four proteins from three RNAs. Virology 97:256–265

Perez-Bercoff R, Gander M (1978) In vitro translation of mengovirus RNA deprived of the terminally-linked (capping?) protein. FEBS Letters 96:306–312

Perler F, Efstratiadis A, Lomedico P, Gilbert W, Kolodner R, Dodgson J (1980) The evolution of genes: the chicken preproinsulin gene. Cell 20:555–566

Perricaudet M, Akusjärvi G, Virtanen A, Pettersson U (1979) Structure of two spliced mRNAs from the transforming region of human subgroup C adenoviruses. Nature 281:694–696

Perricaudet M, le Moullec J-M, Tiollais P, Pettersson U (1980) Structure of two adenovirus type 12 transforming polypeptides and their evolutionary implications. Nature 288:174–176

Person A, Beaud G (1978) Inhibition of host protein synthesis in vaccinia virus-infected cells in the presence of cordycepin (3'-deoxyadenosine). J Virol 25:11–18

Person A, Ben-Hamida F, Beaud G (1980) Inhibition of 40S Met-tRNA$_f^{met}$ ribosomal initiation complex formation by vaccinia virus. Nature 287:355–357

Persson H, Jörnvall H, Zabielski J (1980) Multiple mRNA species for the precursor to an adenovirus-encoded glycoprotein: identification and structure of the signal sequence. Proc Natl Acad Sci USA 77:6349–6353

Petersen NS, McLaughlin CS (1973) Monocistronic messenger RNA in yeast. J Mol Biol 81:33–45

Piatak M, Ghosh PK, Reddy VB, Lebowitz P, Weissman SM (1979) Complex structures and new surprises in SV40 mRNA. In: Cummings DJ, Borst P, Dawid IB, Weissman SM, Fox CF (eds) ICN/UCLA Symposium: extrachromosomal DNA. Academic Press, New York, pp 199–215

Pinck L, Franck A, Fritsch C (1979) Formation of ribosome-RNA initiation complexes with alfalfa mosaic virus RNA 4 and RNA 3. Nucleic Acids Res 7:151–166

Post LE, Nomura M (1980) DNA sequences from the *str* operon of *Escherichia coli*. J Biol Chem 255:4660–4666

Quintrell N, Hughes SH, Varmus HE, Bishop JM (1980) Structure of viral DNA and RNA in mammalian cells infected with avian sarcoma virus. J Mol Biol 143:363–393

Ramabhadran TV, Thach RE (1980) Specificity of protein synthesis inhibitors in the inhibition of encephalomyocarditis virus replication. J Virol 34:293–296

Reddy VB, Ghosh PK, Lebowitz P, Weissman SM (1978a) Gaps and duplicated sequences in the leaders of SV40 16S RNA. Nucleic Acids Res 5:4195–4213

Reddy VB, Thimmappaya B, Dhar R, Subramanian KN, Zain BS, Pan J, Ghosh PK, Celma ML, Weissman SM (1978b) The genome of simian virus 40. Science 200:494–502

Reddy VB, Ghosh PK, Lebowitz P, Piatak M, Weissman SM (1979) Simian virus 40 early mRNA's. I. Genomic localization of 3′ termini and two major splices in mRNA from transformed and lytically infected cells. J Virol 30:279–296

Richards K, Guilley H, Jonard G, Hirth L (1978) Nucleotide sequence at the 5′ extremity of tobacco-mosaic-virus RNA. 1. The noncoding region (nucleotides 1–68). Eur J Biochem 84: 513–519

Richards RI, Wells JRE (1980) Chicken globin genes. Nucleotide sequence of cDNA clones coding for the α-globin expressed during hemolytic anemia. J Biol Chem 255:9306–9311

Richards RI, Shine J, Ullrich A, Wells JRE, Goodman HM (1979) Molecular cloning and sequence analysis of adult chicken β globin cDNA. Nucleic Acids Res 7:1137–1146

Robertson JS (1979) 5′ and 3′ terminal sequences of the RNA genome segments of influenza virus. Nucleic Acids Res 6:3745–3757

Robertson MA, Staden R, Tanaka Y, Catterall JF, O'Malley BW, Brownlee GG (1979) Sequence of three introns in the chick ovalbumin gene. Nature 278:370–372

Rose JK (1978) Complete sequences of the ribosome recognition sites in vesicular stomatitis virus mRNAs: recognition by the 40S and 80S complexes. Cell 14:345–353

Rose JK (1980) Complete intergenic and flanking gene sequences from the genome of vesicular stomatitis virus. Cell 19:415–421

Rosenberg M, Paterson BM (1979) Efficient cap-dependent translation of polycistronic prokaryotic mRNAs is restricted to the first gene in the operon. Nature 279:696–701

Rowekamp W, Poole S, Firtel RA (1980) Analysis of the multigene family coding the developmentally regulated carbohydrate-binding protein discoidin-I in D. discoideum. Cell 20:495–505

Rowlands DJ (1979) Sequences of vesicular stomatitis virus RNA in the region coding for leader RNA, N protein mRNA, and their junction. Proc Natl Acad Sci USA 76:4793–4797

Sagot J, Beaud G (1979) Phosphorylation in vivo of a vaccinia-virus structural protein found associated with the ribosomes from infected cells. Eur J Biochem 98:131–140

Sakano H, Maki R, Kurosawa Y, Roeder W, Tonegawa S (1980) Two types of somatic recombination are necessary for the generation of complete immunoglobulin heavy-chain genes. Nature 286:676–683

Salerno-Rife T, Rutgers T, Kaesberg P (1980) Translation of Southern bean mosaic virus RNA in wheat embryo and rabbit reticulocyte extracts. J Virol 34:51–58

Salomon R, Bar-Joseph M, Soreq H, Gozes I, Littauer UZ (1978) Translation in vitro of carnation mottle virus RNA: regulatory function of the 3′-region. Virology 90:288–298

Salvato MS, Fraenkel-Conrat H (1977) Translation of tobacco necrosis virus and its satellite in a cell-free wheat germ system. Proc Natl Acad Sci USA 74:2288–2292

Sangar DV, Rowlands DJ, Harris TJR, Brown F (1977) Protein covalently linked to foot-and-mouth disease virus RNA. Nature 268:648–650

Sangar DV, Black DN, Rowlands DJ, Harris TJR, Brown F (1980) Location of the initiation site for protein synthesis on foot-and-mouth disease virus RNA by in vitro translation of defined fragments of the RNA. J Virol 33:59–68

Sawicki DL, Kääriäinen L, Lambek C, Gomatos PJ (1978) Mechanism for control of synthesis of Semliki Forest virus 26S and 42S RNA. J Virol 25:19–27

Schaffer FL, Ehresmann DW, Fretz MK, Soergel ME (1980) A protein, VPg, covalently linked to 36S calicivirus RNA. J Gen Virol 47:215–220

Schaffner W, Kunz G, Daetwyler H, Telford J, Smith HO, Birnstiel ML (1978) Genes and spacers of cloned sea urchin histone DNA analyzed by sequencing. Cell 14:655–671

Schroeder HW, Liarakos CD, Gupta RC, Randerath K, O'Malley BW (1979) Ribosome binding site analysis of ovalbumin messenger ribonucleic acid. Biochemistry 18:5798–5808

Schrom M, Bablanian R (1979) Inhibition of protein synthesis by vaccinia virus. I. Characterization of an inhibited cell-free protein synthesizing system from infected cells. Virology 99: 319–328

Seeburg PH, Shine J, Martial JA, Baxter JD, Goodman HM (1977) Nucleotide sequence and amplification in bacteria of structural gene for rat growth hormone. Nature 270:486–494

Seidman JG, Max EE, Leder P (1979) A κ-immunoglobulin gene is formed by site-specific recombination without further somatic mutation. Nature 280:370–375

Setzer DR, McGrogan M, Nunberg JH, Schimke RT (1980) Size heterogeneity in the 3' end of dihydrofolate reductase messenger RNAs in mouse cells. Cell 22:361–370

Shatkin AJ (1976) Capping of eucaryotic mRNAs. Cell 9:645–653

Shatkin AJ, Both GW (1976) Reovirus mRNA: transcription and translation Cell 7:305–313

Sherman F, McKnight G, Stewart JW (1980a) AUG is the only initiation codon in eukaryotes. Biochim Biophys Acta 609:343–346

Sherman F, Stewart JW, Schweingruber AM (1980b) Mutants of yeast initiating translation of iso-l-cytochrome c within a region spanning 37 nucleotides. Cell 20:215–222

Shih DS, Kaesberg P (1976) Translation of the RNAs of brome mosaic virus: the monocistronic nature of RNA1 and RNA2. J Mol Biol 103:77–88

Shih DS, Dasgupta R, Kaesberg P (1976) 7-Methyl-guanosine and efficiency of RNA translation. J Virol 19:637–642

Shine J, Dalgarno L (1974) The 3'-terminal sequence of Escherichia coli 16S ribosomal RNA: complementarity to nonsense triplets and ribosome binding sites. Proc Natl Acad Sci USA 71:1342–1346

Shine J, Czernilofsky AP, Friedrich R, Bishop JM, Goodman HM (1977) Nucleotide sequence at the 5' terminus of the avian sarcoma virus genome. Proc Natl Acad Sci USA 74:1473–1477

Siddell SG, Smith AE (1978) Polyoma virus has three late mRNA's: one for each virion protein. J Virol 27:427–431

Skehel JJ (1972) Polypeptide synthesis in influenza virus-infected cells. Virology 49:23–36

Skup D, Millward S (1980a) Reovirus-induced modification of cap-dependent translation in infected L cells. Proc Natl Acad Sci USA 77:152–156

Skup D, Millward S (1980b) mRNA capping enzymes are masked in reovirus progeny subviral particles. J Virol 34:490–496

Slightom JL, Blechl AE, Smithies O (1980) Human fetal $^G\gamma$- and $^A\gamma$-globin genes: complete nucleotide sequences suggest that DNA can be exchanged between these duplicated genes. Cell 21:627–638

Smith AE (1977) Cryptic initiation sites in eukaryotic virus mRNAs. In: Clark BFC (ed) Gene expression. Federation of European Biological Societies Symposium Vol. 43. Oxford, Pergamon Press, pp 37–46

Smith M, Leung DW, Gillam S, Astell CR, Montgomery DL, Hall BD (1979) Sequence of the gene for iso-l-cytochrome c in Saccharomyces cerevisiae. Cell 16:753–761

Soeda E, Arrand JR, Griffin BE (1980) Polyoma virus DNA: complete nucleotide sequence of the gene which codes for polyoma virus capsid protein VP1 and overlaps the VP2/VP3 genes. J Virol 33:619–630

Somogyi P, Dobos P (1980) Virus-specific RNA synthesis in cells infected by infectious pancreatic necrosis virus. J Virol 33:129–139

Sonenberg N, Morgan M, Merrick WC, Shatkin AJ (1978) A polypeptide in eukaryotic initiation factors that crosslinks specifically to the 5'-terminal cap in mRNA. Proc Natl Acad Sci USA 75:4843–4847

Sonenberg N, Trachsel H, Hecht S, Shatkin AJ (1980) Differential stimulation of capped mRNA translation in vitro by cap binding protein. Nature 285:331–333

Soreq H, Nudel U, Salomon R, Revel M, Littauer UZ (1974) In vitro translation of polyadenylic acid-free rabbit globin messenger RNA. J Mol Biol 88:233–245

Spritz RA, DeRiel JK, Forget BG, Weissman SM (1980) Complete nucleotide sequence of the human δ-globin gene. Cell 21:639–646

Stanley J, Rottier P, Davies JW, Zabel P, Van Kammen A (1978) A protein linked to the 5' termini of both RNA components of the cowpea mosaic virus genome. Nucleic Acids Res 5: 4505–4522

Stanners CP, Francoeur AM, Lam T (1977) Analysis of VSV mutant with attenuated cytopathogenicity: mutation in viral function P, for inhibition of protein synthesis. Cell 11:273–281

Steitz JA (1979) Genetic signals and nucleotide sequences in messenger RNA. In: Biological Regulation and Development. Vol. 1. Gene Expression (Ed. R.F. Goldberger). New York, Plenum Press, pp 349–399

Steitz JA, Jakes K (1975) How ribosomes select initiator regions in mRNA: base pair formation between the 3' terminus of 16S rRNA and the mRNA during initiation of protein synthesis in *Escherichia coli*. Proc Natl Acad Sci USA 72:4734–4738

Stern DF, Kennedy SIT (1980a) Coronavirus multiplication strategy. I. Identification and characterization of virus-specified RNA. J Virol 34:665–674

Stern DF, Kennedy SIT (1980b) Coronavirus multiplication strategy. II. Mapping the avian infectious bronchitis virus intracellular RNA species to the genome. J Virol 36:440–449

Stewart JW, Sherman F, Shipman NA, Jackson M (1971) Identification and mutational relocation of the AUG codon initiating translation of iso-1-cytochrome c in yeast. J Biol Chem 246: 7429–7445

Stoltzfus CM, Kuhnert LK (1979) Evidence for the identity of shared 5'-terminal sequences between genome RNA and subgenomic mRNA's of B77 avian sarcoma virus. J Virol 32:536–545

Subramanian KN (1979) Segments of simian virus 40 DNA spanning most of the leader sequence of the major late viral messenger RNA are dispensable. Proc Natl Acad Sci USA 76:2556–2560

Sures I, Lowry J, Kedes LH (1978) The DNA sequence of sea urchin (S. purpuratus) H2A, H2B and H3 histone coding and spacer regions. Cell 15:1033–1044

Sures I, Levy S, Kedes LH (1980) Leader sequences of *Strongylocentrotus purpuratus* histone mRNAs start at a unique heptanucleotide common to all five histone genes. Proc Natl Acad Sci USA 77:1265–1269

Swinkels P, Bol JF (1980) Limited sequence variation in the leader sequence of RNA 4 from several strains of alfalfa mosaic virus. Virology 106:145–147

Tanaka T, Wool IG, Stöffler G (1980) The effect of antibodies against *Escherichia coli* small ribosomal subunit proteins on protein synthesis by rat liver ribosomes. J Biol Chem 255:3832–3834

Taniguchi T, Weissmann C (1978) Site-directed mutations in the initiator region of the bacteriophage Qβ coat cistron and their effect on ribosome binding. J Mol Biol 118:533–565

Testa D, Chanda PK, Banerjee AK (1980) Unique mode of transcription in vitro by vesicular stomatitis virus. Cell 21:267–275

Török I, Karch F (1980) Nucleotide sequences of heat shock activated genes in Drosophila melanogaster. I. Sequences in the regions of the 5' and 3' ends of the hsp 70 gene in the hybrid plasmid 56H8. Nucleic Acids Res 8:3105–3122

Trachsel H, Sonenberg N, Shatkin AJ, Rose JK, Leong K, Bergmann JE, Gordon J, Baltimore D (1980) Purification of a factor that restores translation of vesicular stomatitis virus mRNA in extracts from poliovirus-infected HeLa cells. Proc Natl Acad Sci USA 77:770–774

Treisman R (1980) Characterisation of polyoma late mRNA leader sequences by molecular cloning and DNA sequence analysis. Nucleic Acids Res 8:4867–4888

Tsujimoto Y, Suzuki Y (1979) The DNA sequence of Bombyx mori fibroin gene including the 5' flanking, mRNA coding, entire intervening and fibroin protein coding regions. Cell 18:591–600

Valenzuela P, Gray P, Quiroga M, Zaldivar J, Goodman HM, Rutter WJ (1979) Nucleotide sequence of the gene coding for the major protein of hepatitis B virus surface antigen. Nature 280:815–819

Valenzuela P, Quiroga M, Zaldivar J, Rutter WJ, Kirschner MW, Cleveland DW (1981) The nucleotide and corresponding amino acid sequences encoded by α tubulin and β tubulin mRNAs. Nature 289:650–655

Van de Voorde A, Contreras R, Rogiers R, Fiers W (1976) The initiation region of the SV40 VP1 gene. Cell 9:117–120

Van Ooyen A, Van den Berg J, Mantei N, Weissmann C (1979) Comparison of total sequence of a cloned rabbit β-globin gene and its flanking regions with a homologous mouse sequence. Science 206:337–344

van Ormondt H, Maat J, van Beveren CP (1980) The nucleotide sequence of the transforming early region E1 of adenovirus type 5 DNA. Gene 11:299–309

van Steeg H, Pranger MH, van der Zeijst B, Benne R, Voorma HO (1979) In vitro translation of Semliki Forest virus 42S RNA. FEBS Letters 108:292–298

Villa-Komaroff L, Guttman N, Baltimore D, Lodish HF (1975) Complete translation of poliovirus RNA in a eukaryotic cell-free system. Proc Natl Acad Sci USA 72:4157–4161

Villarreal LP, White RT, Berg P (1979) Mutational alterations within the simian virus 40 leader segment generate altered 16S and 19S mRNA's. J Virol 29:209–219

Wallis JW, Hereford L, Grunstein M (1980) Histone H2B genes of yeast encode two different proteins. Cell 22:799–805

Warrington RC, Wratten N (1977) Differential action of L-histidinol in reovirus-infected and uninfected L-929 cells. Virology 81:408–418

Weatherall DJ, Clegg JB (1979) Recent developments in the molecular genetics of human hemoglobin. Cell 16:467–479

Weber LA, Hickey ED, Nuss DL, Baglioni C (1977) 5'-Terminal 7-methylguanosine and mRNA function: influence of potassium concentration on translation in vitro. Proc Natl Acad Sci USA 74:3254–3258

Weber LA, Hickey ED, Baglioni C (1978) Influence of potassium salt concentration and temperature on inhibition of mRNA translation by 7-methylguanosine 5'-monophosphate. J Biol Chem 253:178–183

Weiss SR, Varmus HE, Bishop JM (1977) The size and genetic composition of virus-specific RNAs in the cytoplasm of cells producing avian sarcoma-leukosis viruses. Cell 12:983–992

Wengler G, Beato M, Wengler G (1979a) In vitro translation of 42S virus-specific RNA from cells infected with the flavivirus West Nile virus. Virology 96:516–529

Wengler G, Wengler G, Gross HJ (1979b) Replicative form of Semliki Forest virus RNA contains an unpaired guanosine. Nature 282:754–756

Westaway EG (1977) Strategy of the flavivirus genome: evidence for multiple internal initiation of translation of proteins specified by Kunjin virus in mammalian cells. Virology 80:320–335

Wienand U, Feix G (1978) Electrophoretic fractionation and translation in vitro of poly(rA)-containing RNA from maize endosperm. Eur J Biochem 92:605–611

Williams JG, Kay RM, Patient RK (1980) The nucleotide sequence of the major β-globin mRNA from Xenopus laevis. Nucleic Acids Res 8:4247–4258

Wilson JT, Wilson LB, Reddy VB, Cavallesco C, Ghosh PK, deRiel JK, Forget BG, Weissman SM (1980) Nucleotide sequence of the coding portion of human α globin messenger RNA. J Biol Chem 255:2807–2815

Wittek R, Cooper JA, Barbosa E, Moss B (1980) Expression of the vaccinia virus genome: analysis and mapping of mRNAs encoded within the inverted terminal repetition. Cell 21:487–493

Wolgemuth DJ, Yu H-Y, Hsu M-T (1980) Studies on the relationship between 5' leader sequences and initiation of translation of adenovirus 2 and simian virus 40 late mRNAs. Virology 101:363–375

Yakobson E, Prives C, Hartman JR, Winocour E, Revel M (1977) Inhibition of viral protein synthesis in monkey cells treated with interferon late in simian virus 40 lytic cycle. Cell 12:73–81

Yang RCA, Wu R (1979) BK virus DNA sequence coding for the amino-terminus of the T-antigen. Virology 92:340–352

Young RA, Hagenbüchle O, Schibler U (1981) A single mouse α-amylase gene specifies two different tissue-specific mRNAs. Cell 23:451–458

Zain S, Sambrook J, Roberts RJ, Keller W, Fried M, Dunn AR (1979) Nucleotide sequence analysis of the leader segments in a cloned copy of adenovirus 2 fiber mRNA. Cell 16:851–861

Zemell R, Burstein Y, Schechter I (1978) Initiator methionine residues at the NH$_2$-termini of the two precursors of MOPC-41 immunoglobulin light chain. Eur J Biochem 89:187–193

Ziff EB, Evans RM (1978) Coincidence of the promoter and capped 5' terminus of RNA from the adenovirus 2 major late transcription unit. Cell 15:1463–1475

Zuckermann M, Manor H, Parker J, Kamen R (1980) Electron microscopic demonstration of the presence of amplified sequences at the 5'-ends of the polyoma virus late mRNAs. Nucleic Acids Res 8:1505–1519

Zweerink HJ, Joklik WK (1970) Studies on the intracellular synthesis of reovirus-specified proteins. Virology 41:501–518

Priming of Influenza Viral RNA Transcription by Capped Heterologous RNAs

ROBERT M. KRUG*

1   Introduction 125

2   Background 126
2.1 The Host Nuclear RNA Polymerase II is Required for Viral RNA Transcription in the
     Infected Cell 126
2.1.1 Experimental Basis for the Primer RNA Hypothesis 126

3   Capped RNAs Serve as Primers for Influenza Viral RNA Transcription in Vitro . . 127

4   Priming Activity of an RNA Does Not Require Hydrogen Bonding With the Template
     vRNA 129

5   Postulated Mechanism for the Priming of Influenza Viral RNA Transcription . . . 131

6   Identification of the 5′-Terminal Fragment(s) of mRNAs That Initiale Influenza
     Viral RNA Transcription 132

7   Identification of a Cap-dependent Endonuclease in Influenza Virions That Cleaves
     Capped RNAs at Purine Residues Near the 5′-Terminus 135

8   Capped Fragments Generated by Cleavage at A Residues Are Preferentially Utilized
     as Primers to Initiate Transcription 138

9   Mechanism of Priming of Influenza Viral RNA Transcription in Vitro by Capped
     RNAs 139

10   Inhibition of Influenza Viral RNA Transcription by Uncapped RNAs 141

11   Priming by Capped Cellular RNAs Also Occurs in Vivo 142

12   The α-Amanitin-Sensitive Step in Influenza Virus Replication: Synthesis of Capped
     Cellular RNA Primers 145

13   Possible Implications for Cellular Transcription 146

References 147

1 Introduction

Influenza virus is a negative-stranded RNA virus, i.e., the viral messenger RNA (mRNA) is complementary to the genome RNA (which is segmented), and the virion contains the enzyme system which transcribes the genome RNA into the viral mRNA. This virus employs a unique mechanism for the initiation of the synthesis of its mRNA. Specifically, the virion-associated transcriptase system needs to cannibalize capped heterologous

* Molecular Biology and Genetics Unit of the Graduate School, Memorial Sloan-Kettering Cancer
  Center, New York, N.Y. 10021, USA

RNAs, i.e., eukaryotic cellular mRNAs and/or their precursors, in order to synthesize the viral mRNA. This process involves the clipping off by a virion-associated endonuclease of a small piece of the eukaryotic mRNA near its 5'-end, followed by the utilization of this RNA fragment as a primer to initiate the synthesis of the viral mRNA. The methylated cap structure (m^7GpppNm, where Nm = 2'-O-methylated nucleoside) found at the 5'-end of all mammalian cellular mRNAs is part of the RNA fragment that is used as primer and transferred from the cellular to the viral mRNA, and this cap structure is absolutely necessary for the viral nuclease and the priming reaction. In fact, the 5'-methylated cap structure is more stringently required for priming influenza viral mRNA synthesis than for the process in which it had previously been shown to play a role, the translation of mRNAs in cell-free systems. This mechanism for viral mRNA synthesis explains why influenza virus requires the functioning of the host-cell nuclear RNA polymerase II in order to replicate: newly synthesized host mRNAs and/or their precursors are needed as primers for viral mRNA synthesis.

Here, I will first briefly outline the results that led to the discovery that capped RNAs act as primers for influenza viral RNA transcription. I will then describe in more detail the experiments that established the mechanism of this RNA-primed reaction in vitro and those that deal with the priming reaction occurring in the infected cell.

2 Background

2.1 The Host Nuclear RNA Polymerase II Is Required for Viral RNA Transcription in the Infected Cell

One important feature which distinguishes influenza virus from other nononcogenic RNA viruses is that the functioning of the host nuclear DNA-dependent RNA polymerase II is required for virus replication. Actinomycin D and α-amanitin (a specific inhibitor of RNA polymerase II) inhibit virus replication (*Barry* et al. 1962; *Rott* and *Scholtissek* 1970; *Mahy* et al. 1972). In mutant cells containing an α-amanitin-resistant RNA polymerase II, virus replication was also resistant to this drug (*Lamb* and *Choppin* 1977; *Spooner* and *Barry* 1977), thereby definitively establishing that the host RNA polymerase II is required for virus replication. This host function is required for viral RNA transcription, even primary transcription, i.e., the transcription carried out by the inoculum virus. When added at the beginning of infection, actinomycin D or α-amanitin inhibit primary transcription (*Mark* et al. 1979; *Barrett* et al. 1979). In contrast, neither of these drugs inhibit viral RNA transcription in vitro catalyzed by the virion-associated transcriptase (*Chow* and *Simpson* 1971; *Penhoet* et al. 1971). Thus, in an apparent paradox, these drugs inhibit the functioning of the virion transcriptase when it is introduced into the cell to carry out primary transcription, but not when it is assayed in vitro.

2.1.1 Experimental Basis for the Primer RNA Hypothesis

The influenza virion-associated transcriptase exhibits only a very low amount of activity in vitro when assayed under conditions similar to those employed with other negative-stranded viruses like vesicular stomatitis virus (*Chow* and *Simpson* 1971; *Bishop* et al. 1971). The addition of specific dinucleoside monophosphates, however, strongly stimulates influenza viral RNA transcription in vitro (*McGeoch* and *Kitron* 1975; *Plotch* and *Krug* 1977). ApG is the most effective dinucleotide, stimulating transcription about 100-fold, followed closely by GpG (*Plotch* and *Krug* 1977). GpC is the only other dinucleotide with significant stimulatory activity. These dinucleotides act as primers to initiate chains, and the resulting viral RNA transcripts contain poly A and function as viral mRNAs in cell-free systems (*Plotch* and *Krug* 1977; *Bouloy* et al. 1978). On the basis of these results, we proposed that viral RNA transcription in vivo also requires a primer, but that the in vivo primer is not a dinucleotide but rather an RNA synthesized by RNA polymerase II (*Plotch* and *Krug* 1977, 1978). This would explain why α-amanitin inhibits viral RNA transcription in vivo but not in vitro.

The viral mRNAs isolated from the infected cell contain a 5'-terminal methylated cap structure (*Krug* et al. 1976). The caps were found to be heterogeneous: most contained methylated adenosine as the penultimate base (m^7GpppAm and m^7Gpppm^{6}Am), and some contained methylated guanosine at this position (m^7GpppGm). However, capping and methylating enzymes were not detected in the virion (*Plotch* et al. 1978). To assay for these activities, dinucleotide primers containing di- and triphosphate 5'-ends, like ppApG and pppApG, were used since the vaccinia virus and reovirus capping enzymes require at least a diphosphorylated 5'-end (*Martin* and *Moss* 1976; *Moss* et al. 1976; *Furuichi* et al. 1976). Because of these results, we proposed that the 5'-cap found on in vivo viral mRNAs is derived from the primer RNAs synthesized by the host RNA polymerase II (*Plotch* et al. 1978).

3 Capped RNAs Serve as Primers for Influenza Viral RNA Transcription in Vitro

Primer RNAs were first identified in rabbit reticulocyte extracts, where they were shown to be globin mRNAs (*Bouloy* et al. 1978). β-globin mRNA, purified by polyacrylamide gel electrophoresis, stimulated viral RNA transcription about 80-fold and, on a molar basis, was about 1000 times more effective as a primer than ApG. Thus, maximal stimulation of transcription occurred with about 0.2 μ*M* β-globin mRNA (*Bouloy* et al. 1978), whereas with ApG a concentration of about 0.2 m*M* was needed (*Plotch* and *Krug* 1977). Other capped eukaryotic mRNAs were also found to be extremely effective primers (*Bouloy* et al. 1978, 1979; *Plotch* et al. 1979). The viral RNA transcripts primed by these eukaryotic mRNAs were effectively translated into virus-specific proteins in cell-free systems (*Bouloy* et al. 1978).

The 5'-terminal methylated cap structure was shown to be required for priming activity. Only capped mRNAs were active as primers. Removal of the m^7G of the cap of a mRNA by chemical (β-elimination) or enzymatic (tobacco acid pyrophosphatase) treatment eliminated all priming activity, and this activity could be restored by recapping the β-eliminated mRNA using vaccinia virus guanylyl and methyl transferases (*Plotch* et al. 1979). The cap must contain methyl groups, since reovirus mRNAs with 5'-GpppG ends were not active as primers (*Bouloy* et al. 1979). Each of the two methyl groups in the cap, the 7-methyl on the terminal G and the 2'-O-methyl on the penultimate base, strongly influenced the priming activity of an mRNA (*Bouloy* et al. 1980). Of particular interest was the effect of the 2'-O-methyl group. To demonstrate the importance of this group, several plant viral RNAs containing the monomethylated cap 0 structure, m^7GpppG were used. Brome mosaic virus (BMV) RNA 4 stimulated influenza viral RNA transcription only about 10–15 percent as effectively as globin mRNA. After enzymatic methylation of the 2′-O-group of the penultimate base (G) of the cap of BMV RNA 4, its priming activity was greatly increased, about 14-fold. Qualitatively similar results were obtained with other plant viral RNAs: priming activity increased 3- to 20-fold following 2′-O-methylation.

This is the first instance in which the 2′-O-methyl group of the cap has been shown to have a strong and clear-cut effect on a specific function of an mRNA. In cell-free translation systems, the absence of the 2′-O-methyl group in the cap has little or no effect on the ability of an mRNA to be translated (*Shih* and *Kaesberg* 1973; *Muthukrishnan* et al. 1976, 1978). Indeed, the cap is not actually required for translation. Removal of the terminal m^{7}G of the cap or the absence of both methyl groups in the cap only reduces the efficiency of translation; and, in fact, some naturally occurring uncapped RNAs, like picornavirus RNA and satellite tobacco necrosis RNA, are efficiently translated (*Shatkin* 1976). Consequently, the fully methylated cap 1 structure, m^{7}Gppp Nm, which is found in all mammalian cellular mRNAs and most animal viral mRNAs (*Shatkin* 1976), is more stringently required for priming influenza viral RNA transcription than for translation in cell-free systems.

To demonstrate that the cap of the primer mRNA was transferred to the viral mRNA during in vitro transcription, a globin mRNA primer was prepared that contained ^{32}P only in its cap [prepared by enzymatically recapping β-eliminated globin mRNA in the presence of (α-^{32}P) GTP and unlabeled S-adenosylmethionine] (*Plotch* et al. 1979). After transcription in the presence of this primer mRNA and unlabeled nucleoside triphosphates, the resulting viral mRNA segments were shown to contain ^{32}P-labeled cap structures. As the initial approach for determining whether sequences in addition to the cap were transferred, the size of the globin mRNA-primed viral mRNA segments was compared to that of the ApG-primed segments (*Plotch* et al. 1978). The latter segments initiate exactly at the UC sequence at the 3′-end of the virion RNA (vRNA) segments (*Skehel* and *Hay* 1978; *Robertson* 1979). Gel electrophoretic analysis indicated that the globin mRNA-primed viral mRNA segments were 10–15 nucleotides larger than the ApG-primed segments (*Plotch* et al. 1979). This method of analysis indicated that the viral mRNA segments primed by other capped eukaryotic mRNAs were also about 10–15 nucleotides larger (*Bouloy* et al. 1979). Thus, approximately the same number of nucleotides, about 10–15, plus the cap, were transferred from globin and other mRNA primers.

These studies did not allow the identification of which bases of a primer mRNA were transferred. To accomplish this, globin mRNA was labeled in vitro with ^{125}I to high specific activity, thereby labeling the C residues, and this globin mRNA was used as a primer in the presence of unlabeled nucleoside triphosphates (*Robertson* et al. 1980). The ^{125}I-labeled region transferred to each of the viral mRNA segments had the same T1 ribonuclease and pancreatic ribonuclease fingerprints, indicating that the same region of the globin mRNA primer was transferred to each of the segments. The predominant sequence transferred, comprising 75% of the total, was identical to the first 13 nucleotides (plus the cap) at the 5′-terminus of β-globin mRNA, which has the sequence (*Lockard* and *RajBhandary* 1976): m^{7}Gpppm^{6}AmpC(m)pApCpUpUpGpCpUpUpUpUpGpApCp. . .

Because only the C residues were labeled with ^{125}I, it could not be concluded with certainty that all 13 5'-terminal nucleotides were transferred from β-globin mRNA. The results, however, certainly indicated that the β-globin mRNA donated at least the first eight, but no more than the first 14,5'-terminal bases to the viral mRNAs. It was almost certain that the . . .UUUU. . . sequence (residues 9–12) originated from β-globin mRNA since there are no A residues in the common 12-base 3'-terminal sequence of the eight vRNA segments (3'-UCGUUUUCGUCC. . .) (*Skehel* and *Hay* 1978; *Robertson* 1979), the templates for transcription. Thus, these data indicated that the predominant sequence transferred from α-globin mRNA includes the first 12, 13 or 14 5'-terminal nucleotides.

Minor ^{125}I-labeled RNase T1-resistant oligonucleotides were also found in the viral mRNAs. Fourteen percent of the RNase T1 products were the sequences CUUUGp, CUUGp, CUGp and CGp, which could be presumed to derive their C and U residues from β-globin mRNA (residues 8–11) and which must have obtained their G residue by transcription. Similarly, $m^7Gpppm^6AmC(m)AGp$, containing 11% of the ^{125}I label, clearly must have derived its $m^7Gpppm^6AmC(m)p$ from β-globin mRNA; it could have derived its next A residue either from the β-globin mRNA or as a result of transcription, and must have obtained its G residue as a result of transcription. Thus, 14% and 11% of the time 5'-terminal, cap-containing pieces of β-globin mRNA 8–11 bases, and 2–3 bases in length, respectively, were transferred. It was also concluded that these pieces, as well as the predominant 12–14 nucleotide piece, were linked to G as the first base transcribed.

4 Priming Activity of an RNA Does Not Require Hydrogen-bonding With the Template vRNA

In terms of understanding the mechanism of priming, it was necessary to determine whether the priming RNA must contain a sequence complementary to the common 3'-end of the vRNA templates. In one approach to this problem, it was determined whether 5'-terminal fragments of natural mRNAs lacking such a complementary sequence were active as primers (*Krug* et al. 1981). Fragments of globin mRNA generated by partial alkali or ribonuclease T1 digestion were found to be effective primers. After fragmention with alkali, however, there was about a 30% loss of priming activity. This was almost certainly due to ring-opening of the terminal m^7G by alkali (*Shatkin* 1976), because the fragments generated by ribonuclease T1 digestion were four- to eight-fold more effective as primers on a molar basis than the intact globin mRNA. To determine the exact nucleotide length of the 5'-terminal fragments, globin mRNA and 2'-O-methylated alfalfa mosaic virus (AlMV) RNA 4 (each labeled with ^{32}P in the cap) were fragmented by partial alkali digestion, and the fragments of various chain lengths from each of these RNAs were resolved by gel electrophoresis and tested for priming activity (Figs. 1A, 1B). With both these RNAs, 5'-fragments as short as 14–23 nucleotides long were effective primers. In fact, with AlMV RNA 4, fragments of this size were more active per 5'-termini than larger-size fragments. Since 5'-terminal fragments 14–23 nucleotides long from either AlMV RNA 4 or β-globin mRNA do not contain a sequence complementary to the 3'-end of influenza vRNA (*Koper-Zwarthoff* et al. 1977; *Lockard* and *RajBhandary* 1976; *Skehel* and *Hay* 1978; *Robertson* 1979), the observed stimulation by these fragments could not result from hydrogen bonding between them and the 3'-end of vRNA.

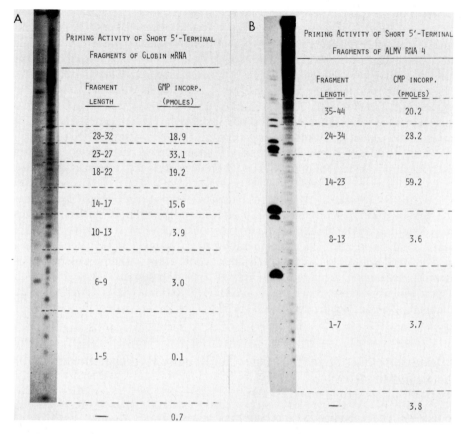

Fig. 1. Priming activity associated with short alkali-generated fragments of globin mRNA (A) and 2'-O-methylated AlMV RNA 4 (B). A mixture of the unlabeled and ^{32}P-cap-labeled RNA was partially digested with mild alkali and subjected to electrophoresis on a 20% acrylamide gel in 7 M urea (right lane in panels A and B). The gel slices containing the indicated fragments were eluted, and each of the fragment preparations was assayed in a transcriptase reaction with (8-^{3}H) GTP (panel A) or (α-^{32}P) CTP (panel B) as labeled precursor. Left lane in panel A: partial T1 RNase digest of ^{32}P-cap-labeled globin mRNA. Left lane in panel B: partial U2 RNase digest of ^{32}P-cap-labeled AlMV RNA 4. From *Krug* et al. (1981)

The same conclusion was obtained using capped ribopolymers as primers (*Krug* et al. 1980). Capped poly A(m^{7}GpppGmC(A)$_n$) and capped poly AU (m^{7}GpppGmC)AU)$_n$) neither of which contain a sequence complementary to the 3'-terminus of vRNA, were about as effective primers as globin mRNA (Table 1). Some, though lower, activity was seen with capped poly U (m^{7}GpppGmC(U)$_n$), even though the 3'-terminal 12-nucleotide sequence common to the eight influenza vRNA segments contain no A residues. Of the various polymers tested as primer, capped poly C (m^{7}GpppGmC(C)$_n$) was the least effective. Thus, while there is some effect of sequence on the efficiency of transcriptase priming by an exogenous capped ribopolymer (see later), there is no requirement for the presence of a sequence complementary to the 3'-end of the vRNA template.

Table 1. Priming Activity of Capped Synthetic Ribopolymers

Experiment[a]	Primer added (pmol)	GMP incorp (pmol)
1	None	1.9
	Globin mRNA (6)	84.4
	Capped poly U (3)	29.1
	Capped poly A (3)	59.1
	Capped poly AU (3)	62.7
2	None	1.1
	Capped poly A (3)	33.0
	Capped poly AG (3)	16.3
3	None	1.2
	Globin mRNA (6)	31.6
	Capped poly AU (3)	27.0
	Capped poly C (3)	5.5

[a] In the three experiments shown, different virus preparations with different specific transcriptase activities (ranging from 14 to 32 nmol GMP incorporated/mg viral protein/h in a globin mRNA-primed reaction) were used. From *Krug* et al. (1980)

In apparent contrast to the situation with capped RNAs as primers, the only dinucleotides that stimulate viral RNA transcription are those that are capable of hydrogen bonding to the 3′-end of the vRNA, namely ApG, GpG, and GpC (*McGeoch* and *Kitron* 1975; *Plotch* and *Krug* 1977). However, it is most likely that priming by these dinucleotides is not the normal mechanism for the initiation of influenza viral RNA transcription because 1. optimal priming by these dinucleotides requires a molar concentration 1000 times higher than that needed for optimal priming by capped RNAs (*Plotch* and *Krug* 1977; *Bouloy* et al. 1978), and 2. the viral mRNAs synthesized in vivo are apparently initiated by capped cellular RNAs (*Krug* et al. 1979; *Caton* and *Robertson* 1980; *Dhar* et al. 1980) (see below). Presumably these dinucleotides allow the transcriptase to avoid the normal initiation step in vitro by providing a high concentration of the initiating G residue in a form in which it can interact with the 3′-end of the vRNA.

5 Postulated Mechanism for the Priming of Influenza Viral RNA Transcription

Based on these results, we postulated a mechanism for the priming of influenza viral RNA transcription by capped RNAs (*Plotch* et al. 1981) (Fig. 2). The capped RNA is cleaved by a virion-associated nuclease to generate one or more 5′-terminal fragments. In the example shown, β-globin mRNA is cleaved at the G residue 13 nucleotides from the 5′-end. Some, or all, of these fragment(s) are the actual primers initiating transcription. In the absence of hydrogen bonding between the primer and vRNA, the stimulation of initiation would result from a specific interaction between the capped RNA fragment and one or more proteins in the transcriptase complex. This specific interaction most likely requires recognition of the 5′-terminal methylated cap structure of the primer, since priming activity requires the presence of this cap structure. As a result of this interaction, the transcriptase acquires the ability to initiate transcription and links a G residue

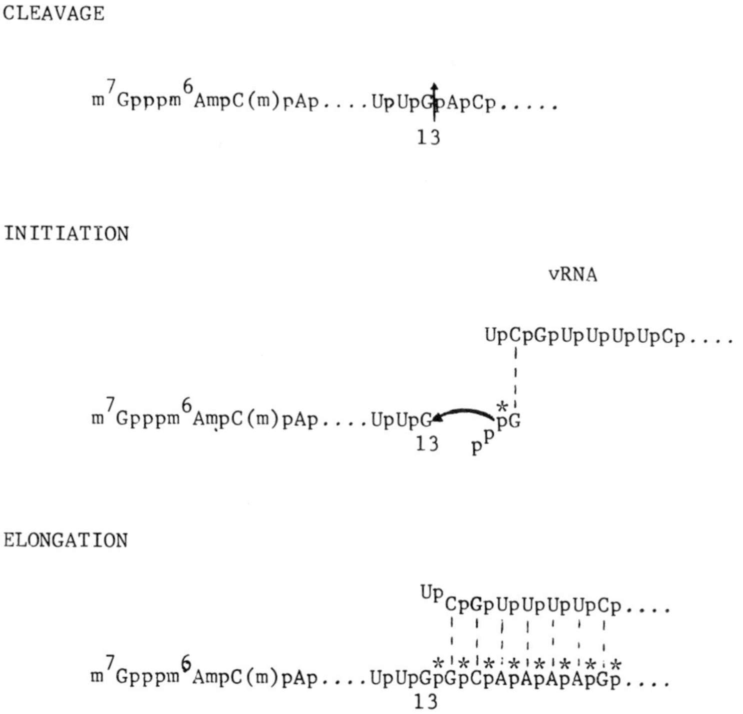

CLEAVAGE

$$m^7 Gpppm^6 AmpC(m)pAp \ldots UpUpGpApCp \ldots$$
$$13$$

INITIATION

vRNA

$$UpCpGpUpUpUpUpCp \ldots$$

$$m^7 Gpppm^6 AmpC(m)pAp \ldots UpUpG \qquad ^* pG$$
$$13 \quad p^p$$

ELONGATION

$$^{Up}CpGpUpUpUpUpCp \ldots$$

$$m^7 Gpppm^6 AmpC(m)pAp \ldots UpUpGpGpCpApApApApGp \ldots$$
$$13$$

Fig. 2. Postulated mechanism for the priming of influenza viral RNA transcription by β-globin mRNA and other capped RNAs. From *Plotch* et al. (1981)

to the 3'-end of the 5'-terminal fragment generated by the nuclease. It is most likely that the incorporation of the initial G residue is directed by the 3'-penultimate C of the vRNA. Elongation of the viral RNA transcripts would then follow. This mechanism predicts the existence of an intermediate in the priming reaction: 5'-terminal fragment(s) cleaved from the mRNA primer. In addition, in a reaction in which the only triphosphate present is GTP, those 5'-terminal fragments that are the actual primers initiating transcription should be linked to a G residue.

6 Identification of the 5'-Terminal Fragment(s) of mRNAs That Initiate Influenza Viral RNA Transcription

The 5'-terminal fragments of globin mRNA that are the actual primers initiating transcription were identified by incubating this mRNA with detergent-treated virus in the presence of (α-^{32}P) GTP as the only ribonucleoside triphosphate (*Plotch* et al. 1981). When the reaction products were analyzed by electrophoresis on 20% acrylamide gels, two major labeled bands were observed in the size range of about 15 nucleotides (Fig. 3). Sequence analysis of band 2 indicated that it was the fragment resulting from cleavage at

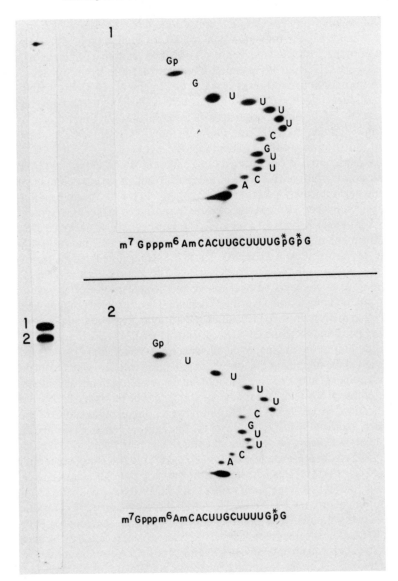

Fig. 3. Identification and sequencing of the 5′-terminal fragments of β-globin mRNA that initiate influenza viral RNA transcription. Globin mRNA was incubated with detergent-treated virus in the presence of (α-^{32}P) GTP and the RNA products were analyzed on a 20% acrylamide gel in 7 M urea. The RNA in bands 1 and 2 was separately eluted, and after β-elimination, was partially digested with alkali. The digest was analyzed by two-dimensional gel electrophoresis. The identity of the 3′-terminal base (Gp) was determined by thin-layer chromatography of the RNase T2 digest of the RNA. From *Plotch* et al. (1981)

the G13 residue of β-globin mRNA (*Lockard* and *RajBhandary* 1976) to which one labeled G residue was added, i.e., m^{7}Gpppm^{6}AmCACUUGCUUUUGpG. This is the species predicted from the postulated mechanism. Thus, the 5′-terminal fragment of β-globin mRNA cleaved at G13 could be presumed to be the actual primer that initiates influenza viral RNA transcription. Band 1 was the same G13 fragment of β-globin mRNA with two G residues added, indicating that more than one G could be added to the primer fragment in the absence of the other ribonucleoside triphosphates. No fragments of α-globin mRNA with 3′-terminal labeled G residues were found, even when the same experiment was performed using purified α-globin mRNA.

When similar experiments were performed using either (α-^{32}P) ATP or (α-^{32}P) UTP as the only ribonucleoside triphosphate in the transcriptase reaction, no incorporation of label into fragments of globin mRNA was detected. With (α-^{32}P) CTP as the only ribonucleoside triphosphate, however, a single C residue was found linked to the G13 fragment of β-globin mRNA (*Plotch* et al. 1981). In addition, a C residue could also be linked to an α-globin mRNA fragment, the fragment resulting from cleavage at nucleotide G10 (*Baralle* 1977), i.e., m^{7}Gpppm^{6}AmCACUUCUGG. These results suggested that the G residue at the third position from the 3′-end of vRNA (see Fig. 2) most likely directed C incorporation in these reactions, with the G residue at the 3′-end of the primer fragments of α- and β-globin mRNA lining up opposite the 3′-penultimate C of the vRNA template. In the case of α-globin mRNA, the two G residues at the 3′-end of its G10 fragment presumably form hydrogen bonds with the UC at the 3′-end of the vRNA (see Fig. 2), thereby precluding G addition to the fragment and allowing only C addition.

These results led to the prediction that primer fragments of mRNAs which contain any nucleotide other than G at their 3′-ends should not be capable of lining up with the 3′-penultimate C of the vRNA template and hence should not be terminally labeled in the presence of (α-^{32}P) CTP (*Plotch* et al. 1981). If, however, the penultimate C of the vRNA normally acts to direct the incorporation of the first base, a G residue (see Fig. 2), then primer fragments containing nucleotides other than G at their 3′-end should be labeled when incubated in the presence of only (α-^{32}-P) GTP or in the presence of both unlabeled GTP and (α-^{32}P) CTP. This was shown to be the case (*Plotch* et al. 1981), using as primers m^{7}GpppGmC(A)$_n$, m^{7}GpppGmC(AU)$_n$, and AlMV RNA 4 [with the 5′-terminal sequence m^{7}GpppGmUUUUUAUUUUUAAUUU. . . . and no other G residue until position 39 from the 5′-end (*Koper-Zwarthoff* et al. 1977)]. The primer fragments derived from these RNAs [i.e., the fragments labeled in a transcriptase reaction in the presence of only (α-^{32}P) GTP] contained totally, or predominantly, an A residue at their 3′-end. With m^{7}GpppGmC(AU)$_n$, all the primer fragments contained 3′-terminal A and not U, and with AlMV RNA 4, which has the extremely U-rich sequence at its 5′-end noted above, the predominant primer fragment (75–80% of the time) was the cleavage product A13. The minor primer fragments of AlMV RNA 4 were the cleavage products at U11 and U12. Thus, the pattern of G and C incorporation onto the primer fragments derived from these mRNAs (A-terminated) and onto those derived from globin mRNA (G-terminated) indicated that this incorporation is almost certainly directed by the second and third bases at the 3′-end of vRNA: C incorporation only occurred next to a G residue, which was either already present at the 3′-end of the primer fragment or was put there by prior incorporation.

7 Identification of a Cap-dependent Endonuclease in Influenza Virions That Cleaves Capped RNAs at Purine Residues Near the 5′-Terminus

In order to demonstrate the cleavage of a capped RNA directly, without G addition, several capped RNAs containing ^{32}P label only in their 5′-terminal methylated cap structure (m^{7}GpppXm) were used as substrates in the absence of the four ribonucleoside triphosphates (*Plotch* et al. 1981). When cap-labeled A1MV RNA 4 was incubated with detergent-treated virus in the absence of ribonucleoside triphosphates, four capped fragments were predominantly generated (in the size range of the 11–15 nucleotide-long alkali-derived fragments of A1MV RNA 4) (Fig. 4, lane 3). The major species, representing 75–80% of the total, was the cleavage product at A13, i.e., m^{7}GpppGm-UUUUUAUUUUUA, and the minor cleavages were at U11, U12, and A14. The fact that the predominant cleavage in this extremely U-rich region was at an A residue reflects the strong preference by the virion endonuclease for cleavage at purines (see later). These cleavage products were shown to contain a 3′-hydroxyl group (*Plotch* et al. 1981), as expected for primer molecules, and thus they migrated slower than the alkali-derived marker fragments of the same size which contain a 2′, 3′ cyclic phosphate group.

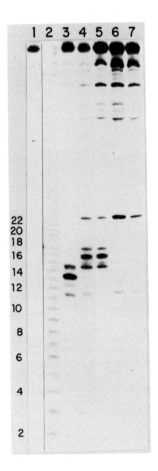

Fig. 4. Identification of a cap-dependent endonuclease in influenza virions that cleaves A1MV RNA 4 at specific positions near its 5′-end. A1MV RNA 4 containing a ^{32}P-labeled cap structure (m^{7}GpppGm) was incubated at 31 °C in the absence of virus (lane 1), or with detergent-treated virus in the absence of ribonucleoside triphosphates (lane 3), or in the presence of 25 µM unlabeled GTP (lane 4 and 5). A1MV RNA 4 containing a ^{32}P-labeled GpppG 5′-end was incubated at 31 °C with detergent-treated virus in the absence of ribonucleoside triphosphates (lane 6) or in the presence of 25 µM unlabeled GTP (lane 7). The phenol-extracted RNA was analyzed by electrophoresis on 20% acrylamide gel in 7 M urea. Lane 2 is the partial alkali digestion products of A1MV RNA containing an m^{7}GpppGm cap, and the numbers on the left refer to the chain lengths of these products, counting the Gm residue as the first base. From *Plotch* et al. (1981)

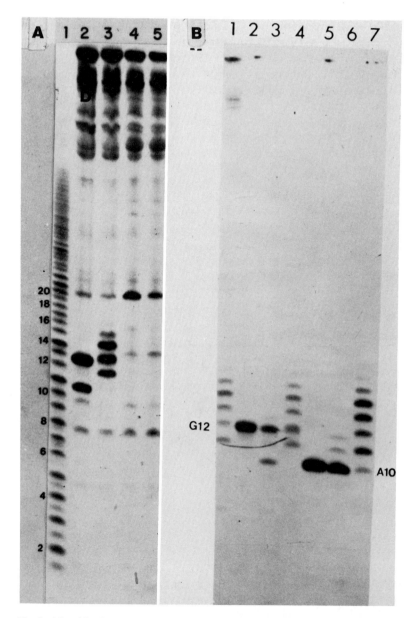

Fig. 5. *A* Specific cleavage of BMV RNA 4 by the influenza virion endonuclease. BMV RNA 4 containing either a ^{32}P-labeled methylated cap structure m^{7}G$\overset{*}{p}$ppGm (lanes 2 and 3) or a ^{32}P-labeled unmethylated cap structure G$\overset{*}{p}$ppG (lanes 4 and 5) was incubated with detergent-treated virus in the absence of ribonucleoside triphosphates (lanes 2 and 4) or in the presence of 25 µM unlabeled GTP (lanes 3 and 5). After incubation, the phenol-extracted RNA was analyzed by electrophoresis on a 20% acrylamide gel in 7 M urea. Lane 1 is the partial alkali digestion product of BMV RNA 4 containing an m^{7}G$\overset{*}{p}$ppGm cap, and the numbers on the left refer to the chain lengths of these products, counting the Gm residue as the first base. From *Plotch* et al. (1981). *B* Ability of fragments cleaved from BMV RNA 4 by the virion endonuclease to be utilized directly as primers for the initiation of transcription in a subsequent incubation with the virus. The fragments cleaved at the A10 residue

The fact that the A13 fragment was utilized as primer could be verified by adding unlabeled GTP to the reaction containing the ^{32}P-cap-labeled A1MV RNA 4 (lanes 4 and 5) (*Plotch* et al. 1981). The A13 fragment disappeared and was replaced by more slowly migrating bands, the mobilities of which were consistent with the addition of one to three G residues to the A13 fragment. The small amount of the U12 fragment generated by the nuclease also disappeared in the presence of GTP, suggesting that it was also used as a primer. No priming by the A14 fragment has been detected. In fact, when the A14 fragment was isolated from a nuclease reaction (done in the absence of GTP) and added to a second reaction (in the presence of GTP), most of the A14 fragment was first cleaved to yield the A13 fragment which was then used as primer (*Krug* and *Broni*, unpublished experiments). This indicates that the transcriptase could only effectively use as primers 5'-terminal fragments 13 nucleotides long or less (plus the cap).

To determine whether specific cleavage of the primer mRNA is dependent on the presence of a methylated cap structure, A1MV RNA 4 containing a 5'-terminal ^{32}P-labeled GpppG blocking group was incubated with detergent-treated virus in the absence (lane 6) or presence (lane 7) of unlabeled GTP (*Plotch* et al. 1981). No primer fragments resulting from cleavage at U12, A13 or A14 were detected and as a result, no bands resulting from the addition of G residues to these cleavage products were produced. A small amount of cleavage at U11 was seen, but no growth of this cleavage product occurred in the presence of GTP. Other, presumably nonspecific cleavages, generating fragments that were not utilized to initiate transcription, occurred at about nucleotide 22 and at nucleotides further from the 5'-end. Most of these cleavages were also seen with the A1MV RNA 4 containing a methylated cap structure. Thus, a methylated cap structure in an RNA is required by the viral endonuclease to generate those specific fragments that serve as primers for viral RNA transcription. This is the only known example of a cap-dependent endonuclease.

The endonuclease has been shown to cleave preferentially at purines (*Plotch* et al. 1981). This was seen most dramatically with BMV RNA 4. With this RNA (containing a ^{32}P-labeled methylated cap structure m^{7}G$\overset{*}{p}$ppGm), two major cleavages occurred (Fig. 5A, lane 2): at nucleotide G12 (*Dasgupta* et al. 1975), i.e., m^{7}GpppGmUAUUAAU-AAUG, and at nucleotide A10 (*Plotch* et al. 1981). No cleavage at U11, however, occurred. In addition, with both α- and β-globin mRNA, cleavage almost certainly occurred primarily, if not entirely, at G residues (G10 with α-globin mRNA and G13 with β-globin mRNA), and with the ribopolymer m^{7}GpppGmC(AU)$_n$, cleavage occurred only at A residues and not at U residues. Even with A1MV RNA 4, which has the extremely U-rich 5'-end noted above, cleavage still occurred preferentially at a purine, the A13 residue. However, with this RNA, some cleavage at the U residues at positions 11 and 12 (and at the A14 residue) also occurred, particularly when larger amounts of the virion endonuclease were used. The ability of the endonuclease to cleave occasionally at U residues would explain why the ribopolymer m^{7}GpppGmC(U)$_n$ exhibits some priming activity

---

and the G12 residue (Fig. 5A, lane 2) were eluted from the gel and purified. The G12 (lanes 2–4) and A10 (lane 5–7) fragments were then separately incubated in the absence of virus (lane 2 and 5), or with detergent-treated virus in the absence of ribonucleoside triphosphates (lanes 3 and 6), or in the presence of 1.0 mM unlabeled GTP (lanes 4 and 7). Lane 1 shows the band pattern obtained when intact BMV RNA 4 containing a m^{7}GpppGm cap structure was incubated with detergent-treated virus in the presence of 1.0 mM unlabeled GTP. From *Plotch* et al. (1981)

(*Krug* et al. 1980). Nevertheless, with most capped RNAs containing a relatively even distribution of purines and pyrimidines near their 5′-end, cleavage most probably occurs almost exclusively at purines.

8 Capped Fragments Generated by Cleavage at A Residues are Preferentially Utilized as Primers to Initiate Transcription

As noted above, BMV RNA 4 was cleaved at both nucleotides A10 and G12, with the latter cleavage usually occurring more frequently (Fig. 5A, lane 2). However, little or no priming by the G12 fragment occurred, whereas the A10 fragment was an effective primer. Thus, when unlabeled BMV RNA 4 was incubated with detergent-treated virus in the presence of (α-^{32}P) GTP, the only primer fragment detected was the A10 cleavage product with one to three G residues added (*Plotch* et al. 1981). The utilization of the A10 fragment as primer could also be shown using ^{32}P-cap-labeled BMV RNA 4 as primer in the presence of unlabeled GTP (Fig. 5A, lane 3): the A10 fragment disappeared, and three more slowly migrating major bands appeared. On the basis of this band pattern, it seemed likely that in the presence of GTP the G12 fragment was cleaved further to yield additional A10 fragment which was then used as primer. Thus, a band corresponding to the G12 fragment was not apparent, and the three bands observed contained more radioactivity than was present in the A10 fragment generated in the absence of GTP (lane 2).

To verify this conclusion, the A10 and G12 fragments were isolated from a nuclease reaction (done in the absence of GTP) and incubated in a subsequent reaction with detergent-treated virus in the absence (Fig. 5B, lanes 3 and 6) and presence (lanes 4 and 7) of GTP (*Plotch* et al. 1981). The A10 fragment was not cleaved further by incubation with the virus in the absence of GTP (lane 6). The faint bands migrating more slowly than the A10 fragment were most probably the result of a low level of G addition to the A10 fragment, due to trace amounts of GTP present in the virus. In the presence of added GTP (lane 7), one to five G residues were linked to this primer fragment, yielding a band pattern nearly identical to that seen when intact cap-labeled BMV RNA 4 was incubated with virus in the presence of GTP (lane 1). This demonstrates that an exogenously added fragment of the proper size and 3′-terminus can serve as primer directly without further modification and that consequently the utilization of an RNA fragment as a primer does not have to be directly coupled to the nuclease reaction that generates that fragment. In contrast to the A10 fragment, some of the G12 fragment was cleaved further in the absence of added GTP (lane 3), yielding the A10 fragment. In the presence of added GTP (lane 4), this cleavage was carried essentially to completion and one to five G residues were added to the resulting A10 fragment. Thus, the preference for the A10 fragment over the G12 fragment was so strong that the G12 fragment was not used directly as primer, but was first converted to the A10 fragment.

The preference for A-terminated fragments extended across different capped RNA species. Thus, the A-terminated fragments of AlMV RNA 4 and BMV RNA 4 were much more efficiently utilized for initiation (G addition) than the G-terminated fragment of globin mRNA (*Plotch* et al. 1981). Preferential utilization of the A-terminated fragments was as much as tenfold.

9 Mechanism of Priming of Influenza Viral RNA Transcription in Vitro by Capped RNAs

These results thus indicate that the priming of influenza viral RNA transcription in vitro by capped RNAs occurs as shown in Figure 6. An endonuclease associated with the transcriptase complex cleaves the capped RNA predominantly, if not entirely, at a purine residue, A or G, 10–13 nucleotides from the 5′-cap. Cleavage at a residue 14 nucleotides from the cap has been found to occur at a low level with one mRNA primer, i.e., the A14 residue of A1MV RNA 4 (*Plotch* et al. 1981). These specific cleavages require the presence of a methylated cap structure in the RNA substrate. After the specific cleavage, the transcriptase preferentially utilizes A-terminated fragments as primers to initiate transcription. Only 5′-fragments 13 nucleotides long or less (plus the cap) are apparently used to initiate transcription. Transcription is initiated by the incorporation of a G residue onto the capped primer fragment. This G incorporation is almost certainly directed by the 3′-penultimate C of the vRNA template. As a consequence of the preference for the utilization of A-terminated fragments, an AGC sequence would preferentially be generated in

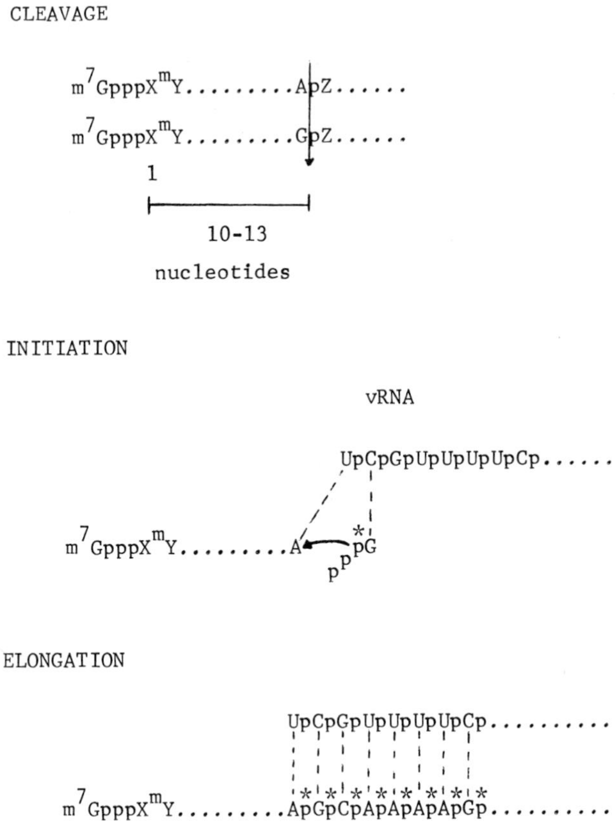

Fig. 6. Mechanism for the priming of influenza viral RNA transcription by capped RNAs

the viral mRNA, complementary to the UCG sequence at the 3'-end of the vRNA. The cleavage and initiation steps are not necessarily coupled, because an appropriate nuclease-generated fragment isolated from one reaction can without any apparent modification directly initiate transcription when added to a second reaction.

The 5'-methylated cap structure is recognized at the cleavage step of the reaction, but as discussed above it was expected that the cap is also recognized at the initiation step, where it would mediate the specific interaction with one or more transcriptase proteins that causes the stimulation of initiation. This expectation has recently been verified. The 5'-terminal A13 fragment of A1MV RNA 4 with a methylated cap structure (m^7GpppGm) was shown to act as a primer directly without prior modification, whereas the same fragment with a GpppG blocking group was inactive (*Ulmanen, Broni* and *Krug,* manuscript in preparation).

Though a specific nucleotide sequence (other than the cap) in an RNA is not required for priming activity (*Krug* et al. 1980), nucleotide sequence does play a role in determining the relative efficiency with which an RNA can prime. Because capped RNA fragments generated by cleavage at A residues initiate transcription more efficiently than fragments cleaved at G residues (*Plotch* et al. 1978), the presence of an A residue 10–13 nucleotides from the 5'-cap should enhance priming activity. In addition, reduced secondary structure was also shown to enhance priming activity (*Krug* et al. 1980). Thus, the priming activity of reovirus mRNA was increased at least three- to fivefold by bisulfite treatment or by replacement of G residues by I residues, two procedures which abolish G-C base-pairing and thereby reduce secondary structure. Diminished secondary structure in a capped RNA, especially in its 5'-terminal region, probably facilitates cleavage of these RNAs by the virion endonuclease. This may be one of the reasons that A1MV RNA 4 (after 2'-O-methylation) has been found to be the best mRNA primer for the influenza viral transcriptase so far examined (*Bouloy* et al. 1978). A similar explanation may hold for the observation that the capped, 5'-terminal, RNase T1-derived fragments of globin mRNA were actually four- to eightfold better primers on a molar basis than intact globin mRNA (*Krug* et al. 1981).

All the steps shown in Figure 6 have been shown to be carried out by purified viral cores which contain four known viral proteins (*Plotch* et al. 1981): the nucleocapsid protein (NP) (60,000 daltons) and the three P (P1, P2, P3) proteins (85–95,000 daltons) (*Rochovansky* 1976; *Inglis* et al. 1976). The NP protein, the predominant viral protein in the core, probably has primarily a structural role, as it is situated along the vRNA chains at approximately 20-nucleotide intervals (*Compans* et al. 1972). The P proteins, representing only about 8% of the total protein in cores (*Inglis* et al. 1976), are most likely the proteins which catalyze transcription. Studies with temperature-sensitive mutants of the WSN influenza A strain indicate that P1 and P3 are required for transcription and that P2 is also involved in viral RNA synthesis (*Krug* et al. 1975; *Palese* et al. 1977). One or more of the P proteins can be presumed to be the cap-dependent nuclease, and one or more the transcriptase. It will be of great interest to establish which P protein(s) carry out these functions and which also recognize methylated cap structures, and to compare this viral cap-recognizing protein(s) to the cellular cap-recognizing protein (24K protein) associated with ribosomes (*Sonenberg* et al. 1979).

10 Inhibition of Influenza Viral RNA Transcription by Uncapped RNAs

Certain uncapped RNAs and ribopolymers have been found to be potent inhibitors of influenza viral RNA transcription primed by globin (or other) mRNAs or by ApG. The same modifications (bisulfite treatment or inosine substitution) that reduced secondary structure and thus increased priming activity of capped reovirus mRNAs converted the uncapped form of these mRNAs from essentially inert species to strong inhibitors of the transcriptase reaction (*Krug* et al. 1980). In addition, one of the requirements for the inhibitory activity of uncapped ribopolymers was the absence of most hydrogen bonding in the ribopolymer. Thus, poly U and especially poly S^4U (4-thiouridylic acid), which probably has less secondary structure than poly U (*Saenger* et al. 1975), were effective inhibitors of viral RNA transcription primed by either globin mRNA (*Krug* et al. 1980) or by ApG (*Krug* et al. 1980; *Smith* et al. 1980). On the other hand, poly AU and poly CG, which have highly ordered secondary structures (*Michelson* et al. 1967), and multistranded poly A – poly U did not inhibit the transcriptase (*Krug* et al. 1981).

Reduced secondary structure by itself, however, was not sufficient for conferring inhibitory activity. Under the conditions of the transcriptase assay (neutral pH, 0.1 M KCl, 5 mM Mg^{2+}), both poly A and poly C should be free of most hydrogen bonding (*Michelson* et al. 1967), yet these two ribopolymers did not inhibit transcription (*Krug* et al. 1980). This suggests that nucleotide specificity may also be involved in inhibition. Such specificity would explain the relative inhibitory activities of poly A, poly AG, and poly G. Both poly A and poly G did not inhibit the transcriptase, whereas poly AG was a potent inhibitor, nearly as good as poly S^4U (*Krug* et al. 1980). Apparently A residues, even if they exist in polymers with little hydrogen-bonding interactions, do not contribute to the inhibitory activity of a ribopolymer, whereas G residues do. It is presumably the localized G-containing regions in poly AG [which should be free of hydrogen bonding (*Michelson* et al. 1967)] that are responsible for the inhibitory activity of this polymer. Because poly G is in the form of multistranded complexes (*Michelson* et al. 1967), its G residues would not be able to cause inhibition. The results obtained with these and other uncapped ribopolymers indicate that U, S^4U, G, and I (but not A and C) apparently contribute to the inhibitory activity of a ribopolymer when these nucleotides are not base-paired in the polymer (*Krug* et al. 1980). These nucleotides contain an oxygen or sulfur, rather than an amino, group at equivalent sites on the purine (6-position) or pyrimidine (4-position) ring.

Inhibition by these uncapped ribopolymers most likely results from their interaction with one or more proteins associated with the transcriptase complex. Poly S^4U and poly AG, the two most effective inhibitors, were found to inhibit the first step in mRNA-primed viral RNA transcription, the endonucleolytic cleavage of the capped mRNA primer (*Plotch* et al. 1981). However, the fact that these ribopolymers also inhibit viral RNA transcription primed by ApG (*Krug* et al. 1980; *Smith* et al. 1980), which does not require the action of the endonuclease, indicates that elongation of chains is also apparently inhibited. A plausible explanation for these results would be that the endonuclease and other transcriptase proteins are tightly associated in a complex so that inhibition of one component also inhibits the other components. Thus, it is not yet certain that poly S^4U and poly AG act directly on the endonuclease protein.

11 Priming by Capped Cellular RNAs Also Occurs in Vivo

Several lines of evidence indicate that influenza viral RNA transcription in the infected cell is also primed by capped cellular RNAs. If such priming occurs in vivo, then the viral mRNA synthesized in the infected cell should contain 10–13 nucleotides at its 5′-end, including the cap, which are not viral coded. This has been established. First, gel electrophoretic analysis indicated that the segments of in vivo viral mRNA, like the segments synthesized in vitro with capped RNA primers, were about 10–15 nucleotides longer at their 5′-end than the ApG-primed in vitro segments (*Krug* et al. 1979). In addition, when ^{3}H-methyl-labeled in vivo viral mRNA was hybridized to vRNA, the 5′-terminal cap structure of the mRNA was not protected against release by pancreatic or T1 RNase digestion (*Krug* et al. 1979). Because many different host capped RNAs should be capable of priming, the initial sequence at the 5′-end of in vivo viral mRNA would be expected to be heterogeneous. Consistent with such heterogeneity, two different bases, Am or Gm, were found at the 5′-penultimate position (*Krug* et al. 1976).

The expected heterogeneity has been directly demonstrated using cloned DNA copies of several of the viral segments. By employing one approach to the cloning of these segments, it was possible to show the heterogeneity at the 5′-end of the in vivo viral mRNAs simply by sequencing one end of the DNA clones. In this approach, DNA complementary to the vRNA segments and DNA complementary to the in vivo viral mRNA segments were separately synthesized using reverse transcriptase, and these two sets of single-stranded DNAs were then annealed to each other (*Lai* et al. 1980; *Caton* and *Robertson* 1980; *Beaton* and *Krug*, manuscript in preparation). The resulting double-stranded DNAs were then cloned into the plasmid pBR322. When the DNA sequences of individual clones corresponding to the 5′-end of the in vivo viral mRNA segments were determined, additional 5′-nonviral nucleotides were detected (*Dhar* et al. 1980; *Caton* and *Robertson* 1979; *Beaton* and *Krug*, manuscript in preparation) (Fig. 7). These additional nucleotides were found in the DNA clones of three different genome segments, using three different influenza virus strains and two different host-cell lines. There was no homology between these different primer sequences (even with the same segment of the same virus strain grown in the same cell), indicating that multiple different host capped RNAs were almost certainly serving as primers.

Because of the in vitro results discussed above, the length of this nonviral nucleotide sequence should be 13 or less. Actually, it would be expected that this length would usually be less then 13, because reverse transcriptase may not copy the in vivo viral mRNA segments completely (including the penultimate base in the 5′-terminal cap). With one exception, the 5′-terminal nonviral sequence was 13 nucleotides long or less. The 5′-sequence of the one exception (the HA clone-Udorn-MDCK cells) (*Dhar* et al. 1980) contains two copies of a 5-nucleotide sequence (AGCAA) complementary to the 3′-end of the vRNA, suggesting that copying errors occurred during the cloning procedure. Errors in the region of the nonviral sequence are not unexpected because the nucleotides in this sequence were unpaired in the original DNA duplex inserted into pBR322, thereby requiring faithful completion of the double strands by bacterial DNA repair enzymes.

Because the 3′-terminal U residue of the vRNA was not always represented by an A residue in the cloned DNAs, it can be concluded that transcription in vivo, like that in vitro, initiates with the G residue complementary to the 3′-penultimate C of the vRNA

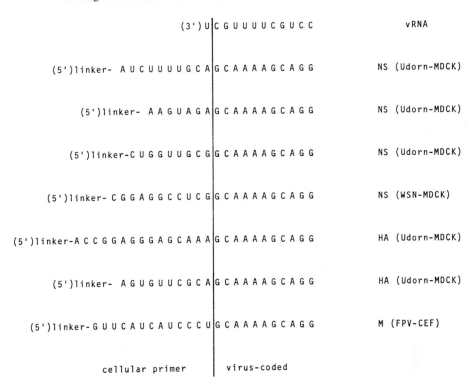

Fig. 7. Host-derived sequences at the 5'-ends of influenza viral mRNA segments determined by direct sequencing of cloned DNA copies of these segments. The cloning method is described in the text. The proteins encoded by the segments that were cloned are indicated on the right: NS (nonstructural protein), HA (hemagglutinin), M (membrane protein). The influenza A virus strain and the cell line used for the preparation of the viral mRNA are indicated in parentheses. The (Udorn-MDCK) data are from *Dhar* et al. (1980), the (FPV-CEF) data are from *Caton* and *Robertson* (1980), and the (WSN-MDCK) data are from *Beaton* and *Krug* (unpublished)

template. Four of the cloned DNAs were found to contain an A residue at the position opposite the 3'-terminal U of the vRNA, and two of the cloned DNAs contained a G at this position. The results are consistent with the demonstrated preference of the virion endonuclease for cleavage at purines and of the transcriptase for initiation with A-terminated primer fragments in vitro (*Plotch* et al. 1981). However, one of the DNA clones (M clone – FPV – CEF) was found to contain a U residue opposite the 3'-terminal U of the vRNA (*Caton* and *Robertson* 1980). Because there are no purine residues 9–13 nucleotides from the 5'-end of the cellular primer sequence for this viral mRNA segment, it can be concluded that the virion endonuclease was forced to cleave at a U residue, as must occur with the $m^7GpppGmC(U)_n$ primer in vitro (*Krug* et al. 1980). This would be expected to be an infrequent event in the infected cell, so that the primer sequence in this DNA clone is most probably not representative of the majority of the primer sequences at the ends of the in vivo viral mRNA segments.

By using an appropriate restriction fragment derived from a cloned DNA as primer for the reverse transcriptase-catalyzed extension of in vivo viral mRNA segments, it should be possible to verify the heterogeneity in the cellular primer sequences and to determine the predominant nucleotide opposite the 3'-terminal U of the vRNA. With this method, the heterogeneity in the cellular primer sequence was verified (*Lamb* and *Lai* 1980; *Caton* and *Robertson* 1980), but the data concerning the nucleotide in in vivo viral mRNA opposite the 3'-terminal U of the vRNA were unclear and conflicting. In one study (*Lamb* and *Lai* 1980), it was concluded that there was an A at this position in the mRNA segment coding for the NS_2 protein, but the sequencing gel in this region of the mRNA was very difficult to read. In another study (*Caton* and *Robertson* 1980), in which the dideoxy-chain termination method of sequencing was used, it was concluded that there was heterogeneity at this position in the mRNA segment coding for the M (membrane) protein. However, there were so many artefactual bands in this sequencing that the nucleotide sequence complementary to the common 3'-end of the vRNA could not be read.

It is important to resolve this issue in order to determine whether the specificities of the virion endonuclease and transcriptase observed in vitro also occur in vivo. It is also important because if an A residue were predominantly found at the position opposite the 3'-terminal U of the vRNA, then it would be conceivable that the same initiation step could be used for the synthesis of both viral mRNA and the full-length transcripts that are the putative templates for vRNA synthesis. The latter transcripts, which comprise only a small fraction of the total viral transcripts in the infected cell, do not have poly A at their 3'-end or a cap structure and host-derived sequence at their 5'-end (*Hay* et al. 1977a, 1980). The synthesis of these transcripts requires the synthesis of one or more virus-coded proteins (*Hay* et al. 1977a). One function of this protein(s) would be to block the termination of transcription (17–22 nucleotides from the 5'-end of vRNA) that occurs during viral mRNA synthesis (*Hay* et al. 1977b). It is not yet known how the full-length transcripts are initiated. One possibility is that the newly synthesized virus-coded protein(s) enable the transcriptase to initiate RNA synthesis without a primer at the 3'-terminal U (instead of at the 3'-penultimate C as occurs during viral mRNA synthesis). If this were the case, these transcripts would have a pppA 5'-terminus. At present, the number of phosphates at the 5'-end of the full-length transcripts is not known (*Hay* et al. 1980). The other alternative is that the same host cell RNA-primed initiation step is used for the full-length transcripts, followed by removal of the host-derived sequence by nucleolytic cleavage. Clearly, this would be feasible only if there were predominantly an A residue opposite the 3'-terminal U of the vRNA, thereby resulting in the proper AGC... sequence at the 5'-end of the full-length transcripts.

Influenza viral mRNAs synthesized in the infected cell contain approximately three m^6A (6-methyladenosine) residues per RNA chain (*Krug* et al. 1976), and one of the three m^6A residues was found to be in the 5'-terminal sequence donated by the host cell RNA primer (*Krug* et al. 1979). Thus, when ^3H-methyl-labeled in vivo viral mRNA was hybridized to vRNA, one of the three m^6A residues was not protected against pancreatic or T1 RNase digestion. It should be noted that six of the seven in vivo primer sequences which have been determined contain at least one A residue (Fig. 7), but none of these in vivo primer sequences contain GAC or AAC, the sequences in which m^6A is found in mRNAs transcribed from cellular or viral DNAs (*Wei* et al. 1976; *Wei* and *Moss* 1977; *Schibler* et al. 1977; *Dimock* and *Stoltzfus* 1977).

It is not known what function, if any, the m^6A residue in the primer sequence serves. This residue is apparently not required for priming, since mRNAs lacking m^6A (e.g.,

AlMV RNA 4) have been found to be effective primers in vitro (*Bouloy* et al. 1978, 1979, 1980). Nevertheless, m^6A could still be recognized by the viral endonuclease and/or transcriptase, thereby increasing the efficiency of priming. The source of this m^6A residue is also not yet known. One possibility is that the cellular capped RNAs used as primers already contain m^6A within the first 13 nucleotides at their 5'-ends. If so, then the influenza viral transcriptase would probably be using a specific subset of cellular mRNAs (and/or their precursors). Though m^6A residues are apparently more frequent toward the 5'-end of eukaryotic mRNAs (*Chen-Kiang* et al. 1979; *Canaani* et al. 1979), it is probably unusual for an m^6A residue to be found within the first 13 nucleotides at the 5'-end. Thus, in 16S and 19S Simian virus 40 mRNAs, two of the three m^6A residues were found in the coding region within about 400 nucleotides from the 5'-end, but little or no m^6A was found in the leader region adjacent to the 5'-cap (*Canaani* et al. 1979). An alternative possibility is that methylation of A residues in the primer region is catalyzed by a viral or cellular enzyme during or after transfer of the primer sequences. No activity capable of methylating internal A residues has so far been detected in purified virions (*Plotch* and *Krug*, unpublished experiments). It is, however, possible that such an activity is associated with transcriptase complexes in the infected cell.

12 The α-Amanitin-Sensitive Step in Influenza Virus Replication: Synthesis of Capped Cellular RNA Primers

Because priming by capped RNAs occurs in vivo as well as in vitro, the α-amanitin-sensitive step required for influenza viral RNA transcription in vivo can be presumed to be the synthesis of capped RNA primers by the host RNA polymerase II. This explanation requires that the influenza viral transcriptase in the infected cell use only newly synthesized, and not preexisting, capped cellular RNAs as primers. This has recently been shown to be the case by the demonstration that the 5'-terminal cap of the viral mRNA, which is donated by the host RNA primer, is synthesized only after and not before infection. Thus, cap structures pulse-labeled after infection with ^3H-methyl methionine, but not those labeled (for long periods) before infection, were found to be incorporated into influenza viral mRNA (*Herz* and *Krug*, manuscript in preparation).

Why should only newly synthesized capped cellular RNAs serve as primers? One possibility is that preexisting capped cellular RNAs are tied up in ribonucleoprotein structures (including polyribosomes) and as a consequence cannot be used by the viral transcriptase. If so, the viral transcriptase would be expected to function near the site of synthesis of capped cellular RNAs in the nucleus. Several lines of evidence are consistent with viral RNA transcription being in the nucleus. Cellular and viral mRNAs synthesized in the nucleus (using DNA templates) contain m^6A (*Desrosiers* et al. 1975; *Furuichi* et al. 1975a; *Lavi* and *Shatkin* 1975; *Perry* et al. 1975; *Moss* and *Koczot* 1976; *Wei* et al. 1976; *Beemon* and *Keith* 1977), whereas the mRNAs of cytoplasmic viruses, including vaccinia virus which contains DNA, lack m^6A (*Wei* and *Moss* 1975; *Furuichi* et al. 1975b; *Abraham* et al. 1975). Consequently, the fact that m^6A residues have been found in internal positions of influenza viral mRNA argues that viral RNA transcription has a nuclear phase. In addition, recent evidence strongly suggests that the two mRNAs specified by the smallest vRNA segment are related to each other by a splicing event, consistent with nuclear transcription (*Lamb* and *Lai* 1980). Finally, experiments measuring the steady state level of viral RNA transcription were interpreted as indicating that the nucleus was the site of at least primary transcription (*Mark* et al. 1979; *Barrett* et al. 1979), the transcription catalyzed by the inoculum transcriptase.

In order to establish the cellular site(s) of viral RNA transcription, the author and his colleagues have devised a new assay for the amount of newly synthesized, or pulse-labeled, viral RNA transcripts in the infected cell (*Herz, Stavnezer* and *Krug*, manuscript in preparation). In this assay, vRNA is covalently linked to small pieces of filter paper, and pulse-labeled infected cell RNA is annealed to the vRNA on these filters. After an extensive washing procedure, pulse-labeled influenza viral RNA transcripts free of labeled cellular RNAs can be quantitated. An important advantage of this assay is that it detects not only intact chains of completed viral RNA transcripts [as detected in the most widely used assay (*Hay* et al. 1977a)], but also nascent transcripts and completed transcripts that may be nicked during cellular fractionation and RNA extraction. Employing this assay and both aqueous and nonaqueous procedures for fractionating cells into nucleus and cytoplasm, it should be possible to establish the cellular site(s) of viral RNA transcription.

13 Possible Implications for Cellular Transcription

The presently available data concerning the transcription of DNA templates (both cellular and viral) make it unlikely that this transcription is initiated by capped RNA primers as occurs in influenza viral RNA transcription (for example, see review by *Ziff* 1980). However, certain features of the reactions catalyzed by influenza viral enzymes may have cellular counterparts. For example, though a cap-dependent endonuclease such as found in influenza virions has not been described in any other viral or cellular system, it is reasonable to ask whether a similar activity can be expected to be found in other systems.

Several possibilities can be suggested. For example, cap recognition may be critical for the step in the processing of heterogeneous nuclear RNA in which the RNA is cleaved near its 5'-terminus to produce fragments (albeit longer than those generated by the influenza virion enzyme) which are subsequently ligated onto 3'-distal regions of the transcript (*Darnell* 1978). With regard to this possibility, it may be significant that an m^6A residue is found in the 5'-terminal sequence of in vivo influenza viral mRNA derived from capped RNA primers, as it has been speculated that m^6A residues may constitute recognition sites for RNA processing or splicing enzymes (*Canaani* et al. 1979; *Chen-Kiang* et al. 1979). Another possible role for a cap-dependent cellular endonuclease may be in mRNA turnover. Since the cap makes mRNAs more resistant to cellular nucleases (*Furuichi* et al. 1977a; *Shimotohno* et al. 1977), the initial removal of the capped 5'-end of an mRNA by a cap-dependent endonuclease would facilitate subsequent RNA degradation. Recent evidence suggests that mRNA turnover may be important in the regulation of the expression of some genes in eukaryotes (*Nevins* and *Winkler* 1980).

If, however, a cap-recognizing endonuclease were found to be unique to influenza virions, then it might be an ideal target for specific antiinfluenza virus drugs, possibly related to the uncapped ribopolymer inhibitors described above. Further investigation of the mechanism of action of this nuclease would therefore be quite useful in facilitating the development of these drugs.

Acknowledgements. The research in the author's laboratory was supported by U.S. Public Health Service Grants CA 08748 and AI 11772.

References

Abraham G, Rhodes DP, Banerjee AK (1975) The 5′ terminal structure of the methylated mRNA synthesized in vitro by vesicular stomatitis virus. Cell 5:51–58

Baralle FE (1977) Structure-function relationship of 5′ non-coding sequence of rabbit α- and β-globin mRNA. Nature 267:279–281

Barrett J, Wolstenholme AJ, Mahy BWJ (1979) Transcription and replication of influenza virus RNA. Virology 98:211–225

Barry RD, Ives DR, Cruickshank JG (1962) Participation of deoxyribonucleic acid in the multiplication of influenza virus. Nature 194:1139–1140

Beemon K, Keith J (1977) Localization of N^6-methyladenosine in the Rous sarcoma virus genome. J Mol Biol 113:165–179

Bishop DHL, Obijeski JF, Simpson RW (1971) Transcription of the influenza ribonucleic acid genome by a virion polymerase. I. Optimal conditions for in vitro activity of the ribonucleic acid dependent ribonucleic acid polymerase. J Virol 8:66–73

Bouloy M, Plotch SJ, Krug RM (1978) Globin mRNAs are primers for the transcription of influenza viral RNA in vitro. Proc Natl Acad Sci USA 75:4886–4890

Bouloy M, Morgan MA, Shatkin AJ, Krug RM (1979) Cap and internal nucleotides of reovirus mRNA primers are incorporated into influenza viral complementary RNA during transcription in vitro. J Virol 32:895–904

Bouloy M, Plotch SJ, Krug RM (1980) Both the 7-methyl and 2′O-methyl groups in the cap of a mRNA strongly influence its ability to act as a primer for influenza viral RNA transcription. Proc Natl Acad Sci USA 77:3592–3596

Canaani D, Kahana C, Lavi S, Groner Y (1979) Identification N^6-methyladenosine containing sequences in Simian Virus 40 RNA. Nucleic Acid Res 6:2879–2899

Caton AJ, Robertson JS (1980) Structure of the host-derived sequences present at the 5′ ends of influenza virus mRNA. Nucleic Acid Res 8:2591–2603

Chen-Kiang S, Nevins JR, Darnell JE (1979) N-6-Methyladenosine in adenovirus type 2 nuclear RNA is conserved in the formation of messenger RNA. J Mol Biol 135:733–752

Chow NL, Simpson RW (1971) RNA-dependent RNA polymerase activity associated with virions and subviral particles of myxoviruses. Proc Natl Acad Sci USA 68:752–756

Compans RW, Content J, Duesberg PH (1972) Structure of the ribonucleoprotein of influenza virus. J Virology 10:795–800

Darnell JE Jr (1978) Implications of RNA-RNA splicing in evolution of eukaryotic cells. Science 202:1257–1260

Dasgupta R, Shih DS, Saris C, Kaesberg P (1975) Nucleotide sequence of a viral RNA fragment that binds to eukaryotic ribosomes. Nature 256:624–628

Desrosiers RC, Friderici KH, Rottman FM (1975) Characterization of Novikoff hepatoma mRNA methylation and heterogeneity in the methylated 5′-terminus. Biochemistry 14:4367–4374

Dhar R, Chanock RM, Lai C-J (1980) Non-viral oligonucleotides at the 5′ terminus of cytoplasmic influenza viral mRNa deduced from cloned complete genomic sequences. Cell 21:495–500

Dimock K, Stoltzfus CM (1977) Sequence specificity of internal methylation in B77 avian sarcoma virus RNA subunits. Biochemistry 16:471–478

Furuichi Y, Morgan M, Shatkin AJ, Jelinek W, Salditt-Georgieff M, Darnell JE (1975a) Methylated blocked 5′-termini in HeLa cell mRNA. Proc Natl Acad Sci USA 72:1904–1908

Furuichi Y, Morgan M, Muthukrishnan S, Shatkin AJ (1975b) Reovirus messenger RNA contains a methylated, blocked 5′-terminal structure: $m^7G(5′)pppGmpCp$. Proc Natl Acad Sci USA 72:362–366

Furuichi Y, Muthukrishnan S, Tomasz J, Shatkin AJ (1976) Mechanism of formation of reovirus mRNA 5′-terminal blocked and methylated sequence, m^7GpppG^mpC. J Biol Chem 251:5043–5053

Furuichi Y, La Fiandra A, Shatkin AJ (1977) 5′ terminal structure and mRNA stability. Nature 266:235–239

Hay AJ, Lomniczi B, Bellamy AR, Skehel JJ (1977a) Transcription of the influenza virus genome. Virology 83:337–355

Hay AJ, Abraham G, Skehel JJ, Smith JC, Fellner P (1977b) Influenza virus messenger RNAs are incomplete transcripts of the genome RNAs. Nucleic Acid Res 4:4197–4209

Hay AJ, Skehel JJ, McCauley J (1980) Structure and synthesis of influenza virus complementary RNAs. Philos Trans R Soc Lond [Biol] 288:341–348

Inglis SC, Carroll AR, Lamb RA, Mahy BWJ (1976) Polypeptides specified by the influenza virus genome. I. Evidence for eight distinct gene products specified by fowl plague virus. Virology 74:489–503

Koper-Zwarthoff EC, Lockard RE, Alzener-Deweerd B, RajBhandary UL, Bol JF (1977) Nucleotide sequence of 5′-terminus of alfalfa mosaic virus RNA 4 leading into coat protein cistron. Proc Natl Acad Sci USA 74:5504–5508

Krug RM, Ueda M, Palese P (1975) Temperature-sensitive mutants of influenza WSN virus defective in virus-specific RNA synthesis. J Virology 16:790–796

Krug RM, Morgan MM, Shatkin AJ (1976) Influenza viral messenger RNA contains internal N^6-methyladenosine and 5′-terminal 7-methyl guanosine in cap structures. J Virology 20:45–53

Krug RM, Broni BB, Bouloy M (1979) Are the 5′ ends of influenza viral mRNAs synthesized in vivo donated by host mRNAs? Cell 18:329–334

Krug RM, Broni BA, LaFiandra AJ, Morgan MA, Shatkin AJ (1980) Priming and inhibitory activities of RNAs for the influenza viral transcriptase do not require base-pairing with the virion RNA template. Proc Natl Acad Sci USA 77:5874–5878

Krug RM, Plotch SJ, Ulmanen I, Herz C, Bouloy M (1981) The mechanism of initiation of influenza viral RNA transcription by capped RNA primers. In: Compans R, Bishop DHL (eds) Negative strand viruses. Elsevier/North Holland, (in press)

Lai C-J, Markoff LF, Zimmerman S, Cohen B, Berndt JA, Chanock RM (1980) Cloning DNA sequences from influenza viral RNA segments. Proc Natl Acad Sci USA 77:210–214

Lamb RA, Choppin PW (1977) Synthesis of influenza virus polypeptides in cells resistant to alpha-amanitin: evidence for the involvement of cellular RNA polymerase II in virus replication. J Virol 23:816–819

Lamb RA, Lai C-J (1980) Sequence of interrupted and uninterrupted mRNAs and cloned full-length DNA coding for the two overlapping nonstructural proteins of influenza virus. Cell 21:475–485

Lavi S, Shatkin AJ (1975) Methylated simian virus 40-specific RNA from nuclei and cytoplasm of infected BSC-1 cells. Proc Natl Acad Sci USA 72:2012–2016

Lockard RE, RajBhandary UL (1976) Nucleotide sequences at the 5′-terminal of rabbit and globin mRNA. Cell 9:747–760

Mahy BWJ, Hastie ND, Armstrong SJ (1972) Inhibition of influenza virus replication by α-amanitin: mode of action. Proc Natl Acad Sci USA 69:1421–1424

Mark GE, Taylor JM, Broni B, Krug RM (1979) Nuclear accumulation of influenza viral RNA transcripts and the effects of cycloheximide, actinomycin D, and α-amanitin. J Virol 29:744–752

Martin SA, Moss B (1976) mRNA guanylyltransferase and mRNA (guanine-7)-methyltransferase from vaccinia virions. J Biol Chem 251:7313–7321

McGeoch D, Kitron N (1975) Influenza virion RNA-dependent RNA polymerase: stimulation by guanosine and related compounds. J Virol 15:686–695

Michelson AM, Massoulie J, Guschlbauer W (1967) Synthetic polynucleotides. Prog Nucleic Acid Res Mol Biol 6:83–141

Moss B, Koczot F (1976) Sequence of methylated nucleotides at the 5′ terminus of adenovirus-specific RNA. Virol 17:385–392

Moss B, Gershowitz A, Wei C-M, Boone R (1976) Formation of the guanylylated and methylated 5′-terminus of vaccinia virus mRNA. Virology 75:341–351

Muthukrishnan S, Morgan M, Banerjee AK, Shatkin AJ (1976) Influence of 5′ terminal m^7G and 2′-O-methylated residues on messenger ribonucleic acid binding to ribosomes. Biochemistry 15:5761–5768

Muthukrishnan S, Moss B, Cooper JA, Maxwell ES (1978) Influence of 5′-terminal cap structure on the initiation of translation of vaccinia virus mRNA. J Biol Chem 253:1710–1715

Nevins JR, Winkler JJ (1980) Regulation of early adenovirus transcription: A protein product of early region 2 specifically represses region 4 transcription. Proc Natl Acad Sci USA 77:1893–1897

Palese P, Ritchey MB, Schulman JL (1977) P1 and P3 proteins of influenza virus are required for complementary RNA synthesis. J Virol 21:1187–1195

Penhoet E, Miller H, Doyle M, Blatti S (1971) RNA-dependent RNA polymerase activity in influenza virions. Proc Natl Acad Sci USA 68:1369–1371

Perry RP, Kelley DE, Friderici K, Rottman F (1975) The methylated constituents of L-cell messenger RNA: evidence for an unusual cluster at the 5′ terminus. Cell 4:387–394

Plotch SJ, Krug RM (1977) Influenza virion transcriptase: the synthesis in vitro of large, poly-adenylic acid-containing complementary RNA. J Virol 21:24–34

Plotch SJ, Krug RM (1978) Segments of influenza virus complementary RNA synthesized in vitro. J Virol 25:579–586

Plotch SJ, Tomasz J, Krug RM (1978) Absence of detectable capping and methylating enzymes in influenza virions. J Virol 28:75–83

Plotch SJ, Bouloy M, Krug RM (1979) Transfer of 5′ terminal cap of globin mRNA to influenza viral complementary RNA during transcription in vitro. Proc Natl Acad Sci USA 76:1618–1622

Plotch SJ, Bouloy M, Ulmanen I, Krug RM (1981) A unique cap (m^{7}GpppXm)-dependent influenza virion endonuclease cleaves capped RNAs to generate the primers that initiate viral RNA transcription. Cell 23:847–858

Robertson HD, Dickson E, Plotch SJ, Krug RM (1980) Identification of the RNA region trans-ferred from a representative primer, β-globin mRNA, to influenza mRNA during in vitro transcription. Nucleic Acid Res 8:925–942

Robertson JS (1979) 5′ and 3′ terminal nucleotide sequences of the RNA genome segments of influenza virus. Nucleic Acid Res 6:3745–3757

Rochovansky O (1976) RNA synthesis by ribonucleoprotein-polymerase complexes isolated from influenza virus. Virology 73:327–338

Rott R, Scholtissek C (1970) Specific inhibition of influenza replication by α-amanitin. Nature 228:56

Saenger W, Mazumdar SK, Suck D, Manor PC (1975) Parallel and antiparallel homopolymer nucleic acid double helices. In: Sundaralingam M, Rao SJ (eds) Structure and conformation of nucleic acids and protein-nucleic acid interactions. University Park Press, Baltimore, pp 537–555

Schibler U, Kelley DE, Perry RP (1977) Comparison of methylated sequences in messenger RNA and heterogeneous nuclear RNA from mouse L cells. J Mol Biol 115:695–714

Shatkin AJ (1976) Capping of eukaryotic mRNA's. Cell 9:645–653

Shih DS, Kaesberg P (1973) Translation of brome mosaic viral ribonucleic acid in a cell-free system derived from wheat embryo. Proc Natl Acad Sci USA 70:1799–1803

Shimotohno K, Kodama Y, Hashimoto J, Miura K (1977) Importance of 5′-terminal blocking structure to stabilize mRNA in eukaryotic protein synthesis. Proc Natl Acad Sci USA 74:2734–2738

Skehel JJ, Hay AJ (1978) Nucleotide sequences at the 5′ termini of influenza viral RNAs and their transcripts. Nucleic Acids Res 4:1207–1219

Smith JC, Raper RH, Bell LD, Stebbing N, McGeoch D (1980) Inhibition of influenza virion transcriptases by polynucleotides. Virology 103:245–249

Sonenberg N, Rupprecht K, Hecht S, Shatkin AJ (1979) Eukaryotic mRNA cap binding protein: purification by affinity chromatography on Sepharose-coupled m^{7}GDP. Proc Natl Acad Sci USA 76:4345–4349

Spooner LLR, Barry RD (1977) Participation of DNA-dependent RNA polymerase II in replica-tion of influenza viruses. Nature 268:650–652

Wei C-M, Moss B (1975) Methylated nucleosides block 5′ terminus of vaccinia messenger RNA. Proc Natl Acad Sci USA 72:318–322

Wei C-M, Moss B (1977) Nucleotide sequence at the N^6-methyladenosine sites of HeLa cell messenger ribonucleic acid. Biochemistry 16:1672–1676

Wei C-M, Gershowitz A, Moss B (1976) 5′-terminal and internal methylated nucleotide sequen-ces in HeLa cell mRNA. Biochemistry 15:397–401

Ziff EB (1980) Transcription and RNA processing by the DNA tumour viruses. Nature 287:491–499

Origin and Replication of Defective Interfering Particles

Jacques Perrault*

1	Introduction	152
2	General Aspects of Defective Interfering (DI) Particles	153
2.1	Ubiquity of DI in RNA Viruses	153
2.2	Biological and Structural Properties	154
2.3	Role of DI in RNA Virus Persistence	155
3	Genome Rearrangements in DI RNAs	155
3.1	Overview	155
3.2	Vesicular Stomatitis Virus (VSV) DI RNAs	157
3.2.1	General Properties and Types of Molecules	157
3.2.2	Terminal Sequence Complementarity	159
3.2.3	Snap-Back Hairpin Molecules	159
3.2.4	Internal Genome Deletions	161
3.3	Other Negative-Strand Viruses	163
3.3.1	Sendai	163
3.3.2	Influenza	163
3.4	Positive-Strand Viruses	165
3.4.1	Togaviruses	165
3.4.2	Picornaviruses	168
3.5	Double-Strand Viruses	169
4	Origin of DI RNAs	170
4.1	Host Cell Effects on the Generation of DI RNAs	170
4.2	The Unlikely Provirus Hypothesis	173
4.3	Purposeful Error-Prone Virus Polymerase	174
4.3.1	Terminal Sequence Complementarity and the Copy-Back Model	174
4.3.2	Genesis of Internal Deletions and Complex Genome Rearrangements	177
4.3.3	General Model	178
5	Replication and Interfering Properties of DI RNAs	181
5.1	Host Cell Modulation	181
5.2	Transcriptional and Translational Activities of DI RNAs	182
5.3	Conserved Replication and Encapsidation Origins	185
5.4	Interference Mechanisms of VSV DI	187
5.4.1	Replicase Competition and Terminal Sequence Complementarity	187
5.4.2	Additional Parameters Affecting VSV DI Interference	190
5.5	Interference Mechanisms of Other RNA Virus DI	192
6	DI of DNA Viruses – Brief Overview	194
7	Concluding Remarks	195
References		196

* Department of Microbiology and Immunology, Washington University School of Medicine, St. Louis, Missouri 63110, USA

1 Introduction

Defective interfering virus (DI) particles represent a major controlling element of virus replication. They are constantly generated at low levels by infectious virus and only amplify to interfering levels when the parent helper virus is abundant. This autointerference phenomenon, as it was called when first discovered, is achieved by rearrangements and deletions of the standard virus genome such that the resulting "incomplete form" of the virus can preferentially replicate.

Studies on all aspects of DI have greatly expanded in the last decade. This interest stems not only from their characteristic attenuating properties but from their role in the establishment and maintenance of persistent viral infections. I shall limit myself in this review mostly to a discussion of recent findings regarding DI of RNA viruses. At the present time much less is known about the properties and biological importance of DI of DNA viruses (see review by *Huang* and *Baltimore* 1977) and except for a brief overview of their current status (Section 6) they will not be discussed in detail.

It is generally agreed that RNA viruses (with the exception of retroviruses) lack the ability to integrate double-stranded DNA copies or fragments of their genome into eucaryotic host cell chromosomes (see discussion Section 4.2). RNA viruses may therefore rely on alternative mechanisms of attenuation, such as DI, to achieve long term virus-host cell association. An additional important facet of these DI is that their generation apparently involves recombination directly at the RNA level. The relationship, if any, between this type of genomic rearrangement and other recombinational events in RNA viruses is of obvious importance. Furthermore, the possible mechanistic and/or evolutionary relationship between RNA recombination in viruses and gene splicing in eucaryotic mRNAs is intriguing.

This review will first introduce the reader to general aspects of DI structure and function, followed by a detailed survey of our current information regarding genome sequence rearrangements in DI of RNA viruses. The remainder of the article will attempt to integrate this information within a framework of hypotheses and models to account for the origin and preferential replication of DI RNAs. We will omit from discussion the retroviruses and the plant RNA viruses because of difficulties in defining DI operationally in these groups. Multiple interactions between endogenous and exogenous, defective, and nondefective retroviruses often obscure a straightforward DI phenomenon, although some reports lend support to such a concept (*Huang* and *Baltimore* 1977; *Estis* and *Temin* 1979; *Canaani* and *Aaronson* 1980). Plant RNA viruses on the other hand are often multipartite systems with two or three distinct particles, all of which are necessary for infectivity. In addition, until the recent advent of protoplast cultures, simple direct tests of interference by purified particles in synchronously infected cells have been impossible. Nevertheless, some reports of defective plant viruses are consistent with their being called DI (see *Huang* 1973; *Atabekov* 1977) and future studies may well uncover a more common occurrence.

Several reviews on the subject of DI have been published in recent years. For a general comprehensive description of DI (both RNA and DNA) and their properties the reader is referred to *Huang* and *Baltimore* (1977). The more recent review of *Holland* et al. (1980) discusses both the structure and biological properties of DI and focuses on their role in virus persistence. Detailed reviews of DI in particular virus groups have also appeared: poliovirus, *Cole* (1975); rhabdoviruses, *Reichmann* and *Schnitzlein* (1979); togaviruses, *Stollar* (1979, 1980); arenaviruses, *Pedersen* (1979); influenza, *Nayak* (1980); and virus-like particles of yeast (*Bruenn* 1980). Short review articles on selected properties of vesicular stomatitis virus (VSV) DI are also included in the CRC volume series on Rhabdoviruses (*Faulkner* and *Lazzarini* 1980; *Reichmann* and *Schnitzlein* 1980; *Kang* 1980).

2 General Aspects of Defective Interfering (DI) Particles

2.1 Ubiquity of DI in RNA Viruses

Table 1 presents an updated list of RNA viruses reported to generate DI. It is obvious from this table that all serious attempts to generate DI in any RNA virus group

Table 1. Occurrence of DI in RNA Viruses

Virus group	Member name	References[a]
Negative strand		
Rhabdo	Vesicular stomatitis, rabies, bovine ephemeral fever, others	*Reichmann* and *Schniztlein* (1979)
Paramyxo	Sendai	*Kolakofsky* (1979)
	Newcastle disease	*Roman* and *Simon* (1976)
	Measles	*Rima* et al. (1977)
	Mumps	*Norval* (1979)
Orthomyxo	Influenza, fowl plague	*Nayak* (1980)
Arena	Lymphocytic choriomeningitis, Amapari, Parana, Pichinde	*Pedersen* (1979)
	Tacaribe	*Gimenez* and *Compans* (1980)
Bunya	Bunyamvera	*Kascsak* and *Lyon* (1978)
	LaCrosse	*Bishop* and *Shope* (1979)
	Turlock	*Schnurr* and *Hardy* (1980)
Positive strand		
Picorna	Poliovirus	*Lundquist* et al. (1979)
	Mengovirus	*McClure* et al. (1980)
Calici	Feline calicivirus	*Schaffer* (1979)
Toga	Sindbis, Semliki Forest, West Nile	*Stollar* (1979)
	Japanese encephalitis	*Schmaljohn* and *Blair* (1977)
Corona	Mouse hepatitis	*Robb* and *Bond* (1979)
Double strand		
Reo	Reovirus	*Ahmed* and *Fields* (1981)
Orbi	Bluetongue virus of sheep	*Verwoerd* et al. (1979)
Fungal	Yeast-killer, others	*Bruenn* (1980)
Other	Infectious pancreatic necrosis virus	*MacDonald* and *Yamamoto* (1978)

[a] The references listed are either recent review articles or publications wherein earlier work on the particular DI is described. For a list of the earliest reports describing DI in various virusgroups the reader is referred to *Huang* and *Baltimore* (1977)

(retroviruses not considered) have so far been successful. No exceptions have yet been reported and it therefore appears to be a general rule.

The methods employed for detecting and purifying DI have been reviewed recently (*Huang* and *Baltimore* 1977) and will not be detailed here. In general, biological cloning of a virus leads to the disappearance of most or all DI in a given working stock. During passage at high multiplicities of infection any newly arising or preexisting DI particle replicates because of complementation by helper virus. The population of virions eventually becomes mostly DI because the latter replicate preferentially and inhibit the growth of the standard virus.

The ease with which DI are produced varies widely in different virus groups. For example, high titer cloned stocks of VSV and influenza virus can produce large amounts of DI in as little as two or three undiluted passages. In contrast, at least 20 or so serial passages are needed to detect significant amounts of poliovirus DI. There is no simple way to predict the ease with which a particular RNA virus will produce DI since many different factors are involved. These include growth conditions, multiplicities of infection, the host cell, relative rates of standard virus replication and DI enrichment, virus strain differences, and intrinsic rates of DI generation.

2.2 Biological and Structural Properties

As defined by *Huang* and *Baltimore* (1970, 1977) the criteria for the definition of DI are as follows: 1. Antigenic similarity to standard virus, 2. requirement for homologous parent virus as helper for replication, 3. preferential replication of DI over standard virus (also called enrichment), and 4. interference with the replication of the standard virus. So far, all DI examined critically contain deletions in a part of the genome essential for infectivity. However, as pointed out before (*Huang* and *Baltimore* 1977) it is possible to imagine point mutations which might fall within the limits of these criteria.

The structural similarity between standard virus and DI extends to overall shape and size in viruses with icosahedral symmetry such as picornaviruses and reoviruses. In most of these cases, DI contain less total RNA than the parent virus and can sometimes be separated by density gradient centrifugation. In VSV and other rhabdoviruses, the length of the particle RNA governs the overall size of the bullet-shaped viruses, and since DI contain shorter RNAs they are easily separated by size from the standard virus. In more pleiomorphic viruses, such as influenza and measles virus, DI tend to be smaller than the standard particle but the variability in size of the virion population as a whole makes it difficult to achieve clean separation (for a discussion of DI sizes and sedimentation properties, see *Huang* and *Baltimore* 1977).

In general, the requirement for helper virus as well as interfering activity is limited to the homologous parent or to serologically related strains. The nature of the helper function supplied by the standard virus varies in different virus systems. For example, the VSV standard virus almost always provides all five virus-coded proteins for replication and encapsidation of a DI RNA template which does not code for any translation products. In poliovirus, however, the standard virus helper, at least in some cases, provides the missing capsid proteins to a DI RNA which gives rise to all other virus translation products (see Section 5.2). The enrichment and interfering properties of DI also vary in different virus systems, but these are subject to important modulations by the host cell. These effects are described in more detail below (Sections 4.1 and 5.1).

Since DI are not antigenically distinct from their parent virus, their biological properties are attributable to the genome deletions they contain. DI interference with standard
genome replication is an intracellular phenomenon occurring after virus penetration but
generally early during the growth cycle. It is not mediated by interferon or other host-cell
coded products, and is distinct from the heterologous type of interference often observed
when two different viruses infect the same host cell. There is no evidence, so far, indicating that an aberrant virus-coded translation product is reponsible for the interfering or
preferential replication properties of DI. In the best studied systems, it appears that some
property of the DI template RNA itself leads to an altered interaction with the polymerase activities replicating the viral polynucleotides.

2.3 Role of DI in RNA Virus Persistence

This topic which has recently been reviewed in detail (*Holland* et al. 1980) is briefly discussed here because it underlines the importance of understanding the mode of action of
DI. The pioneering studies of *Holland* and *Villarreal* (1974) provided the first clear
evidence for a DI requirement in establishing stable VSV carrier cell cultures in vitro.
Since then, *Holland* and colleagues, as well as many other laboratories, employing
several different RNA viruses, have also shown a requirement for DI in the establishment and/or maintenance of persistent infections in cell culture. Other factors, such as
interferon and ts virus mutants, are also likely to play a role but it is clear that the attenuating properties of DI, either alone or in conjunction with these other factors, allow host
cells to survive an otherwise cytocidal infection.

Two important facts regarding DI and virus persistence need be mentioned here.
First, the overall structure and apparent biological activity of DI recovered from persistently infected cell cultures or animals appear very similar if not identical to DI generated
by high multiplicity passages in permissive cell lines (*Holland* et al. 1980). Second, DI
appear to act as a selection pressure for rapid and extensive mutational drift of standard
virus during long term persistence (*Holland* et al. 1979; *Wechsler* et al. 1979). This is exemplified by the rapid emergence of standard virus mutants which are no longer subject to
interference by DI originally employed to establish a persistently infected culture. The
new standard virus, however, is still capable of generating new DI which interfere with its
own growth (see Section 5.4.2). This important phenomenon has now been observed in
several different virus systems: rabies virus (*Kawai* and *Matsumoto* 1977); lymphocytic
choriomeningitis virus (*Jacobson* et al. 1979); VSV (*Horodyski* and *Holland* 1980); Sindbis
virus (*Weiss* and *Schlesinger* 1981); and, at least in part, the "killer" virus-like particles of
yeast (*Kane* et al. 1979; *Bruenn* and *Brennan* 1980). This selective effect of DI on the evolution of RNA viruses in culture may yet harbor an even more important role for these particles in nature.

3 Genome Rearrangements in DI RNAs

3.1 Overview

Single-strand RNA viruses of animals are classified as positive-strand if the encapsidated
RNA molecule is infectious by itself, i.e., corresponds to a functional mRNA molecule.

Negative-strand viruses on the other hand carry the opposite strand, and are strictly dependent on viral transcriptase enzymes packaged within the virions to initiate the infectious cycle (*Baltimore* 1971). Similarly, double-stranded RNA viruses also depend on a particle-bound transcriptase for infectivity (*Shatkin* and *Sipe* 1968).

Many of our current concepts regarding the origin and replication of DI are derived from the VSV system which has been studied in most detail. This rhabdovirus serves as a model for negative-strand viruses in general, and in particular for paramyxoviruses which employ a very similar if not identical strategy for replication. DI of the paramyxovirus Sendai closely resemble VSV DI in their genome structure (see below). No details of genomic sequence rearrangements in DI are known for other important rhabdoviruses, such as rabies or paramyxoviruses, or for measles, mumps, and Newcastle disease virus.

The only other negative-strand virus group where DI have been characterized in some detail at the molecular level is the orthomyxovirus (influenza) group. Current cloning and sequencing studies of the eight virion RNA segments of the influenza genome are paving the way for rapid progress in the characterization of DI RNAs generated in this group.

Biological studies of arenavirus DI have been carried out for more than a decade but little is yet known about the nature of genome sequences in their RNAs (the standard genome consists of two viral RNA segments). This virus group shows a propensity for establishing persistent infections both in cell culture and in the animal. Lymphocytic choriomeningitis virus (LCM) causes life long infections in mice, and evidence for DI involvement in this natural disease, as well as in persistently infected cell cultures, is strong (reviewed by *Pederson* 1979, and *Holland* et al. 1980).

The remaining negative-strand virus group is a relatively newly defined and large family of arboviruses, the Bunyaviruses, and again detailed characterization of DI RNA species is lacking (the standard genome consists of three segments). An important aspect of this group (also shared by most togaviruses and some rhabdoviruses and reoviruses) is the ability to grow both in vertebrate and invertebrate host cells. The possible role of DI in the natural transmission cycle of arboviruses is yet to be explored.

In the positive-strand RNA virus groups, both togavirus and picornavirus DI have been studied in some detail. Except for one preliminary report (see Table 1) on the occurrence of DI in the newly defined caliciviruses, nothing else is known regarding DI in this group. The remaining positive-strand virus family, the coronaviruses, are just beginning to attract the attention of molecular virologists and no definitive identification of DI have yet been reported.

Among the double-strand RNA viruses, the best studied DI system is the yeast killer virus (see review by *Bruenn* 1980), although the realization that these viruses generate DI has only surfaced recently (Table 1). Reovirus DI were discovered relatively early but they have not been characterized extensively. The salmonid infectious pancreatic necrosis virus (IPNV), which contains two double-strand RNA segments, is also known to generate DI RNAs which have not been characterized at the molecular level. In both reovirus and IPNV, DI do appear to be involved in persistence (*Holland* et al. 1980; *MacDonald* and *Kennedy* 1979).

3.2 Vesicular Stomatitis Virus (VSV) DI RNAs

3.2.1 General Properties and Types of Molecules

Several laboratories have contributed to determining the size, cistronic origin, and structure of VSV DI RNAs. I will mention here the main conclusions from these earlier studies (for details, see review by *Reichmann* and *Schnitzlein* 1979) and discuss the more recent work on the recombinant sites in these DI RNAs.

VSV DI RNAs range from approximately 10 to 60% of the standard VSV genome size which is about 11 kb long. Each DI particle RNA is packaged as a single molecule within a helical ribonucleoprotein the length of which is determined by the size of the RNA. This structural feature, as mentioned before, is responsible for the ease with which the shorter truncated particles can be purified free from standard virus. In general, a given clonal isolate of standard virus gives rise to one or a few major DI species after a few passages at high multiplicities of infection. A DI band of a particular size can be isolated directly from a sucrose velocity sedimentation gradient, and amplified in a second cycle of infection with DI-free standard virus.

A large number of independently isolated VSV DI have been studied in various laboratories over the last decade. A uniform system of nomenclature has recently been proposed to clarify the relationship between the different isolates (*Reichmann* et al. 1980). As a result, VSV DI previously known by names such as tsG31 ST (ts = temperature sensitive, G = Glasgow isolate of Indiana VSV strain, 31 = mutant number designation of group III complementation group, ST = short truncated or T particle) have now been renamed VSI tsG31 *DI 0.10* (5′, 65%), where VSI stands for VSV Indiana strain, tsG31 as above, *0.10* for the fractional length of the DI RNA molecule in comparison to the standard genome, and (5′, 65%) for derivation from the 5′-end of the genome and percentage level of self-annealing. This system has not yet been adopted widely, and may in some cases lead to confusion (such as more than one new designation for the same isolate passed on to different laboratories). To avoid ambiguity in this review, I will refer to particular isolates by both old and new names (if the latter is already in use in the literature) and point out particular situations where uncertainties exist.

In contrast to standard virus, VSV DI sometimes package mixtures of minus- and plus-strand polarity RNAs (*Roy* et al. 1973; *Perrault* and *Leavitt* 1977a). The minus strands are apparently always in excess except in the case of the so-called snap-back DI RNAs where the plus and minus strands are covalently-linked as a hairpin molecule (*Lazzarini* et al. 1975; *Perrault* 1976; *Perrault* and *Leavitt* 1977a). Why VSV DI sometimes package some plus strands in addition to minus strands is not entirely clear but it is likely to be related to the structural features at the ends of their RNAs (see Section 3.2.2).

All VSV DI RNAs examined so far contain virus-coded nucleotide sequences only. At least five different structural types of molecules have been reported to date (Fig. 1). In addition, these fall into two classes on the basis of transcriptional ability (*Perrault* and *Semler* 1979; see also Section 5.2).

The standard VSV genome is transcribed both in vivo and in vitro (catalyzed by the endogenous virion polymerase) into five monocistronic mRNAs, each coding for one of the five virus proteins (see Section 5.2 for a more detailed discussion of VSV transcription). The base sequence of all of the noncoding and a large proportion of the coding

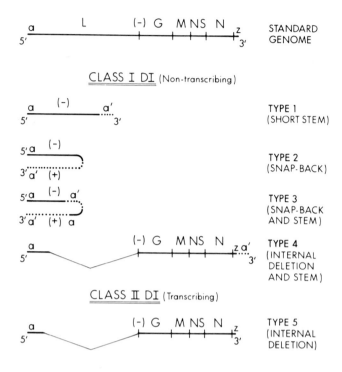

Fig. 1. Types of genomic sequence rearrangements in VSV DI. The standard virus minus-strand genome (about 11 kb), coding for five genes (L, G, M, NS, and N), is illustrated at the top of the figure. Short stretches of genome terminal sequences, 45–70 nucleotides at the 5′-end and 50 nucleotides at the 3′-end, are represented by the letters 'a' and 'z' respectively. Dotted lines indicate plus-strand sequences and a′ stands for a complementary copy of sequence a. The light solid lines in types 4 and 5 show deleted regions of the genome

regions are now known (*Keene* et al. 1978; *McGeoch* and *Turnbull* 1978; *Semler* et al. 1979; *Rowlands* 1979; *McGeoch* and *Dolan* 1979; *McGeoch* 1979; *Rose* and *Iverson* 1979; *Keene* et al. 1980; *Schubert* et al. 1980; *Rose* 1980; *Rose* et al. 1980a, b). The replication of the genome involves the synthesis of a full-size plus strand which then serves as template for minus-strand replication *(Wagner* 1975).

A variety of studies employing different approaches have shown that the majority of VSV DI RNAs (class I, types 1–3 in Fig. 1) contain a contiguous segment from the 5′-end of the standard genome. The evidence for this comes from hybridization to individual VSV mRNAs (*Leamnson* and *Reichmann* 1974; *Stamminger* and *Lazzarini* 1974; *Schnitzlein* and *Reichmann* 1976; *Schnitzlein* and *Reichmann* 1977a) and comparative oligonucleotide maps, which show that the smaller DI RNAs are subsets of the larger ones and correspond to sequences within the L cistron (*Clewly* et al. 1977; *Kang* et al. 1978a; *Clewly* and *Bishop* 1978; *Clerx-Van Haaster* et al. 1980). In addition, the presence of the exact 5′-terminal sequence of the standard genome in various DI RNAs was established through analysis of terminal complementarity and base sequencing studies described in the following section.

3.2.2 Terminal Sequence Complementarity

The hallmark of the most abundant class of VSV DI RNAs (class I, Fig. 1) is the presence of inverted complementary terminal sequences not found in the standard genome. The first evidence for this structural feature came from electron microscopic observations of circular DI RNAs with characteristic small panhandles or stems in VSV (*Perrault* 1976; *Perrault* and *Leavitt* 1977b) and in the paramyxovirus Sendai (*Kolakofsky* 1976). Isolation of the complementary VSV stem sequences from a short VSV DI (tsG31 ST, referred to as *DI 0.10* in the new nomenclature), following digestion of the single-stranded portion of the molecules with ribonuclease, yields a uniform size duplex molecule originally estimated to be approximately 60 bp in length (*Perrault* and *Leavitt* 1977b), and now known to be 53 bp long (*S.T. Nichol* and *J. Perrault* unpublished). By labeling the 5'-ends of these duplex stem molecules, or the 5'-end of the standard genome RNA, and using these probes in various hybridization experiments with unlabeled preparations of the same RNAs or other VSV DI RNAs the following conclusions were reached: 1. the 5'-end sequence of the standard genome and the DI RNAs are identical for the length of the duplex stems; 2. the 3'-end sequence of the DI RNAs (one strand of the duplex stem molecules) is not present within the minus strand of the standard genome; 3. this short extragenomic sequence at the 3'-ends of DI RNAs corresponds to the 3'-end of the complementary plus strand of the standard genome (*Perrault* et al. 1978). The extragenomic origin of these sequences was also suggested in other studies by the appearance of two unique oligonucleotides in T1 ribonuclease-digested DI RNAs, one of which appears to be derived from the 3'-end since it binds to a borate-affinity column (*Freeman* et al. 1978).

   Several studies determining the base sequence corresponding to the ends of the VSV genome and its DI RNAs have confirmed the validity of the above conclusions. These include: 1. direct RNA sequencing of endogenous VSV particle polymerase products (see Section 5.2), which represent complementary copies of the 3'-end of DI RNAs (*Semler* et al. 1978; *Schubert* et al. 1978), or the 3'-end of the standard genome (*Colonno* and *Banerjee* 1978a); 2. direct RNA sequencing of the 3'-end of the standard genome and a number of DI RNAs (*Keene* et al. 1978; *Keene* et al. 1980); 3. cDNA sequencing of the 3'-end of the standard genome (*McGeoch* and *Dolan* 1979; *Rowlands* 1979); 4. direct RNA sequencing of the 5'-ends of the DI RNAs (*Schubert* et al. 1979; *Schubert* et al. 1980) and of the standard genome (*Semler* et al. 1979). The results from these sequencing studies are summarized in Figure 2. The standard genome of the VSV Indiana serotype shows a limited terminal sequence complementarity (14 out of the first 17 terminal residues). This limited complementarity undoubtedly accounts for the inability to isolate stable double-stranded stem structures from the standard VSV Indiana RNA. The terminal sequences of the VSV Indiana DI RNAs examined so far (excluding snap-back molecules discussed below) are capable of forming a unique size stable duplex varying from 45 to 70 bp in different isolates. A similar situation presumably holds true for the New Jersey VSV strains and some of its DI RNAs but in this case the limited terminal complementarity of the standard genome extends to the first 20 bases and gives rise to a stable duplex (*Keene* et al. 1979). For a discussion of the possible sequence specificities involved in generating DI RNA stem sequences see Section 4.3.1 below.

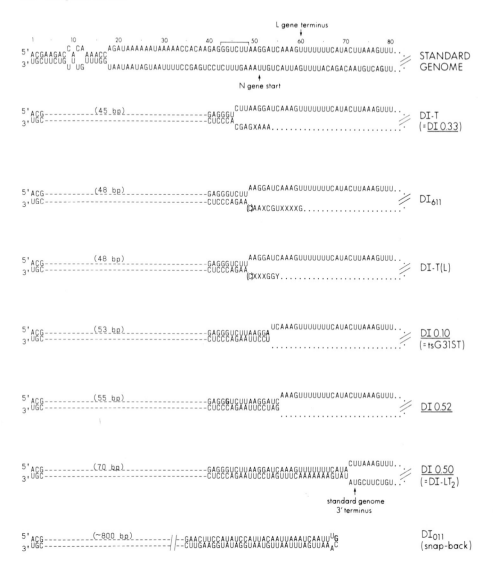

Fig. 2. Terminal sequences of VSV standard and DI RNAs. The dashed lines indicate complementarity of terminal DI RNA sequences, with the 5′-end sequence identical to that of the standard genome. The nucleotide sequence following the stem structure at the 3′-ends of the DI RNAs is not known beyond the few bases indicated (except for DI₀₁₁ and DI 0.50). Residues in parentheses are tentative assignments whereas 'x' stands for undetermined. The putative promoter sequence at positions 43–48 from the 5′-end of the standard genome is indicated by a bracket. The sources of the various DI RNA sequences are as follows: DI-T, DI₆₁₁, and DI-T(L), *Schubert* et al. (1979); *DI 0.10, S. Nichol* and *J. Perrault*, unpublished; *DI 0.52, Hagen* and *Huang* (1981) and D. *Rao* and *A.S. Huang*, personal communication; *DI 0.50, Keene* et al. (1981a, b); DI₀₁₁, *Schubert* and *Lazzarini* (1981)

3.2.3 Snap-Back Hairpin Molecules

This kind of VSV DI RNA (Class I, types 2 and 3 in Fig. 1) was discovered independently in two laboratories by virtue of the odd behaviour of the molecules following denaturation protocols (*Lazzarini* et al. 1975; *Perrault* 1976). They appear to instantly snap-back into a double-stranded configuration after disruption of all hydrogen bonding by heat and/or denaturing solvents. If the molecules are first treated with ribonuclease to remove any putative single-stranded regions, they can then be denatured into separate plus and minus strands each equal to about one-half of the original mass of the molecule. Electron microscopic and nuclease studies further indicated that these molecules contain little single-stranded character and are most likely hairpin molecules obtained on deproteinization of a single-stranded ribonucleoprotein complex.

Further extension of these studies showed that snap-back hairpin type molecules of different sizes are relatively common in VSV DI isolates, and like most other VSV DI RNAs correspond to unique subsets of the L cistron (*Perrault* and *Leavitt* 1977a; *Schubert* et al. 1979; *Keene* et al. 1979). Analysis of the 5'- (*Johnson* and *Lazzarini* 1977a) and 3'-terminal residues (*Keene* et al. 1977) as well as more extensive hybridization and sequence analysis of the prototype DI_{011} snap-back RNA (*Schubert* et al. 1979) established that the molecules consist of a contiguous 5'-end segment of the L gene (minus strand) linked covalently at its own 3'-end to a plus strand complement of this same segment. Very recently, *Schubert* and *Lazzarini* (1981) determined the "turn-around" sequence which links the minus and plus strands of DI_{011} RNA (Fig. 2). This sequence bears no obvious relationship to other VSV DI RNA terminal sequences. It is, however, symmetrical such that breakage of a single phosphodiester bond between a G and C residue yields a perfectly base-paired duplex (estimated to be about 860 bp long).

Electron microscopic observations also indicated that ribonuclease-treated snap-back molecules (single-stranded region removed) are capable of circle and concatemer formation (*Perrault* and *Leavitt* 1977b). On this basis it was suggested that intact snap-back molecules contain inverted complementary sequences at both ends of the duplex. Hybridization studies and partial sequence determinations carried out in the author's laboratory have confirmed that this is indeed the case for DI tsG31 MT snap-back RNA but not so for DI_{C5ST} (*S.T. Nichol* and *J. Perrault* unpublished). The latter DI is most likely identical to DI_{011} of *Lazzarini* and colleagues since it was grown independently in the two laboratories from the same standard virus inoculum stock originating from a five times consecutively plaqued clone (*Holland* personal communication). There are therefore two distinct types of snap-back VSV DI RNAs (Fig. 1). The exact base sequence of the "turn-around" region in the tsG31 MT DI has not yet been determined. The ability of a small proportion of the ribonuclease treated DI_{C5ST} RNA duplex preparation to circularize or form large concatemers (*Perrault* and *Leavitt* 1977b) may have been due to contamination with other DI RNAs or to some unexplained property of these molecules. For a discussion of the possible origins of snap-back molecules, see Sec. 4.3.1 and 4.3.3.

3.2.4 Internal Genome Deletions

As mentioned previously the majority of VSV DI RNAs contain sequences contiguous with the 5'-end of the standard genome except for a short stretch at their 3'-ends. Early studies, however, showed one important exception. The HR (heat resistant) VSV Indiana strain gave rise to at least one LT (long truncated particle) DI preparation which maps at the 3'-end of the standard genome (see *Reichmann* and *Schnitzlein* 1979).

Furthermore, this HR-LT isolate is unusual in that it interferes heterotypically with the standard VSV New Jersey virus (see Section 5.4.1 below).

In addition, this HR-LT DI transcribes the four VSV mRNAs proximal to the 3'-end of the standard genome both in vitro (*Colonno* et al. 1977) and in vivo (*Chow* et al. 1977; *Johnson* and *Lazzarini* 1977b, 1978). This strongly suggests that the template HR-LT RNA contains the exact 3'-end terminal sequence of the infectious parent virus up to and including the G gene. However, high resolution gel analysis of denatured RNA species (*Perrault* and *Semler* 1979), as well as electron microscopic analysis (*Epstein* et al. 1980), revealed the presence of at least two types of molecules in the HR-LT isolate. Hybridization studies with the separated RNAs (*Perrault* and *Semler* 1979), using end-labeling techniques and DI RNA stems (corresponding to the 5'-end of the standard genome) led to the following conclusions: 1. the larger of the two HR-LT RNA species examined, denoted VSI HR ATCC *DI 0.50*, contains stems, approximately 65 bp long, which are derived from the 5'-end of the standard genome and its complement, as in other VSV DI RNAs previously examined; 2. the smaller (by about 10%) of the two HR-LT RNA species, denoted VSI HR ATCC *DI 0.46*, does not contain stem structures and its ends are identical to the original 5'- and 3'-end sequences of the standard genome, thus corresponding to an internal deletion; 3. the larger *DI 0.50* RNA also contains all or almost all of the sequences derived from the 3'-end of the standard genome present in the smaller *DI 0.46* RNA, and therefore also contains an internal genome deletion (see Fig. 1).

Epstein et al. (1980), using a different approach, reached many of the same conclusions regarding the two species of RNA in their preparations of the HR-LT DI. Only the larger species, denoted in their study DI-LT$_2$ (probably identical to *DI 0.50*), is capable of circularization suggesting stem structures. Sequencing techniques in addition revealed that both forms retain the 5'-end of the genome, but only the shorter linear species, denoted DI-LT$_1$ (probably identical to *DI 0.46*), retains the parental 3'-terminal sequence. A third study by *Clerx-Van Haaster* et al. (1980) also strongly suggests the presence of internal deletions in their HR-LT isolate, which was not characterized in terms of the number of RNA species present, but clearly shows conservation of T1 oligonucleotides from both the 3'- and 5'-ends of the standard genome.

In addition to the structural features described above, *Perrault* and *Semler* (1979) suggested, on the basis of hybridization studies, that *DI 0.50* RNA might contain the exact 3'-end sequence of the standard genome a short distance inward from its own 3'-end. This important feature was recently confirmed and extended by *Keene* et al. (1981a, b), who directly sequenced the 3'-end of their DI-LT$_2$ RNA and showed it to be an exact complement of the 5'-end of the standard genome for 70 nucleotides, followed by one noncoded A residue, and then immediately followed by the standard genome 3'-end sequence. The implications of these findings regarding polymerase activities in DI and standard VSV are discussed in Section 5.2 below.

Size estimates of the 5'-end standard genome segment conserved in the different HR-LT isolates from different laboratories vary considerably. *Perrault* and *Semler* (1979) estimated approximately 200 nucleotides for *DI 0.46* RNA, and approximately 500 nucleotides for *DI 0.50* RNA. *Epstein* et al. (1980) reported 320–350 nucleotides for their DI-LT$_1$, and possibly about 860 nucleotides for DI-LT$_2$ (the revised length estimate of the DI$_{011}$ hybridization probe). *Chanda* et al. (1980) suggested approximately 450 nucleotides on the basis of duplexes generated by nuclease digestion of a full-length RNA transcript of their HR-LT isolate [denoted VSI HR ATCC *DI 0.67*(3') in their study] annealed to the standard genome RNA. It is not clear at the present time whether these differences reflect imprecision in the methods employed, or possibly variable size RNAs in the isolates of HR-LT DI. It should be noted here that all HR-LT stocks analyzed in the above studies were originally derived from the same isolate (*Petric* and *Prevec* 1970). The passage history in different laboratories, however, may have enriched for one or more given RNA species or generated additional genomic rearrangements. As discussed below (see Section 5.4.1) it is already clear that some DI can preferentially replicate as compared to others.

3.3 Other Negative-Strand Viruses

3.3.1 Sendai

The standard genome of the paramyxovirus Sendai is about 15 kb long and serves as template for the synthesis of six monocistronic mRNAs in vivo or in vitro (*Choppin* and *Compans* 1975; *Kingsbury* 1977). Its replication strategy is very similar to that of VSV. The earliest characterization of Sendai DI RNAs showed that they are smaller than standard virion RNA (sedimenting at 19S and 25S in contrast to 50S for standard RNA), are negative in polarity, and behave similarly to previously characterized VSV DI RNAs (*Kingsbury* et al. 1970; *Kingsbury* and *Portner* 1970). No further work on the properties of Sendai DI RNAs was published until several years later when they gained major importance in being the first reported to form circular molecules (*Kolakofsky* 1976).

A series of reports from *Kolakofsky* and colleagues have since provided several details of Sendai DI RNA structure, many of which shortly preceded and/or paralleled the developments in the similarly organized VSV system. In particular, Sendai DI RNAs were shown to contain stem structures approximately, 110–150 bp in length, which can be isolated by ribonuclease digestion (*Leppert* et al. 1977). As in the case of VSV (see Section 3.2.2 above) the 3'-end sequence of the DI RNAs is not found in the standard genome but represents a complementary copy of the 5'-end sequence common to both standard and DI particle RNAs (*Leppert* et al. 1977). Furthermore, the sequences of at least two DI particles RNAs, approximately 1200 and 2600 bases long, were shown to be contiguous with sequences at the 5'-end of the standard genome (except for the small stretch at the 3'-end represented in the stem structure). The length of independently generated Sendai DI RNAs was also examined under denaturing conditions and found to vary from about 670 to 7100 nucleotides (*Kolakofsky* 1979). So far, the genomic rearrangements observed in Sendai RNAs are analogous to those seen in VSV.

3.3.2 Influenza

Although the earliest biological studies on the generation of DI were carried out with influenza virus (*von Magnus* 1954) much less is known about their molecular biology than in the VSV system. This was in part due to the lack of a system for growing large amounts of influenza DI and difficulties in separating them from infectious virus (see review by *Nayak* 1980). More recent studies have employed cell lines which yield large amounts of virus and which can be infected under controlled conditions producing either standard virus only, or highly enriched DI preparations (*Lenard* and *Compans* 1975; *Nayak* et al.

1978; *Janda* et al. 1979; *Nakajima* et al. 1979). In addition, a direct biological assay system based on infectious center reduction was recently developed for quantitating influenza DI (*Janda* et al. 1979).

Early reports indicated that influenza DI contain reduced amounts of the larger viral RNAs (*Duesberg* 1968; *Choppin* and *Pons* 1970; *Nayak* 1972). However, further characterization of these RNAs did not progress until recent years when it was shown unambiguously that influenza virus is composed of eight RNA gene segments (*Palese* 1977; *Scholtissek* 1978). Three laboratories then reported the presence of extra small RNAs specific for influenza DI preparations (*Nayak* et al. 1978; *Crumpton* et al. 1978; *Nakajima* et al. 1979). Further studies showed that standard virus free from small RNAs can be isolated, and that such standard virus clones consistently generate DI-containing small RNAs on further serial passage (*Nayak* et al. 1978; *Janda* et al. 1979; *Ueda* et al. 1980).

The genomic content of single DI particles in influenza is not known. The loss of plaque-forming ability in undiluted passages of the virus did not correlate well with the loss of large RNA segments in at least one study (*Bean* and *Simpson* 1976). *Nayak* et al. (1978) attributed the decrease of infectivity to the nonspecific loss of one or more of the four largest viral RNA segments. Additional studies showed variability in reduction of these fragments in DI generated from different standard virus clones (*Janda* et al. 1979). Recently, *Pons* (1980) reported a good correlation between loss of segment 1 and loss of plaque-forming ability. *Crumpton* et al. (1981), on the other hand, find no such simple relationship. Further studies are needed to clarify these differences. Interfering ability, however, is directly correlated with the presence of virus ribonucleoproteins containing small RNAs (*Janda* and *Nayak* 1979), and shows small UV target size compared to infectivity (*Nayak* et al. 1978).

The replication strategy of influenza differs significantly from that of VSV and paramyxoviruses. In contrast to the latter, influenza does not code for enzymes capable of directly capping its mRNAs. Instead, the virions contain a nuclease (most likely virus coded) which cleaves small cap-containing fragments (10–14 nucleotides long) from the 5'-ends of host mRNAs in vivo (or added to in vitro reactions with purified virus) and uses these as primers to initiate transcription at the 3'-ends of the gene segments. This dependence on capped host mRNAs undoubtedly accounts for the requirement of a functional host RNA polymerase II for influenza virus replication (for a recent review of influenza transcription priming see *Krug* et al. 1981). Transcription of each gene segment also terminates about 20–30 residues from the 5'-end of the templates followed by polyadenylation. Thus, as in VSV, some yet uncharacterized regulatory switch must occur during virus growth to allow synthesis of full-size negative-strand templates. In addition, influenza is so far the only true RNA virus which produces spliced mRNAs, most likely using the host nuclear enzymes (*Lamb* and *Lai* 1980).

The influenza DI RNAs so far examined are negative-strand molecules (*Davis* and *Nayak* 1979). Reported sizes vary from as little as approximately 100 nucleotides for the smallest avian fowl plague virus RNAs (*Crumpton* et al. 1978) to molecules possibly as large as about 1200 nucleotides (slightly larger than virion segment 7) for the WSN strain of influenza (*Janda* et al. 1979). The sequence relationship between DI RNAs and individual virion RNA segments was studied by oligonucleotide fingerprinting (*Nakajima* et al. 1979; *Davis* and *Nayak* 1979; *Ueda* et al. 1980) and direct RNA sequencing (*Davis* et al. 1980). In all cases studied, the small RNAs are derived from one or the other of the three large polymerase genes (P_1, P_2 or P_3). In some instances, one or more extra oligonucleotides not present in the virion segment of origin are observed. The most extensive study (*Davis* and *Nayak* 1979) showed that oligonucleotides from different size DI RNAs, originating from the same virion segment, are either completely overlapping or only partially overlapping. The latter observation led to the suggestion that some of these DI RNAs might correspond to internal deletions within genome segments. *Ueda* et al. (1980) also reported that two small RNAs originating from the same P_1 gene share none of the large unique oligonucleotide spots from this segment. Paradoxically, only one of these RNAs is associated with a reduction of the P_1 gene segment while the other shows a reduction of the P_2 gene. Only one report (*Crumpton* et al. 1979) has claimed that influenza DI RNAs might also originate from segments other than the P genes, but the interpretation of the oligonucleotide maps is clouded by the fact that the analysis was carried out with mixtures of RNA segments.

Sequence determination of the first 13 bases of the 5′-end and the first 12 bases at the 3′-end of the P genes (these sequences are essentially identical in all virion segments) and three DI RNAs (derived from P_1) show complete homology (*Davis* et al. 1980). These results clearly establish the presence of internal genome deletions in at least these three DI RNAs which are all derived from the same standard virus clone. Whether this is the case for most or all influenza DI RNAs remains to be established. Very recently, *Nayak* and colleagues (personal communication) determined the complete sequence of a cloned double-stranded DNA copy derived from the smallest of these three influenza DI RNAs (409 bp long). The bases flanking the site of internal deletion (very near the middle of the molecule) bear no homology to the consensus sequence for a splice site in eucaryotic mRNAs including the splice junction of the NS_2 mRNA derived from virion segment 8 of influenza virus (*Lamb* and *Lai* 1980). The implications of these recent findings are discussed in Section 4.3.2.

3.4 Positive-Strand Viruses

3.4.1 Togaviruses

All of the information available on the standard genome sequences represented in togavirus DI originates from studies of two alphaviruses, Sindbis (SV) and Semliki Forest virus (SFV) (for detailed review on all aspects of togavirus DI, see *Stollar* 1979 and 1980). The standard genome of these viruses (about 13 kb long) is capped at the 5′-end, polyadenylated at the 3′-end, and contains one active site near its 5′-end for the translation of a non-structural protein precursor. In addition, a subgenomic 26S RNA (about 4.2 kb long), which contains the translation initiation site for a structural protein precursor, is synthesized in infected cells. This subgenomic RNA corresponds to a contiguous segment at the 3′-end of the genome and its synthesis most likely results from internal initiation on a complementary negative-strand RNA copy of the full-size genome (*Dubin* et al. 1979; *Pettersson* et al. 1980). The latter also serves as a template for the synthesis of progeny RNA (see reviews by *Kääriäinen* and *Soderlund* 1978, and *Kennedy* 1980). The complete nucleotide sequence of the 26S mRNA of both SFV and SV was recently determined (*Garoff* et al. 1980a, b; *Rice* and *Strauss* 1981; *Ou* et al. 1981). The sequence results show unambiguously that the genome length RNA and the subgenomic 26S RNA share identical sequences extending to the 3′-terminus (*Ou* et al. 1981). The mechanism of gene expression in this virus group is seemingly more complex than that seen in rhabdo- or paramyxoviruses. This feature is perhaps responsible for the greater complexity of structures seen in togavirus DI RNAs.

The first reports on the nature of togavirus DI RNAs described the appearance of novel RNA species in cells infected with high passage SV (*Shenk* and *Stollar* 1972; *Weiss* and *Schlesinger* 1973; *Eaton* and *Faulkner* 1973). DI RNAs of SFV were first analyzed by *Bruton* and *Kennedy* (1976). Several different size species of DI RNAs are observed in both SV and SFV grown in vertebrate or invertebrate cell lines. These range from about 1.7 kb to about 10 kb (*Johnston* et al. 1975; *Kowal* and *Stollar* 1980). Other published values for both SV and SFV DI RNAs fall between these extremes (see *Stollar* 1979). Interestingly, several laboratories reported that larger DI RNAs decrease progressively in size as serial undiluted passage of virus stocks is continued (*Johnston* et al. 1975; *Guild* et al. 1977; *Stark* and *Kennedy* 1978). The implication of these findings in relation to interference with standard virus replication is discussed below (see Section 5.5).

The polarity of SV and SFV DI RNAs was determined by hybridization experiments with various combinations of particle RNAs and single- and double-stranded RNAs isolated from infected cells (*Weiss* et al. 1974; *Bruton* et al. 1976; *Guild* et al. 1977), as well as oligonucleotide mapping (*Kennedy* 1976; *Kennedy* et al. 1976; *Dohner* et al. 1979). These studies showed that the DI RNAs are polyadenylated, positive strands, and contain virus-coded sequences only.

The hybridization and oligonucleotide studies also served to establish maps of the genome sequences represented in the various DI RNAs. A common theme in all of these is conservation of both 5'- and 3'-end sequences of the standard genome, although in some cases, one of the conserved ends appears to be very small in size (*Weiss* et al. 1974; *Kennedy* et al. 1976). Based on comparison of unique oligonucleotides in DI RNAs vs standard RNA, and the relative map position of these oligonucleotides, the sequence arrangement shown in Figure 3a was proposed for SFV DI RNAs (*Kennedy* 1976; *Stark* and *Kennedy* 1978). On the basis of RNA-RNA hybridization studies, and assuming a simple internal deletion, *Guild* and *Stollar* (1977) proposed the arrangement shown in Fig. 3b for SV DI RNAs.

The studies discussed so far indicate a somewhat larger representation of standard genome sequences derived from the 5'-end in various togavirus DI RNAs. In contrast to this, a SV DI RNA, about one-fifth the size of the genome, was shown to contain sequences originating mostly from the 3'-end of the standard genome, with only a short 5'-end sequence of undetermined size (*Weiss* et al. 1974; *Kennedy* et al. 1976).

It seems clear from the above studies that many togavirus DI RNAs represent internal deletions of the standard genome. However, some published reports suggested more complex situations and recent analysis of one particular SFV DI shows this to be the case. On the basis of oligonucleotide maps, both *Stark* and *Kennedy* (1978) and *Dohner* et al. (1979) suggested the presence of two or more noncontiguous internal deletions in at least one DI RNA from SFV and SV respectively (see Fig. 3a). Furthermore, although the report of *Kennedy* (1976) indicated molar yields of oligonucleotides from SFV DI RNAs, *Dohner* et al. (1979) reported wide variations in these yields for the one SV DI RNA examined.

Pettersson and colleagues (personal communication) have now determined the detailed sequence organization of one SFV DI RNA as deduced from a molecular cloned double-stranded DNA copy (about 1650 bp long). The results obtained show

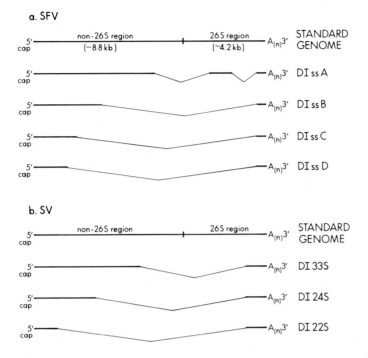

Fig. 3. Proposed sequence organization of alphavirus DI RNAs. The solid lines represent conserved regions of the genome whereas light lines indicate deleted portions. Evidence for more complex sequence rearrangements is discussed in the text

three repeat sequences 484 nucleotides long, with a small insert sequence between two of these, as well as within one of the repeats. All the sequences of this clone appear to be derived from within the 5'-two-thirds of the standard genome (non-26S RNA sequences) except for a stretch of 106 identical residues at the 3'-ends of both the standard and DI RNA. The cloned DNA copy was obtained from a heterogeneous mixture of DI RNAs sedimenting at about 18S in a sucrose gradient. S1 nuclease mapping experiments, however, showed that this cloned DNA contains a faithful and uninterrupted complementary copy of at least one SFV DI RNA in this mixture. The preparation of DI RNAs was obtained following the tenth high multiplicity passage of a standard SFV stock which already showed the presence of DI RNAs at passage four. The cap-containing T1 oligonucleotides of this "18S" RNA mixture were also found to be heterogeneous with the general sequence cap-AU(AU)$_n$CAUG, where n = 4 to 8 (*Pettersson* 1981). This cap sequence is different from that reported for both standard and 26S SFV RNAs, i.e., cap-AUG and cap-AUUG respectively (*Wengler* et al. 1979; *Pettersson* et al. 1980). Therefore, the exact 5'-end terminal sequence of the standard genome is apparently not conserved in some of these DI molecules (the heterogeneity of the DI 5'-cap sequences, however, could conceivably be generated by a nontemplated mechanism). The cap sequences of two SV DI RNAs were recently reported to resemble, at least in part, the cap sequences of standard virus in one case and that of 26S subgenomic RNA in the other (*Kowal* et al. 1980). The above results clearly show that extensive genome rearrangements, including deletions, duplications, insertions and possibly others, can occur during the genesis of togavirus DI RNAs. Future experiments should clarify whether the heterogeneity and more complicated rearrangements of these DI RNAs evolve from simpler forms during multiple passages of virus stocks (see discussion Section 4.3.2).

3.4.2 Picornaviruses

Only two picornaviruses, poliovirus, and mengovirus were reported to generate DI (*Cole* et al. 1971; *McClure* et al. 1980). The relative difficulty in generating such particles (by long term passage at high multiplicities of infection) is unusual in comparison to other RNA viruses. The reasons for this are unclear but may be related to relatively low levels of interference and to the choice of host cell which appears to influence the production of picornavirus DI (*McClure* et al. 1980; see also Section 4.1). Poliovirus live vaccines also do not generally contain DI (*McClure* et al. 1980) in contrast to previous suggestions (*McClaren* and *Holland* 1974).

Almost all of the molecular studies of picornavirus DI were carried out with the type I Mahoney poliovirus strain originating from the same laboratory (*Cole* et al. 1971; *Nomoto* et al. 1979; *Lundquist* et al. 1979). The standard genome of poliovirus (approximately 7500 nucleotides long) is covalently-linked to a small virus-coded protein, VPg, at its 5'-end and is polyadenylated at its 3'-end. It contains a major initiation site for synthesis of a large polyprotein precursor ($\sim$ 200,000 daltons mol. wt.) near its 5'-end, and possibly a second initiation site of unknown location and coding potential (*Celma* and *Ehrenfeld* 1975). The standard genome is the only mRNA so far detected intracellularly and is replicated via synthesis of a full-size complementary RNA copy (for a review of picornavirus gene expression and replication see *Agol* 1980 and *Kitamura* et al. 1980). The complete sequence of the type I Mahoney poliovirus genome has recently been determined (*E. Wimmer,* personal communication).

The studies of *Cole* and colleagues (*Cole* et al. 1971; *Cole* and *Baltimore* 1973a, b, c) on the nature of poliovirus DI RNA led to the following conclusions: 1. the three independent isolates of DI particles studied all contain RNAs differing slightly from each other in size and are about 15% smaller than the standard genome; 2. about 87% of the standard genome sequences are conserved in the DI RNAs isolated, as determined by competition hybridization experiments with the replicative form of the standard genome; 3. deleted portions of the standard genome correspond to sequences coding for capsid polypeptides (mapping towards the 5'-end of the genome), since cells infected with DI particles in the absence of standard virus give rise to translation products missing only about one-third of the capsid protein precursor. The latter observation was confirmed and extended in subsequent studies (*Humphries* et al. 1979; *Lundquist* et al. 1979; *Phillips* et al. 1980). The findings of *Villa-Komaroff* et al. (1975) also suggested that poliovirus DI RNAs correspond to internal deletion since the DI RNA-directed polyprotein precursor synthesized in vitro contains the same initiation tryptic peptide as found for standard virus RNA. Furthermore, *Humphries* et al. (1979) showed that DI RNA contains the additional in vitro protein initiation site discovered earlier for the standard genome. The latter investigators also demonstrated that DI RNA can serve as template for the synthesis of VPg in vivo.

Further studies on the map location of internal deletions in poliovirus DI RNAs were carried out using a variety of methods. *Nomoto* et al. (1979) employed three methods: 1. limited digestion with ribonuclease III to produce large fragments of standard and DI

RNAs (map order deduced from the presence or absence of poly A); 2. comparison of oligonucleotide fingerprints; and 3. electron microscopy of RNA-RNA heteroduplex molecules formed by annealing DI RNA and standard genome replicative form molecules. These studies confirmed that the deletions in all three DI RNA preparations originally isolated by Cole and colleagues are in the 5'-terminal half of the standard genome, and are all missing the same four unique oligonucleotides. In addition, the report showed that the RNA molecules in one of the DI preparations are about 12% shorter than the genome but are somewhat heterogeneous since the location and extent of individual deletions in heteroduplex molecules varied (located approximately 1300 to 3100 bases from the 5'-end). A more detailed electron microscopic study of heteroduplex molecules from poliovirus DI RNAs generated from the same poliovirus strain, and possibly representing independent isolates (the standard virus, however, was not cloned) provided further evidence for heterogeneity (*Lundquist* et al. 1979). The deletions in this case were shown to be about 16% of the standard genome but were found to be located anywhere from about 500 to about 3800 bases from the 5'-end. Some of the deletions examined are not contiguous and represent double and even triple deletions (still adding to the same 16% or so overall deletion). It was also noted that the DI RNA population is not static on further passage but differs in the relative amounts of individual species suggesting a basis for the extensive heterogeneity observed.

Although several laboratories experienced great difficulty in generating DI in picornaviruses, other than the poliovirus strain mentioned in the studies above, the results of *McClure* et al. (1980) suggested that this problem may in part result from the small size of the deletions generated in most cases. The deletions detected in two different clinical isolates of poliovirus and a laboratory stock of mengovirus are reproducibly in the range of 4–6%, whereas even stocks cloned twice consecutively from the poliovirus strain employed in all previous studies, repeatedly give rise to the larger deletions. As pointed out by a number of authors (*Cole* 1975; *Lundquist* et al. 1979; *McClure* et al. 1980) it is likely that packaging restraints govern which size molecules are eventually encapsidated in picornavirus DI and this may explain the differences in deletion sizes for the different virus strains (see Section 5.3). The map locations of the small picornavirus deletions have not yet been determined. The poly(C) tract of mengovirus (approximately 100 residues in length), located near the 5'-end of the genome, is conserved in its DI RNA (*McClure* et al. 1980).

The marked population heterogeneity of picornaviruses DI RNAs has somewhat complicated a more detailed analysis of the recombination sites in these molecules. Molecular cloning of DNA copies from these genomes will undoubtedly be reported soon and rapid progress is likely to follow.

3.5 Double-Strand Viruses

Reovirus was the first double-strand virus reported to generate DI (*Nonoyama* et al. 1970). Members of the reovirus group contain ten double-strand RNA segments each coding for a unique viral gene protein. Each segment is completely transcribed by the virion-associated transcriptase into a capped plus-strand mRNA which in turn serves as template for synthesis of the double-stranded progeny RNA (*Joklik* 1980). *Nonoyama* and *Graham* (1970) reported that five independent clones of type 3 reovirus each give rise to

DI lacking the largest virion segment now known to code for the λ_3 polymerase component. *Schuerch* et al. (1974) using ts mutants of type 3 reovirus reported that one of these generates DI with virion segment 3 missing, whereas another generates DI with both segments 1 and 3 missing. The same two virion segments were again implicated in DI recovered from infected animals (*Spandidos* and *Graham* 1976) and persistently infected cell cultures (*Ahmed* and *Graham* 1977). Aside from some transcriptional aspects (see Section 5.2) no further detailed molecular studies have yet been carried out with these various DI isolates. In particular, efforts should be made to look for small RNA segments which might represent internal deletions within gene segments analogous to influenza virus DI. Two such possible internally deleted segments have recently been observed by *Ahmed* and *Fields* (1981). The "light defective" particles obtained from persistently infected cells might also contain such RNAs (*Ahmed* and *Graham* 1977).

Virus-like particles in fungi are considered to be bona fide viruses although they lack the criterion of infectivity (see review by *Bruenn* 1980). The well-characterized yeast double-stranded *Saccharomyces cerevisiae* virus (ScV) contains two genome segments, L and M, separately encapsidated. The virus was shown to give rise to smaller RNAs in suppressive yeast strains (*Vodkin* et al. 1974; *Tzen* et al. 1974). Since the smaller RNAs appear to replace the M segment whenever present in the same cytoplasm, they are considered analogous to DI (*Bruenn* and *Kane* 1978; *Fried* and *Fink* 1978). The L genome fragment, about 4500 bp long, codes for the major capsid protein and the M segment, about 1800 bp long, codes for the "killer toxin" (*Bostian* et al. 1980). For a detailed discussion of the relationship between sensitivity to toxin, synthesis of toxin, and segregation of suppressive sensitive strains, the reader is referred to *Bruenn* (1980).

The size of the various ScV DI RNAs observed ranges from about 540 to 1500 bp. All of these are derived from M, as demonstrated by comparative oligonucleotide fingerprint analysis (*Bruenn* and *Kane* 1978; *Kane* et al. 1979), by electron microscopic heteroduplex analysis (*Fried* and *Fink* 1978), and by 3'-end sequence analysis (*Bruenn* and *Brennan* 1980). All of the DI RNAs examined conserve sequences from both the 5'-and 3'-ends of the M RNA segment and are thus internal genome deletions. Some of these appear to regularly give rise to tandemly duplicated molecules. The sequences flanking the deletion sites have not yet been determined.

Although relatively little is known regarding the replication strategy of ScV (it is probably somewhat similar to reovirus) this system is attractive for DI studies because well defined gene mutations, some of which map in the host nucleus, specifically affect the replication of the M virus segment. In addition, this system represents an extreme case of virus persistence since transmission occurs only during mating. Other less well studied fungal virus systems also share properties similar to ScV and most likely produce similar DI RNAs (*Bruenn* 1980).

4 Origin of DI RNAs

4.1 Host Cell Effects on the Generation of DI RNAs

The passage number at which virus yields become greatly diminished, as a result of DI production, not only varies widely for different viruses, but also for the same virus grown in different host cells. This general phenomenon could result a priori from a host effect on the de novo generation of DI from standard virus and/or from modulation of the amplification properties of DI. Many published studies on this subject are somewhat confusing because they have not attempted to differentiate between these two alternatives. Effects on DI generation (this term will be used throughout this article to denote the events which give rise de novo to a DI RNA molecule, either from a standard virus genome or from a previously existing DI molecule) are understandably much more difficult to measure.

Obviously, many different types of molecules with particular genome sequence rearrangements could be generated at low frequencies during virus replication. The ones that concern us, however, are only those which are capable of amplification, i.e., replication and enrichment. Claims that DI generation per se is specifically altered by the host must obviously eliminate explanations involving replication and/or interference effects. The latter two processes are clearly affected by the host cell and are discussed in Section 5.1.

The only DI system in which some attempt was made to measure the de novo rate of DI generation is that of VSV. *Holland* et al. (1976b) estimated this to be about 10^{-7} to 10^{-8} per infectious particle replication in baby hamster kidney (BHK_{21}) cells. This estimate was made possible because of the apparent random nature of individual DI particle generation. Whenever a given VSV plaque clone is grown to a seed stock containing more than about 10^7 to 10^8 plaque forming units (pfu) per ml, it invariably gives rise to the same array of DI species even if independent high multiplicity passage series are carried out. However, if the initial virus plaque (containing about 10^6 pfu or less) is not grown to a seed stock first, but used directly to initiate independent series of undiluted passages, a different array of DI RNA species appears in each case (*Holland* et al. 1976a). This crucial observation shows that, in addition to the rather random character of DI generation, many of the VSV DI RNA molecules amplified, whether large or small, possess similar interfering and replicating properties.

Others have reported that single VSV clones have a genetic capacity to regularly generate the same DI species in a given cell type (*Reichmann* et al. 1971; *Kang* et al. 1978a). However, these studies were carried out with VSV pools already contaminated with seed quantities of DI and the results therefore do not support a viral genetic basis for the type of VSV DI generated (*Holland* et al. 1980). A similar randomness in the type of DI generated from clonal virus pools is also observed with influenza DI (*Janda* et al. 1979) and Sendai DI (*Kolakofsky* 1979).

A possible host effect on the frequency of VSV DI generation was also noted by *Holland* et al. (1976a) who showed that a particular HeLa cell line fails to produce DI after 27 serial undiluted passages and does not replicate added DI generated in BHK_{21} cells. Only very few DI were detected in the HeLa lysates by subsequent amplification in BHK_{21} cells. This effect, however, is also consistent with a low amplification rate.

Stark and *Kennedy* (1978) likewise reported lack of SFV DI production in the same HeLa cell line after more than 200 serial passages. More recently, *McClure* et al. (1980) showed lack of mengovirus DI production specific for this same host cell. SFV DI or mengovirus DI grown in other hosts, however, were reported to replicate well in this HeLa host. These results are therefore suggestive of specific effects at the generation level. Curiously, *Kang* and *Tischfield* (1978) also claimed that a human cell line is capable of suppressing the production of VSV DI in eight karyotypically different human-mouse hybrid cell lines, without influencing the replication of DI produced in other host cells.

This is not, however, a general property of human cell lines, since poliovirus DI can be generated in the HeLa cell line mentioned above (*McClure* et al. 1980), and SFV DI can also be generated in a different strain of HeLa cells (*Stark* and *Kennedy* 1978). Moreover, HeLa cells can produce VSV DI at times but unpredictably so (*Holland* et al. 1978; *J. Perrault* and *P. Schnarr*, unpublished).

Igarashi and *Stollar* (1976) were unable to find evidence for the production of SV DI during serial undiluted passage in *Aedes albopictus* cells. Later work showed, however, that alphavirus DI are produced in persistently infected mosquito cells (*Eaton* 1977). They also accumulate on serial passage if a longer incubation time is used (*King* et al. 1979) or if individual clonal cell populations are first selected for high virus yield (*Logan* 1979; *Stollar* 1979; *Holland* et al. 1980; *Tooker* and *Kennedy* 1981). VSV DI are also generated in high yields from mosquito cells (*Gillies* and *Stollar* 1980a). It thus seems probable that arboviruses in general are also capable of generating DI in invertebrate hosts.

A more striking and direct role for the host cell in the generation of VSV DI was proposed by *Kang* and *Allen* (1978) and *Kang* et al. (1978b). These authors claimed that pretreatment of a variety of vertebrate host cells for 24 h with actinomycin D completely abolishes the generation of VSV DI even after 12 undiluted passages, whereas control cells show a large accumulation of DI by two or three passages. No interference activity could be detected even though, as shown previously and confirmed in this study, actinomycin D has no effect on VSV standard or DI particle replication. These data clearly suggest that a cellular factor, requiring renewed transcription and possibly translation within 24 h, is essential for the generation of VSV DI. Unfortunately, these important claims have not been confirmed despite serious effort by a number of other laboratories (*Youngner* et al. 1981; *Reichmann*, personal communication; *Horodyski* and *Holland*, personal communication; *J. Perrault* and *P. Schnarr*, unpublished).

The various rates of DI accumulation in different host cells observed for VSV (*Huang* and *Baltimore* 1970; *Coward* et al. 1971; *Potter* and *Stewart* 1976; *Kang* et al. 1978a; *Youngner* et al. 1981), paramyxoviruses (*Kingsbury* and *Portner* 1970; *Roman* and *Simon* 1976), influenza (*Choppin* 1969; *De and Nayak* 1980), and togaviruses (*Darnell* and *Koprowski* 1974; *Stark* and *Kennedy* 1978) are difficult to assess in terms of DI generation versus amplification because all of the above studies were initiated with virus stocks already contaminated with seed quantities of DI. Furthermore, replication rates and interference levels were not measured independently of generation. Most or all the above host effects could thus be explained on the basis of a cellular influence on the amplication properties of DI RNAs (see Section 5.1).

An interesting observation analogous to a host effect on DI production was also reported by *Winship* and *Thacore* (1979). Undiluted passage of VSV in African green monkey kidney cells results in DI production but the latter are not present if the cells are first infected by Shope fibroma virus (ShFV) in the presence of hydroxyurea which inhibits the poxvirus replication without affecting VSV synthesis. Yields of infectious VSV are similar under both conditions suggesting a specific effect on DI production. As in previous cases, however, the results can most likely be explained by effects on DI replication and/or interference. Nevertheless, this system offers a promising approach in attempting to identify a putative host cell factor(s) specifically affecting VSV DI RNA replication.

A possible host cell effect on the kind of SFV DI RNA produced, rather than the general frequency at which DI are generated, was also reported by *Stark* and *Kennedy*

(1978). As mentioned previously (Section 3.4.1) larger togavirus DI RNAs appear to decrease progressively in size on continued passage. In the case of SFV, the decrease in size is consistent with a sequential series of deletions leading to subsets of smaller DI RNAs up to a "limit size" DI. In the pig kidney cell line (PK-15), the smallest DI RNA detected does not undergo the two additional deletions observed regularly in other host cells, even when passaged 32 times beyond the "limit passage". A possible interpretation is that this host cell lacks factors necessary for generating these deletions. Alternatively, the host cell could influence the selection of preexisting DI RNAs as observed in other systems (see Section 5.1).

Overall, the evidence presented above indicates that the host cell could sometimes influence the frequency and possibly the nature of DI generated de novo. However, it is impossible to rule out that all these effects occur at the level of DI amplification subsequent to their initial appearance. The weight of the evidence strongly argues that the nature of various DI molecules is more directly under virus than host cell control. The genetic make-up of an infectious virus might therefore be expected to influence directly the nature and/or rate of DI generation. Surprisingly, very few studies have addressed themselves specifically to this question. The claims regarding a standard virus clonal influence on the type of VSV DI produced and the probable alternative explanation have been discussed above already. *McClure* et al. (1980) on the other hand reported that only one of the four distinct isolates of poliovirus type 1 examined does not produce DI in HeLa cells. Furthermore, characteristic deletion sizes in DI RNAs from each of two isolates are reproducibly obtained in this same cell line even after repeated cloning to eliminate previously existing DI. These observations, which could be explained by several genetic differences between the isolates in terms of generation, could also be due to differences in stability of capsids containing the shorter RNAs. These studies further illustrate the difficulties encountered in trying to pinpoint the basis for differences in DI accumulation observed in different virus-host systems.

4.2 The Unlikely Provirus Hypothesis

Before discussing specific models for the generations of DI RNAs, it is important to consider first whether such recombination events could possibly occur at the DNA level. One laboratory in particular has published a number of reports claiming that several negative-strand RNA viruses, including measles, VSV, simian virus 5, LCM, and possibly influenza, as well as two positive-strand togaviruses, SV and tick-borne encephalitis, can integrate DNA copies of their genome into various host cells (*Zhdanov* and *Parvanovich* 1974; *Zhdanov* et al. 1974; *Zhdanov* 1975; *Gaidamovich* et al. 1978). The evidence for this claim is based mostly on DNA transfection experiments (giving rise to recoverable infectious virus) and detection of cellular DNA copies of the virus genome with labeled nucleic acid probes. A similar claim of DNA transfection using cells infected with the respiratory syncytial paramyxovirus (RSV) was also reported (*Simpson* and *Inuma* 1975). Three different mechanisms were suggested to account for these observations: 1. a gene product interaction between a negative- or positive-strand virus and a latent retrovirus; 2. a cellular reverse transcriptase-mediated integration event (*Zhdanov* 1975); or 3. a mutational or recombinational event (with a retrovirus genome or cellular genome) yielding an RNA virus variant with reverse transcriptase activity (*Furman* and *Hallum* 1973; *Simp-*

son and *Inuma* 1975). Although these ideas are intriguing possibilities, the weight of currently available evidence strongly argues against these claims.

This counterevidence includes DNA transfection attempts with cells persistently infected by VSV, RSV, SV, LCM, measles, mumps, influenza, and rabies (*Holland* et al. 1976c; *Igarashi* et al. 1977; *Pringle* et al. 1978) as well as attempts to detect proviruses by hybridization experiments with DNA from cells persistently infected with VSV, SV, measles, and rubella (*Holland* et al. 1976c; *Friedman* and *Costa* 1976; *Igarashi* et al. 1977; *Haase* et al. 1977; *Norval* 1979). The experiments of *Holland* et al. (1976c), in particular, are noteworthy in that the VSV carrier culture was well characterized, with essentially all cells remaining infected for over two years, and at the limit of detection contained less than one DNA provirus copy per 40 cells. Earlier claims of provirus DNA copies (detected by hybridization) in the yeast ScV system (*Shalitin* and *Fischer* 1975; *Vodkin* 1977) have also been refuted (*Wickner* and *Liebowitz* 1977; *Hastie* et al. 1978).

It is clear from the above studies that classic RNA viruses can associate with host cells for long periods of time without recourse to DNA integration. However, it is not possible to rule out that, under special and rare circumstances, an integration phenomenon can take place. It will be interesting to see whether biologically active proviral DNA copies of these RNA viruses can be constructed in the future by genetic manipulation in vitro. At the present time, we can safely assume that the deleted genomes in DI of RNA viruses are generated by events occurring at the RNA level, at least under most circumstances.

4.3 Purposeful Error-Prone Virus Polymerase

4.3.1 Terminal Sequence Complementarity and the Copy-Back Model

The very nature of DI RNAs suggests strongly that they originate from low frequency events during the replication or transcription of standard virus RNAs. Although we can view these events as "errors" in contrast to the dominant "fidelity" of the replication process, they are as purposeful as any other type of mutations in biological systems.

It is important to note here that trivial explanations for the generation of DI RNAs, such as RNA chain scission or premature termination during synthesis, are insufficient by themselves to explain the conservation of genomic ends or the presence of inverted terminal complementarity. Thus, fragmentation of VSV ribonucleoproteins by sonication, or chemical mutagenesis and UV irradiation of standard virus, does not lead to DI production (*Holland* et al. 1976a).

The unexpected features of terminal sequence complementarity in VSV and Sendai DI RNAs (see Section 3.2.2 for details) provide the strongest argument for the involvement of virus polymerases in the origin of DI RNAs. These observations led both *Kolakofsky* and colleagues (*Leppert* et al. 1977), and *Huang* (1977) to propose a "template-switching" and "copy-back" model for DI generation in negative-strand viruses (Fig. 4). The essential feature of this model is a viral replicase detaching from its template (while remaining attached to the nascent chain), and then binding back near the 5'-end of the nascent chain to initiate copying in the reverse direction. Since most VSV and all Sendai DI RNAs examined so far retain a large fragment from the 5'-end of the standard genome, it is assumed that such a copy-back event would occur during synthesis of minus strands.

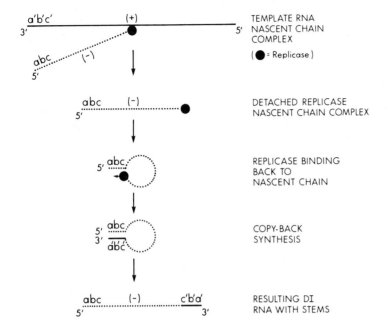

Fig. 4. Kolakofsky-Huang copy-back model for the generation of DI RNAs. The terminal sequences abc and their complement c′b′a′ in the resulting DI RNAs can anneal to each other (after isolation from the ribonucleoprotein template structure) to give rise to characteristic panhandles or stems

The Kolakofsky-Huang model raises some interesting questions regarding specificities of the "fall-off" sites on the template as well as the "resumption" sites of synthesis on the nascent chains. So far, only short stem structures (45–70 bp) or large hairpin snapback molecules have been observed in VSV and Sendai DI RNAs (see Figs. 1 and 2). This suggests strongly that only sites close to the ends of nascent molecules are competent for resumption of copy-back synthesis. In contrast, judging from the extensive variability in size of the 5′-end standard genome segment conserved in various VSV and Sendai DI RNAs, the fall-off points may well be relatively random at least to a point about halfway down the genome. In this context, it should be remembered that replication of both plus and minus strands of rhabdo- and paramyxoviruses takes place on helical nucleocapsid templates. The tightly bound proteins of these templates may be displaced locally and transiently during RNA synthesis but "naked" RNA molecules are not detectable during RNA replication (*Soria* et al. 1974; *Hill* et al. 1979). Furthermore, the nascent chains are very rapidly assembled with newly synthesized core proteins. This protein association appears to completely protect the RNA from ribonuclease digestion (*Hill* et al. 1979) and extends to within at least 5 bases from both ends of Sendai DI particle nucleocapsids (*Lynch* and *Kolakofsky* 1978). Core protein-template RNA interactions may thus play a major role in replicase fall-off and resumption sites. The VSV and Sendai polymerases undoubtedly recognize some nucleotide sequence features but there would seem to be little chance for dependence on an extensively base-paired secondary structure in the template. With this in mind, we can now examine possible nucleotide sequence specificities of the copy-back model.

Lazzarini and co-workers have provided a large share of the information available regarding sequences flanking the recombination sites in VSV DI RNAs. On the basis of their data on three independently isolated DI RNAs *Schubert* et al. (1979) proposed a specific RNA polymerase resumption site near the 5'-end of VSV genomic RNA. The sequence 5'-GGUCUU-3', at positions 43 to 48 from the 5'-end of the standard genome (see Fig. 2) is also present at positions 4–9 at the 3'-ends of all DI RNAs (except *DI 0.46* = DI-LT$_1$) and at the 3'-end of standard genome plus strands. This hexamer sequence may thus be at least part of a putative promoter recognition site.

To account for the small differences in the precise location of the copy-back site (positions 45, 48, and 48 in the three DI RNAs examined in their study) *Schubert* et al. (1979) suggested two possibilities: 1. nucleotides copied just prior to replicase fall-off are, sometimes by chance, complementary to those adjacent to the polymerase recognition site; and 2. slippage of the RNA polymerase can occur in analogy to procaryotic promoter sites (see *Rosenberg* and *Court* 1979). In addition, a more general form of this model was proposed allowing inter- as well as intramolecular changes in template which could also explain internal deletions (see Section 4.3.2 and 4.3.3).

The copy-back model, with the added features of random fall-off and sequence specific resumption sites of synthesis, would seem to offer a coherent explanation for the origin of terminal sequence complementarity and internal deletions in DI RNAs. However, more recent work in the VSV system casts some doubt on the universal applicability of this model. Stem lengths in more recently characterized VSV DI RNAs (see Fig. 2) are somewhat longer (53, 55, and 70 bp) than the ones previously studied. The proposed resumption site for copy-back synthesis may therefore be less localized than anticipated. Furthermore, the sequence of the "turn-around" region in the snap-back DI$_{011}$ (*Schubert* and *Lazzarini* 1981) which can be equated with the resumption site in this DI RNA, bears no homology at all to the putative VSV polymerase promoter (Fig. 2).

A quite different model was proposed by *Schubert* and *Lazzarini* (1981) to explain the origin of DI$_{011}$. The features of this model include the following: 1. replication complexes (synthesizing minus strands) contain more than one nascent chain; 2. individual replicase molecules move at variable speed along the template allowing a faster one to "tailgate" a slower one; 3. the trailing polymerase switches templates and starts synthesis (independent of the putative VSV promoter site) on the daughter strand attached to the leading polymerase; 4. this strand switching takes place exactly symmetrically at the replication fork. It should be noted here that the origin of the snap-back RNA structure proposed by *Perrault* and *Leavitt* (1977b) for type 3 molecules (Fig. 1) does not require any significant deviation from the original copy-back model. As pointed out by *Leppert* et al. (1977), the replicase-nascent chain complex of a replicating DI RNA could copy back on itself starting near the 3'-end of the nascent chain to give rise to snap-back molecules with inverted repeat sequences.

In addition to the unique origin proposed for DI$_{011}$ RNA, yet a third model was suggested by *Keene* et al. (1981a, b) to account for the origin of stems in the unusual VSV DI-LT$_2$ (also called *DI 0.50*, see Figs. 1, 2). This model proposes the same specific promoter sequence recognition for resumption of synthesis, but differs from earlier models in that template switching occurs when a nascent minus strand terminates at residue 70, and resumes copying starting at the exact 3'-end of a second minus-strand genome template.

A complementary copy of this newly generated molecule would thus correspond to a genome-size minus strand with a 70-bp stem structure. The deletion event is viewed as a separate process taking place either before or after the template switch just described. The critical difference here is that resumption of synthesis occurs at the opposite end of a minus strand and involves the very terminal residue rather than an internal site. The origin of the uncoded extra A residue in position 71 is not explained but, as pointed out by the authors, the VSV polymerase is known to insert noncoded A residues in transcripts (*Colonno* and *Banerjee* 1978a; *Herman* et al. 1978).

In summary, the origin of terminal sequence complementarity in both VSV and Sendai DI RNAs is generally thought to occur by some sort of strand-switching event during polymerization. The essential features of this concept originate from the Kolakofsky-Huang copy-back model. However, attempts at explaining specificities in terms of sequence at resumption sites of synthesis, or in terms of particular strand selection, suggest that the models proposed so far may be too restrictive conceptually. Different mechanisms are perhaps involved in generating individual DI RNA species such as DI_{011} (= C5 ST) and DI-LT$_2$ (= *DI 0.50*) as opposed to other DI RNAs. However, it is probably more useful to consider a more general model which encompasses all structural features observed so far in all virus DI RNAs (see Section 4.3.3).

4.3.2 Genesis of Internal Deletions and Complex Genome Rearrangements

Internal genome deletions are now known to exist in DI RNAs of both negative- and positive-strand viruses as well as double-strand viruses (see Section 3). This type of genome rearrangement is thus observed more commonly than copy-back sequences which so far are restricted to rhabdo- and paramyxoviruses where they clearly predominate. This situation perhaps reflects unique polymerase and/or template properties of the latter virus groups.

One possible mechanism for the generation of internal deletions in DI RNA is that of splicing by host cell enzymes involved in the synthesis of mRNAs. The majority of animal RNA viruses, however, replicate exclusively in the cytoplasm. Nevertheless occasional accessibility of viral RNA templates to such enzymes (perhaps during cell division or after virus induced damage to the cell nucleus) cannot be ruled out. As mentioned previously (Section 3.3.2) the sequences flanking the simple internal deletions in the one influenza DI RNA examined bear no homology to the eucaryotic "consensus-type" splice sequences. The extensively rearranged SFV DI RNA also mentioned before (Section 3.4.1) also lacks such sequences at the recombinant sites (*Pettersson*, personal communication). It seems likely then that RNA viruses have evolved a "splicing mechanism" (breakage and ligation of RNA molecules) of their own, or rely on other mechanisms to achieve similar results. It is interesting to note here the parallel between genesis of internal genome deletions in DI RNAs and the long-standing and unresolved question of the mechanism responsible for genetic recombination of the nonsegmented picornaviruses genome (see discussion in next Section).

Only a few brief mentions of a possible involvement of a breakage-and-reunion, or "splicing" scheme, in the generation of internal deletions in DI RNAs have appeared in the literature (*Cole* 1975; *Lundquist* et al. 1979; *Kang* 1980; *Clerx-Van Haaster* et al. 1980). On the other hand, several authors suggested models which involve some sort of transcriptive or replicative error during viral RNA synthesis. These include: "copy-choice" of

RNA fragments (*Cole* 1975), or undefined templates (*Lundquist* et al. 1979) in poliovirus; recombination during transcription of alphavirus RNAs whose ends might be juxtaposed by virtue of terminal sequence complementarity (*Kennedy* 1976); replicase fall-off and reattachment at a distal point in the alphaviruses (*Guild* and *Stollar* 1977); similar resumption of synthesis at a specific site homologous to the VSV promoter sequence (*Schubert* et al. 1979); dissociation and reassociation of ScV (virus-like particle of yeast) transcriptase at some internal sequence (*Kane* et al. 1979); and looping out of the template and copying across a replication fork for VSV (*Kang* 1980). All of these suggestions are obviously variations on the same theme and reflect the preference of most authors for DI RNA generation based on "errors" during polymerization. Only the model of *Schubert* et al. (1979) suggests a sequence specificity in the resumption site of synthesis. A possible specificity in the fall-off sites for VSV polymerase (a short purine-rich stretch) was also suggested (*Keene* et al. 1980). Detailed sequence information on various DI RNAs is likely to accumulate very rapidly in the next few years (or even by the time this review is published). As in the case of procaryotic recognition sequences, the pattern of specificities if any may only become apparent by comparison of a large number of putative sites.

A more complex type of DI RNA rearrangement is the case of VSV DI *0.50* (= DI -LT$_2$) discussed in Section 3.2.4 (see also Figs. 2, 3). This DI RNA was most probably generated by two separate and distinct events, one resulting in an internal deletion and the other in a copy-back sequence (*Perrault* and *Semler* 1979; *Keene* et al. 1981a, b). The order in which these events might have occurred is interesting in this case because a VSV DI RNA with a simple internal deletion only was shown to possess very different biological properties (see Sections 5.2 and 5.4.1).

Multiple internal deletions (two or three) in the same DI RNA molecule were also reported in poliovirus and alphaviruses (see Sections 3.4.1 and 3.4.2). The heterogeneity in the position of the deletion in poliovirus DI is also interesting because it may reflect a relative lack of sequence specificity in the fall-off and resumption sites of synthesis within this particular region of the genome.

An additional instance of extensive rearrangement in a DI RNA is the peculiar case of the SVF DI examined by *Pettersson* and colleagues (Section 3.4.1). This particular rearrangement may not be representative of the majority of DI RNAs found in their heterogeneous mixture of species but nevertheless this information suggests caution in generalizing from the simpler DI RNA structures discussed so far, especially in togaviruses. Obviously, this SFV DI RNA has undergone multiple recombinational events most likely in succession. It is not immediately clear, how it acquired the tandem triplicate repeat structure or the various small inserts. However, if one assumes that the viral polymerase is responsible for this, then one is forced to hypothesize an even greater flexibility in template termination sites, as well as choice of strands and sequence specificity for resumption sites, than hitherto suspected. The general model of DI RNA generation presented in the next section does in fact attempt to remove many of the constraints inherent in previous proposals.

4.3.3 General Model

Several of the ideas advanced by many different workers regarding DI RNA generations can be incorporated in a more general view of these mutational events. Central to this view is the concept of promiscuous fall-off and resumption of synthesis by a viral polymerase-nascent chain complex. The copy-back model of Kolakofsky and Huang, for example, which first captured the essence of DI RNA generation, can then be viewed as one of many possible ways this process can take place. Stems, snap-back RNAs, internal genome deletions, repeats, inserts, and other rearrangements yet to be discovered, can all be accounted for by what can be called, the "leaping replication complex model" (see Fig. 5). Furthermore, an extension of this model also suggests a mechanism for recombination between homologous standard virus RNAs (see below.).

The essential features of the "leaping replication complex" model are as follows:
1. *Interrupted synthesis* – the generation of a recombinant site in DI RNAs (bringing together previously noncontiguous regions of a genome) does not involve ligation but interrupted synthesis of a plus or minus strand by the viral polymerase complex followed by resumption of synthesis at a different site.
2. *Variable choice of secondary templates* – the resumption site can be on the same template strand, or on the nascent chain carried by the leaping polymerase complex, or perhaps less frequently on a different viral template RNA which is not part of the original replicating complex.

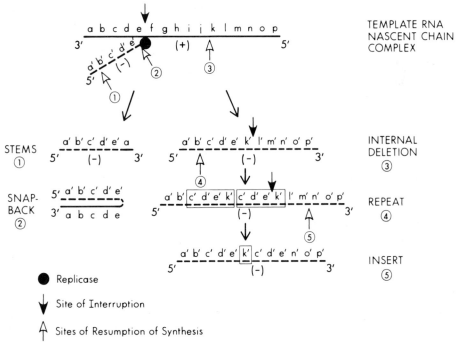

Fig. 5. A general model for the generation of DI RNA genome rearrangements. Five distinct types of minus-strand genome rearrangements are illustrated. The first two correspond to copy-back synthesis (see Fig. 4) resulting in either simple stems or snap-back molecules (see text, Section 4.3.1). The three other types of genomic rearrangements are illustrated on the right side of the figure as a succession of events (only the resulting minus strands are drawn for simplicity). Resumption of synthesis downstream from the interruption site leads to an internal deletion whereas resumption upstream produces a repeat sequence. A second deletion event results in an apparent insert sequence (k') flanked by repeats (c' d' e'). Further deletion event(s) can also result in apparent inserts not flanked by repeat sequences (not shown)

3. *Specificity of sites on secondary templates* – the viral polymerase-nascent chain complex can resume synthesis at variable sites of a secondary template (or the same template) with specificities and frequencies determined both by base sequence and viral nucleoprotein template properties (the contribution of each depending on the particular virus system).

As shown diagrammatically in Figure 5, resumption of synthesis on the nascent chain near its 5′-end, generates copy-back DI with small stems, while resumption near its 3′-end gives rise to snap-back RNAs. Similarly, resumption of synthesis on the same template strand further downstream from the termination site produces an internal deletion, whereas leaping back to a site upstream from the termination gives rise to a repeat sequence. Furthermore, an apparent insert sequence flanked by repeats can easily be generated starting from a simple deletion followed in succession by a repeat event and a further deletion event. The model is drawn in Figure 5 with a nascent minus strand only for the sake of simplicity. However, in some or all virus systems the leaps could occur within any replicating viral RNA complexes, DI or standard, regardless of polarity (but of course within the confines of the 5′- to 3′-rules of synthesis). Moreover, the model can also be drawn with circular replicating complexes and/or with more than one nascent chain per template. A leap from one replication complex to a different template not involved in the original termination event has also been suggested for VSV *DI 0.50* (see Section 4.3.1), although in this case the structure can equally well be explained by a copy-back event following complete reading of an internally deleted DI RNA template.

It is obvious that, in its most general form, the "leaping replication complex" hypothesis allows for an immense variety of structural rearrangements. It emphasizes the rather promiscuous abilities of viral replicase complexes to terminate and resume synthesis at a large variety of sites, in contrast to specifying events unique to the generation of each DI RNA molecule. The model does make one clear prediction, i.e., all DI RNAs must conserve at least one end sequence of the standard genome corresponding to the segment copied before interruption of synthesis. It should be remembered, however, that only those molecules capable of accumulating at the expense of standard viral RNA templates, i.e., possessing both the ability to replicate and interfere with standard virus synthesis, qualify as DI RNAs. Thus, the origin of these molecules is intimately tied to a discussion of the minimal template requirements for preferential replication (see Section 5.3, 5.4, and 5.5).

Before leaving the subject of the promiscuous leaping polymerase complex, I should point out that if one or more leaps occur symmetrically between two standard virus RNA molecules of the same polarity, but carrying different point mutations, the result is homologous genetic recombination in the classical sense (copy-choice scheme). Recombination frequencies as high as about 2% between point mutations on the same RNA molecule (as opposed to genetic reassortments between separate segments) can be observed in picornaviruses (*Cooper* 1977; *Romanova* et al. 1980) but have remained undetected in other RNA viruses. It seems likely that such recombination does indeed occur with all true RNA viruses but its frequency may be easily masked by high levels of spontaneous mutations (*Domingo* et al. 1978; *Semler* and *Holland* 1979; *Flamand* 1980; *Bruenn* and *Brennan* 1980; *Nottay* et al. 1981), frequent reversion at other sites (*Ramig* and *Fields* 1979; *Murphy* et al. 1980), and high levels of gene product complementation in polyploid particles (*Pringle* 1977). It is interesting to note that a scheme very similar to the leaping polymerase complex model described above was previously entertained as a possibility to explain genetic recombination in picornaviruses (*Cooper* 1977).

5 Replication and Interfering Properties of DI RNAs

5.1 Host Cell Modulation

Many of the studies discussed in relation to possible host effects on the de novo generation of DI (Section 4.1) can also be interpreted in terms of influence on DI replication and/or interference. I will discuss here only selected aspects of the previously mentioned reports as well as some additional studies which more directly implicate host control over DI amplification.

Perrault and *Holland* (1972a) suggested the existence of "low vs high interference" cells with regard to VSV DI replication. The basis for this distinction was suggested by the observation that VSV DI (from BHK_{21} cells) interfere much more strongly with standard virus replication in some hosts, such as BHK_{21}, HeLo, and chick embryo fibroblast (CEF) cells, versus others such as MDCK, PK-15, and MDBK cells. This variable interference potential of DI was also shown to be independent of their replication since they did replicate well in the "low interference" cells. A host cell factor(s) modulating the relative affinities of the viral replicase for standard and DI template was suggested as a possible explanation.

Huang (1977) also reported that VSV DI interference is stronger in fibroblast cells from young as opposed to old mice. This observation, which may be related to the ease with which VSV and rabies DI are produced in newborn versus adult mouse brain (*Holland* and *Villarreal* 1975) further suggests that the state of cell differentiation may affect DI interference.

The study of *Holland* et al. (1976a) also uncovered a different host cell effect on DI function. In this case, VSV DI (from BHK_{21} cells) strongly interfered with standard virus replication in HeLa cells but without concomitant replication. This result implies that DI replication per se is not necessary for expression of interference. As discussed previously, however, this same HeLa cell line does not always behave in this way (see Section 4.1). The same report from Holland's laboratory, as well as others (*Lunger* and *Clark* 1977; *Kang* et al. 1978a) also demonstrated that different host cells selectively amplify a different array of VSV DI from a VSV stock already containing seed quantities of DI. This result emphasizes the intricate relationship between replication of particular DI and putative host cell factors.

Turning to other virus systems, we can also find evidence for host cell modulation of DI amplification. *Crumpton* et al. (1981) very recently reported the selection of a different array of avian influenza DI RNAs in CEF versus BHK cells when starting with the same CEF-grown virus inoculum. Surprisingly, when the CEF-grown virus is switched to mouse L cells no change occurs in the DI RNA pattern but virion segment 6, and to a lesser degree segment 5, are reduced. The significance of these results is unclear since host factors related to permissiveness for viral growth may also be involved.

In the togavirus system, *Levin* et al. (1973) reported that SFV DI produced in CEF cells display more interference in mouse cells than in the cell of origin. Similarly, SV DI from BHK cells do not interfere or replicate in *Aedes albopictus* cells (*Stollar* et al. 1975; *Eaton* 1975; *Igarashi* and *Stollar* 1976). *Kascsak* and *Lyons* (1978) reported that Bunyamvera virus DI (from BHK_{21} cells) show stronger interference in BHK_{21} and Vero cells than in MDBK or *A. albopictus* cells. The same type of phenomenon was also reported for BHK_{21}-grown mengovirus DI which interfere more strongly in HeLa than BHK_{21}

cells (*McClure* et al. 1980). Similarly LCM virus DI interfere more strongly in BHK than in MDCK cells (*Dutko* and *Pfau* 1978).

The studies cited above strongly support the view that DI replication and/or interference with standard virus is subject to host control. A recent study by *Gillies* and *Stollar* (1980b), however, illustrates additional complexities in the interaction of DI with host cells. When VSV DI produced in *A. albopictus* cells are tested for interference with standard virus growth, they do so only with standard virus growing in the mosquito cells but not in BHK cells. In contrast, BHK-grown VSV DI interfere equally well with standard virus in both BHK and *A. albopictus* cells. When each DI preparation is grown for one additional passage in the heterologous cell types, the pattern of interference is reversed. These results strongly suggest that DI particles can be phenotypically modified by the host cell in such a way as to influence their interference properties. It is interesting to note that the earlier studies cited above may also involve undetected phenotypic alterations. The biochemical nature of this host modification(s), however, remains unclear.

How the host cell affects DI RNA replication specifically is unknown. Standard virus RNA replication is undoubtedly affected by the host cell as illustrated by the many instances of intracellular restriction of virus RNA replication, as well as the occurrence of host range mutants. The host cell could exert a direct influence on the viral RNA replicase, for example, by providing subunits as in the RNA bacteriophages (*Blumenthal* and *Carmichael* 1979). In addition or alternatively, a more indirect influence, such as membrane attachment sites, or availability of substrates, could be hypothesized. Progress in understanding the role of the host cell is likely to be dependent on the future availability of in vitro systems of replication for animal RNA viruses.

5.2 Transcriptional and Translational Activities of DI RNAs

Only two RNA virus DI systems, VSV and poliovirus, have been studied in detail with regard to transcriptional and translational activities. The lack of such activities in most VSV DI is well documented, and is clearly a result of their particular genome sequence rearrangements. In contrast, some poliovirus DI RNAs are efficiently transcribed and translated giving rise to abnormal truncated proteins. The situation in other virus systems is less clear cut because of insufficient relevant data. I shall review here what is known in each of these virus systems since the presence or absence of such activities may be biologically important for DI function.

The transcription of the VSV genome is a highly regulated process which is only partially understood. The five genes are seemingly transcribed by the VSV polymerase as if they were part of a single transcription unit beginning exactly at the 3'-end of the genome. The mandatory order of transcription is also accompanied by an attenuation process which results in stepwise decreasing amounts of gene transcripts as a function of their distance from the 3'-end of the template. It is not clear whether the transcriptase can only begin synthesis at this end of the molecule. In any case, it first gives rise to a 47-nucleotide long, plus-strand leader RNA of unknown function, and then probably continues with a separate initiation or processing event for each gene as it travels down the template. An alternative possibility is that initiation of each gene occurs simultaneously giving rise to very short transcripts, which are then elongated in the mandatory order (*Banerjee* et al. 1977; *Banerjee* 1980; *Testa* et al. 1980). Whatever the mechanism, it is clear that a regulatory function must somehow subvert this transcription process, at some point in time during the virus life-cycle, and allow a polymerase to copy the entire template into a plus strand to serve as an intermediate in replication.

Turning now to VSV DI RNAs it is easy to see that, except for the unique class V DI all such templates lack the standard genome 3'-end sequence at their own 3'-end (see Fig. 2). Furthermore, the first three DI classes (the most common VSV DI) lack a sequence corresponding to the start of any gene. In retrospect, it is not surprising that *Huang* and *Manders* (1972) and *Perrault* and *Holland* (1972b) both reported lack of transcriptase activity in VSV DI both in vitro and in vivo. Likewise, it is also easy to see why the class V DI (*DI 0.46* = DI-LT$_1$) synthesizes four of the five VSV gene transcripts (missing L gene) both in vitro (*Colonno* et al. 1977) and in vivo (*Chow* et al. 1977; *Johnson* and *Lazzarini* 1977b). Moreover, these transcripts are translated into the corresponding VSV proteins. Perhaps more interestingly from the standpoint of the mechanism of VSV transcription, the class IV DI (*DI 0.50* = DI-LT$_2$) is transcriptionally inactive in vitro (*Perrault* and *Semler* 1979; *Keene* et al. 1981a, b) and would presumably be so in vivo as well. This latter finding underlines the importance of a correct "promoter" sequence at the very terminus of the template since this same sequence is found internally in *DI 0.50* but remains functionless.

From the above discussion, and remembering the rule that DI particles contain the same proteins as standard virions, it is not surprising to find that transcriptionally inactive VSV DI nevertheless contain a polymerase activity which synthesizes mRNAs when added to standard virus ribonucleoprotein templates (*Emerson* and *Wagner* 1972). What is more surprising, however, is that the 3'-end of these DI RNAs serves as template for the synthesis of a small 46-nucleotide long, minus-strand leader RNA in vitro (*Reichmann* et al. 1974; *Emerson* et al. 1977; *Semler* et al. 1978; *Schubert* et al. 1978) and in vivo (*Rao* and *Huang* 1979; *Leppert* et al. 1979; *Leppert* and *Kolakofsky* 1980; *Rao* and *Huang* 1980). The significance of this short RNA, which is apparently synthesized abundantly in vivo by the transcriptase rather than the replicase (*Rao* and *Huang* 1980) is unknown (see Section 5.4.1). Perhaps the availability of the VSV core protein N changes RNA synthesis from transcription to replication by binding to such small RNAs (N acting as antiterminator) as suggested by *Leppert* et al. (1979).

The unique transcribing ability of VSV *DI 0.46* (= DI-LT$_1$) offers several additional insights regarding VSV DI interference and replication (see Section 5.4.1). Suffice it to say here, that although this type of DI could play an expanded role in virus infections because it can complement deficient standard virus functions (*Johnson* and *Lazzarini* 1980) and unlike other VSV DI it can kill host cells (*Marcus* et al. 1977), it may only accumulate under rare circumstances since it is very easily outcompeted by the production of other nontranscribing DI, at least in BHK$_{21}$ cells (*Perrault* and *Semler* 1979; *Epstein* et al. 1980).

It is important to note here that *Marcus* and *Sekellick* (1977) also propose that snapback type VSV DI possess the unique ability (not shared by other VSV DI) to induce interferon very efficiently in host cells in the absence of standard virus. The same authors later proposed that such snap-back VSV DI may play a role in the establishment of persistent viral infections (*Sekellick* and *Marcus* 1978). However, other studies indicate a lack of correlation between snap-back VSV DI RNA and interferon induction (*Frey* et al. 1979). Very recently, *Frey* et al. (1981) presented evidence which shows that the variable interferon-inducing capabilities of VSV DI preparations can be directly correlated with small amounts of standard virus contamination.

We can now turn to a brief discussion of poliovirus DI RNAs which, in contrast to VSV DI, appear to be commonly transcribed and translated. These features were uncovered by Cole and colleagues in their initial characterization of poliovirus DI (see review by *Cole* 1975). It should be noted here that the distinction between transcription and replication in picornaviruses is somewhat blurred since the virion RNA and the mRNA are identical in sequence and differ only in that virion RNA contains a 5′-end covalently linked protein, VPg (see review by *Wimmer* 1979).

The ability to separate pure poliovirus DI from their standard virus (by density gradient centrifugation) enabled *Cole* and *Baltimore* (1973a) to test whether such DI can carry out any intracellular functions by themselves. Indeed, the poliovirus DI display all activities normally found for standard virus (similar rates of viral RNA and protein accumulation) except for a deletion of about one-third of the capsid-protein precursor which prevents them from packaging their RNA (*Phillips* et al. 1980). The shortened capsid precursor polypeptide is unstable and is rapidly degraded in infected cells. *Lundquist* et al. (1979) and *Humphries* et al. (1979) observed a very similar situation with their preparation of poliovirus DI. As mentioned previously (see Section 3.4.2) subsequent work showed that the DI RNA conserves the site for initiation of the polyprotein precursor (as well as the additional initiation site of unknown function) found in the standard genome (the exact position of this putative site is still unclear). As pointed out by *Lundquist* et al. (1979), the heterogeneity in the position of the DI RNA internal deletions could conceivably mask the presence of nontranslatable (out of reading frame) molecules. Nevertheless, these authors argued that the poliovirus polymerase may be a cis-acting protein early in infection (due to initial compartmentalization of parental genomes) and therefore only deleted RNA molecules capable of synthesizing a functional polymerase may be amplified. However, earlier experiments of *Cords* and *Holland* (1964) have clearly shown that poliovirus RNA can be readily replicated by a heterologous picornavirus polymerase supplied very early before significant multiplication of the poliovirus template. Since all picornavirus DI deletions so far mapped were all obtained from one particular isolate of poliovirus, there appears to be little basis for predicting that all such deletions should correspond to sequences coding for capsid proteins.

Surprisingly little information is available regarding possible transcriptional and translational activities of togavirus DI RNAs. The situation is somewhat more complicated than the other DI systems described so far because: 1. these are two classes of transcripts in standard virus infections, the full-size genome (indistinguishable in structure so far from the replication product) and the 26S transcript corresponding to the 3′-end one-third of the genome; and 2. togavirus DI RNAs vary greatly as to which genome sequences are deleted (mostly internal deletions). Nevertheless, as in the poliovirus DI system it would seem possible in many cases that togavirus DI RNAs, which are capped and polyadenylated (see Section 3.4.1), conserve a functional initiation site for protein synthesis, in particular the polymerase precursor site, near the 5′-end of the standard genome (the exact position of this site is not yet known). Aberrant nonfunctional proteins large or small, could then be produced and possibly degraded rapidly as in poliovirus DI. Aberrant proteins related to capsid precursor, however, may be much less frequent or nonexistent because the translation initiation site for these is normally cryptic in the full-size genome and is only active in the 26S transcript. Alternatively, the lack of a functional translation initiation site in togavirus DI RNA, may be essential for their interfering property (see Section 5.5).

A few instances of novel uncharacterized proteins in togavirus standard and DI coinfected cells were reported (*Weiss* and *Schlesinger* 1973; *Weiss* et al. 1974; *Guild* and *Stollar* 1975), but as suggested by *Weiss* et al. (1974), these could represent normal precursor molecules or by-products which for unknown reasons accumulate under conditions of interference only. The latter study also presented evidence that their 20S SV DI RNA is not translated in vitro and is probably not associated with polysomes intracellularly. A later study by the same laboratoy showed that no viral translation products can be detected by immunofluorescence techniques in cells infected with SV DI only (*Schlesinger* et al. 1975). *Bruton* et al. (1976) also reported that purified SFV DI are unable to carry out any step in virus multiplication except uncoating, and that SFV DI RNAs are not present on polysomes in coinfected cells. These clearly represent only a few attempts at detecting aberrant transcripts or translation products in togavirus DI infected cells. A more critical search for such products may well turn out to be useful in delineating control regions on the viral templates.

The situation in influenza virus DI RNA has been even less explored with regard to gene expression. The difficulties in obtaining pure DI populations were mentioned previously (Section 3.3.2). In addition, the segmented nature of the genome raises the fascinating question as to how the replication of one or more DI RNA segments, originating from one or more of the P genes, can so profoundly affect the replication of all segments. As in our previous discussion of togavirus DI RNAs, it seems plausible to suspect that a simple internal deletion might allow the transcription and possible translation of the shortened RNA. Aberrant transcripts and/or translation products related to DI RNAs have not yet been looked for in influenza-infected cells. Likewise, no information on this question is available for the segmented reovirus DI system. Pure reovirus DI, missing the L1 segment, were reported to transcribe the remaining nine segments normally both in vitro and in vivo (*Spandidos* et al. 1976). The remaining segments in reovirus DI can function in vivo to provide complementing functions (*Spandidos* and *Graham* 1975) and can undergo genetic reassortment (*Ahmed* and *Fields* 1981). *Bean* and *Simpson* (1976) also reported that influenza DI preparations contain somewhat reduced levels of transcriptase activity (not enough to account for the much greater loss of infectivity) but that all eight virion segments are transcribed. In the light of the more recent results regarding small DI RNAs in influenza and possibly reovirus, it would be rewarding to reexamine this question and determine whether these molecules are active as templates for transcription.

In summary, relatively little is known about gene expression in DI RNAs. This situation reflects the emphasis of past studies on VSV DI which are for the most part genetically inert. This certainly indicates that RNA viruses are not forced to rely on such gene expression from their DI templates in order to achieve interference and control over their own multiplication. Nevertheless, gene expression in DI RNAs of some viruses may be common perhaps without playing a significant role. Such aberrant gene expression in naturally occurring deletion mutants could prove to be useful in elucidating control functions.

5.3 Conserved Replication and Encapsidation Origins

All DI RNAs examined to date conserve one or both end sequences of the standard virus genome. This feature is central to the models for the origin of DI RNAs discussed previously (Section 4.3) and is not unexpected since all true RNA viruses most likely replicate using a virus-coded polymerase initiating synthesis at the very 3'-OH end of viral template molecules. Thus the 3'-end sequences of both plus and minus RNA strands must correspond, at least in part, to replication origin signals (the sequences complementary to these can also be viewed as termination signals although viral RNA replicases could simply continue synthesis to the very end of the template without regard to sequence specificity). In rhabdo- and paramyxoviruses, DI RNAs usually conserve the 3'-end sequence of the intracellular plus-strand complement of the standard genome at the 3'-end of both their plus and minus strands. This feature may in fact be responsible for their interfering properties (see Section 5.4.1 below). Internally deleted DI RNAs obviously conserve both ends. The only possible exception to this rule is the extensively rearranged SFV DI discussed previously (see Section 3.4.1) but this remains speculative until more information regarding the sequence at the 5'-end of the SFV standard genome is obtained.

Some tentative conclusions regarding the minimum size of conserved replication origins can be gathered from DI RNA base sequence data available so far. In VSV, the stem sizes are 45–70 bp long. Since the sequences beyond these recombination sites vary in different molecules (see Fig. 2) it is very likely that the replication origin signal for minus-strand synthesis does not extend beyond the first 45 residues at the 3'-end of the standard genome plus-strand template. The larger stem sizes in Sendai virus (110–150 bp) could conceivably reflect a longer signal sequence, but other explanations, such as a more distally located encapsidation signal (see below) can also be hypothesized. The only influenza DI RNA sequenced to date contains an internal deletion located very near the center of the virion segment of origin (Section 3.3.2) and thus little can yet be said regarding the minimum sequence needed for replication. The SFV DI RNA previously mentioned contains a conserved genome 3'-end sequence segment 106 nucleotides long beyond the poly A tail. It is not clear whether this noncoding segment represents a minimum size for a replication origin (perhaps in addition to the poly A tail) but it is intriguing to note that reverse transcription of the 3'-end of the SFV standard genome shows a very strong stop at residue 104, and a similar stop (not quite as strong) is also found for SV at position 145 (*Ou* et al. 1981). The secondary structure of the template at these positions (perhaps involving partial complementarity with the 5'-end) may determine an important signal for replication. The pattern which emerges from these few examples is that only a relatively short 3'-end sequence (less than 150 nucleotides) is sufficient for recognition as a specific replication origin in RNA viruses. Rapid accumulation of sequence data for a number of DI virus systems in the near future should provide a more refined picture of the minimal requirements for such signals.

DI RNAs must obviously also conserve the sites necessary for encapsidation. A priori these sites could be anywhere on the standard virus genome and not necessarily at the ends. This is exemplified in the case of the plant tobacco mosaic virus RNA where the recognition site for initiating the assembly of its helical ribonucleoprotein is situated about 15% of the way from its 3'-end (*Otsuki* et al. 1977; *Zimmern* 1977). Nevertheless, as mentioned previously (Section 4.3.1) very short nascent strands of the VSV replication complex are rapidly assembled into a helical ribonucleoprotein structure. It is therefore very likely that a capsid protein recognition site is situated very near the 5'-end of the VSV genome. Likewise, VSV standard genome plus strands are always found encapsidated intracellularly and a similar site is probably present at the 5'-end of these plus strands (the two 5'-end sequences are almost identical for the first 20 or so residues, see Fig. 2). Very recently, *Blumberg* et al. (1981) provided strong support for this idea since the small plus- and minus-strand VSV leader RNAs, corresponding to the first 47 and 46 residues at the 5'-ends of genome length molecules, are found in association with the VSV nucleoprotein in vivo. An analogous situation probably holds true for the paramyxoviruses which use a similar strategy for replication. The encapsidation sites for other RNA viruses, however, remain undefined except to the extent that DI RNAs must conserve them to be packaged.

Icosahedral RNA viruses (picornaviruses, togaviruses, reoviruses) appear to have packaging constraints influencing DI RNA selection and these may be more stringent than in helical symmetry viruses. It seems reasonable to speculate that, in addition to conserving a recognition site for initiating nucleocapsid assembly, the overall stability of DI particles must be equal or nearly equal to that of standard virus. In VSV, for example, DI containing RNAs as small as 10% of the genome are stably packaged. In togaviruses, on the other hand, standard size capsids appear to contain multiple copies of smaller DI RNA ($\frac{1}{6}$ to $\frac{1}{2}$ of genome length) which together add up to an RNA content similar to standard virus (*Bruton* and *Kennedy* 1976; *Kennedy* et al. 1976; *Guild* et al. 1977; *Stark* and *Kennedy* 1978). Packaging restraints were also suggested to play a role in DI RNA selection in picornaviruses (*Cole* 1975; *Lundquist* et al. 1979; *McClure* et al. 1980; see also Section 3.4.2). It is possible that specific viral RNA sequences other than the site involved in the initiation of nucleocapsid assembly are in some cases necessary for the construction of biologically stable and functional DI particles.

5.4 Interference Mechanisms of VSV DI

5.4.1 Replicase Competition and Terminal Sequence Complementarity

There are as yet no unifying hypotheses which can explain interference mechanisms by DI of all RNA viruses. This is perhaps not surprising since different RNA virus groups display quite unique strategies for viral replication. Even in the best studied VSV DI system there are probably two distinct interference mechanisms corresponding to two different types of DI and both of these are still poorly understood.

Several years ago, *Huang* and *Baltimore* (1970) suggested that interference by DI might be analogous to the successful replication competition by short fragments of Qβ bacteriophage RNA with full-length RNA during in vitro synthesis (*Mills* et al. 1967). However, it was soon realized that VSV DI RNAs do not compete by virtue of size since the smallest DI are not invariably selected during replication (*Perrault* and *Holland* 1972a; *Holland* et al. 1976a). Moreover, a similar specific interfering ability was observed for all VSV DI regardless of size (*Reichmann* and *Schnitzlein* 1977; *Adachi* and *Lazzarini* 1978). Nevertheless smaller VSV DI RNAs can conceivably be favored for replication over long-term passage in some cases. This phenomenon is quite distinct from the overwhelming and quantitatively similar replicative advantage displayed by different size VSV DI RNAs in a single replication cycle (see also Section 5.4.2 below for a discussion of interference based on size in other RNA virus DI).

Studies by *Stampfer* et al. (1969), *Perrault* and *Holland* (1972b), and *Huang* and *Manders* (1972) established that VSV DI RNAs not only preferentially replicate but are incapable of transcription on their own and do not inhibit primary transcription by input parental virus. Overall reduction of secondary transcription and viral translation products was proposed to result indirectly from inhibition of genome RNA synthesis. These observations led to the suggestion that VSV DI RNAs successfully compete for the VSV replicase by virtue of a higher affinity for the enzyme. In addition, it was proposed that DI RNAs can gain a kinetic advantage in replication by virtue of their availability as templates while the standard genomes are engaged in active mRNA transcription. These general concepts were later strengthened by further quantitative studies of RNA species in standard and autointerfered infections (*Palma* et al. 1974; *Stamminger* and *Lazzarini* 1977) and still remain to date the most probable explanation for interference by the majority of VSV DI. More recently, the discovery of the unique structural property of VSV DI RNAs represented by stems led *Perrault* et al. (1978) to suggest that this particular feature plays a central role in interference.

According to this proposal, the replication origin at the 3'-end of the VSV genome minus strand is recognized by a different replicase than the one playing a similar role at the 3'-end of the plus strand. The two types of replicases were further postulated to differ by the presence or absence of host cell factors. The synthesis of plus and minus DI RNAs can thus be accomplished by the same replicase (the one responsible for minus-strand genome replication) and involves only one kind of recognition event rather than two for standard virus. Furthermore, an additional kinetic advantage is gained if the synthesis or availability of plus-strand genome templates is rate-limiting during standard virus replication. A slightly different model involving only one replicase recognizing a "high affinity" binding site at the 3'-end of standard genome plus strands and a "low affinity" binding site at the 3'-end of standard genome minus strands was suggested by *Huang* et al. (1978). It is also possible to view the preferential replication of these DI RNAs (without invoking differential binding affinities) as a mass effect resulting from two DI RNA templates, with identical 3'-terminal sequences, competing with one standard virus RNA template for a single type of replicase (*Reichmann* and *Schnitzlein* 1979).

These models, which are not mutually exclusive, necessarily remain very speculative at this time since very little is known regarding the mechanism of standard VSV RNA replication. Nevertheless, the importance of stems in governing the replicative advantage of VSV DI RNAs is strongly supported by the observation that the transcribing VSV *DI 0.46*(= DI-LT$_1$), which lacks such complementary end sequences (see Fig. 2), replicates very poorly in the presence of other stem-containing DI RNAs during a single cycle of infection (*Perrault* and *Semler* 1979). This is so even when compared to *DI 0.50*(= DI-LT$_2$) which aside from stems differs only in having a slightly longer 5'-end genome segment. The transcribing VSV *DI 0.46* alone however, appears to interfere as well with standard virus replication as other VSV DI (*Reichmann* and *Schnitzlein* 1977; *Adachi* and *Lazzarini* 1978; *Reichmann* and *Schnitzlein* 1979). Whatever the mechanism of interference might be for this unique *DI 0.46* (see below), it appears to be superceded by the replicative advantage conferred by stems. It is likely also that the mere presence of these end sequences prevents any DI RNA from functioning as a template for mRNA synthesis. This is exemplified by VSV *DI 0.50* which is transcriptionally inert even though it contains all sequences necessary for transcription of four VSV genes (see Sections 3.2.4 and 5.2). This lack of transcription as mentioned above, could be crucial in governing interference.

Aside from preventing transcription, VSV DI stem sequences also serve as template for the synthesis of the short minus-strand leader RNA 46 nucleotides long) in vitro and in vivo (see Section 5.2). This small RNA is found only in very low levels in standard virus-infected cells, but is synthesized in 50-fold or more molar excess over DI RNA template in interfered infections (*Rao* and *Huang* 1979; *Leppert* et al. 1979; *Leppert* and *Kolakofsky* 1980; *Rao* and *Huang* 1980). The efficient synthesis of this minus-strand leader RNA from DI templates led *Rao* and *Huang* (1979) to suggest that it may play a role during interference by binding enzymes or substrates or by blocking specific complementary sequences. As mentioned previously (Section 5.2) a model suggested by *Leppert* et al. (1979) proposes that the availability of the VSV nucleocapsid N protein regulates the switch from transcription to replication by binding to the small plus-strand leader RNA (the 47-nucleotide long RNA copied from the 3'-end of the minus strand genome in vitro and in vivo) and promoting read-through synthesis of plus-strand genome copies past this strong stop signal. If the minus-strand leader RNA plays a similar role for minus-strand genome synthesis, then a decrease in the availability of N protein in interfered infection might account for the accumulation of the small minus-strand leader (*Leppert* et al. 1977; *Leppert* and *Kolakofsky* 1980). These speculations are consistent with the reported transcriptive mode of synthesis of this minus-strand leader (resistant to cycloheximide and enhanced in ts mutants which increase transcription) as well as its lack of association with the N core protein in interfered infections (*Rao* and *Huang* 1980). The latter is in contrast to plus-strand leader which for the most part is assembled into a ribonucleoprotein in standard virus infections (*Blumberg* et al. 1981). It is tempting to speculate that the plus-strand leader RNA synthesized in interfered infections might be rapidly degraded because of lack of N protein, thereby leading to decreased genome RNA synthesis. Whether this is the case or not, the continued study of these small leader RNAs, which represent initiating events in VSV replication, is at present a most promising approach to elucidating the details of DI-mediated interference and VSV genome replication.

As mentioned above, interference by the transcribing VSV *DI 0.46* most likely involves a different mechanism. Aside from the unique structural and replicative features already discussed, a number of additional properties of this DI support this notion. It is the only VSV DI shown to interfere heterotypically with the New Jersey VSV serotype (*Prevec* and *Kang* 1970; *Schnitzlein* and *Reichmann* 1976). The basis for this is unclear but the heterotypic interference is restricted to the Concan subgroup of VSV New Jersey and does not occur with the Hazelhurst subgroup (*Adachi* and *Lazzarini* 1978; *Reichmann* et al. 1978; *Metzel* et al. 1978; see also following Section).

The transcribing VSV DI also displays an unusual inactivation target size. A number of laboratories have shown that VSV DI possess a smaller UV target size for replication and interference than standard virus infectivity (*Holland* et al. 1976a; *Winship* and *Thacore* 1979; *Bay* and *Reichmann* 1979). In the careful quantitative study of *Bay* and *Reichmann* (1979) the target size of interference by various DI particles was found to correspond to the size of the whole molecule. The one exception, however, is the transcribing DI which exhibits a target size equivalent to about 42% of its RNA. In addition, these investigators showed that, in contrast to other VSV DI, the unique transcribing DI interferes with primary transcription of input standard virus in vivo. This DI isolate was shown previously to carry out its own in vivo primary transcription (minus the L gene) as well as some synthesis of DI size plus and minus strands in the absence of helper virus (*Johnson* and *Lazzarini* 1977b). Thus the unusual UV inactivation target size was interpreted as being a compromise between the requirements for replication of its genome and those for interference with primary transcription. These studies were recently further extended by *Bay* and *Reichmann* (1981) who demonstrated that active transcription in vivo by the DI itself is necessary for interference with heterotypic virus primary transcription and standard virus production. It is apparent from these results that the mechanism of interference by this unique DI is complex and involves at least one step of standard virus replication which is not affected by the interference activity of other VSV DI. Unfortunately at this time, the occasional preliminary reports on the isolation of new VSV DI originating from the 3'-end of the standard genome (*Adler* and *Banerjee* 1976; *Reichmann*, personal communication) which might be expected to behave like *DI 0.46* have not yet been confirmed.

5.4.2 Additional Parameters Affecting VSV DI Interference

Several additional aspects of interference by VSV DI need to be mentioned in order to appreciate the complexity of the phenomenon. Most importantly, replication of VSV DI RNAs is not always accompanied by interference. There are at least three distinct situations where this uncoupling can be observed: 1. growth of DI in "low interference" cell lines, 2. adding DI late during the course of standard VSV growth, and 3. support of DI with heterotypic helper virus.

The first of these situations has already been discussed in detail in Section 5.1. The second was noted by *Stampfer* et al. (1969) when they added VSV DI 2.5 h after infection with standard virus. This observation emphasizes that interference involves competition for an early step of virus multiplication (beyond penetration). In this regard it is interesting to note that VSV DI RNAs are rapidly assembled into nucleocapsids but accumulate under conditions of interference in the infected cell. They appear to be more slowly and less efficiently matured to virions than standard virus (*Palma* and *Huang* 1974; *Khan* and *Lazzarini* 1977; *Moyer* and *Gatchell* 1979). This deficiency of DI nucleocapsid budding may be due to insufficient availability of viral membrane proteins (*Moyer* and *Holmes* 1981) although what causes this protein specific deficiency is unknown.

The third case of replication without interference can be observed when Indiana VSV DI are supported by a heterotypic New Jersey VSV helper virus (*Schnitzlein* and *Reichmann* 1977b; *Khan* and *Lazzarini* 1977; *Adachi* and *Lazzarini* 1978). As mentioned before (previous Section) only the unique transcribing VSV Indiana DI causes interference under these conditions. These studies suggest that protein specificities, probably involving interactions between heterotypic polymerase and template ribonucleoproteins, are important in determining the outcome of competition between DI and standard genome RNA. The base sequence divergence between the two serotypes is extensive enough to result in very different T1 oligonucleotide maps (*Clewly* et al. 1977). The protein specificity of interference is further illustrated by the fact that chimeric DI (Indiana VSV DI RNA encapsidated in New Jersey VSV proteins) show a dramatic increase over pure Indiana DI in their interfering ability towards New Jersey standard virus (*Schnitzlein* and *Reichmann* 1977b).

Holland et al. (1976a) also reported a different sort of uncoupling phenomenon whereby VSV DI show strong interference in HeLa cells without apparent replication of biologically active DI ribonucleoproteins in the cytoplasm (pure DI RNA is not biologically active in interference assays). This exceptional case could either involve the replication of biologically inactive DI ribonucleoprotein (unable to interfere in BHK_{21} cells) or point to the existence of yet a different type of interference phenomenon in HeLa cells. The variable behaviour of HeLa cells in terms of DI replication mentioned previously (Section 4.1) however, hampers efforts to study this phenomenon further.

An additional important aspect of VSV DI interference is the question of whether it is an all or none phenomenon at the single cell level. The classical studies of *Bellett* and *Cooper* (1959) showed that, at a constant input multiplicity of standard virus, increasing input concentrations of DI result in an exponential decline of plaque-forming progeny in chick embryo cells at least over two orders of magnitude. These first-order kinetics at low-input concentrations of DI suggest that only one DI particle per infected cell is requir- ed to elicit complete interference. In contrast to this, *Khan* and *Lazzarini* (1977) reported the absence of single-hit inactivation with their VSV DI in BHK_{21} cells using radiolabeled viral RNA quantitation as their assay (massive replication of DI_{011} occurs at low-input DI multiplicities with only marginal interference with standard virus RNA synthesis). These contrasting results could be due to different host cells or virus strains employed, or the nature of the assays. More recently, *Sekellick* and *Marcus* (1980) analyzed plaque-forming virus yields from individual Vero-Green monkey kidney cells infected with standard VSV virus or DI. They concluded that indeed the presence of a single functional DI in a cell is sufficient to inhibit essentially all infectious virus production. However, at higher multiplicities of DI less interference is observed so that many coinfected cells yield inter- mediate levels of infectious virus. In light of the many parameters affecting DI genera- tion, replication, and interference discussed above, it seems reasonable to expect that the all or none interference results obtained represent only one end of the spectrum govern- ing the interaction between standard virus and DI.

A different approach to determining critical parameters in VSV DI interference was also pursued by *Schnitzlein* and *Reichmann* (1977a). These investigators compared nu- cleotide sequence homologies (by hybridization techniques) between one short DI RNA derived from the Glasgow New Jersey VSV isolate (now referred to as subtype Hazelhurst) and the Ogden New Jersey standard virus (now referred to as subtype Concan) with which it interferes efficiently. By this annealing test, the two RNAs are found to share no more than about 230 nucleotides in common (not neces- sarily in a single stretch). Similarly, the transcribing VSV Indiana DI which interferes heterotypically with New Jersey subtype Concan virus (see above) also shares only a small sequence, about 260 nucleotides long, in common with the heterotypic standard virus genome. These homologies are probably related, at least in part, to the highly con- served genomic end sequences of these different VSV serotypes as determined by direct base sequencing (*Colonno* and *Banerjee* 1978b; *Rowlands* 1979; *Keene* et al. 1979; *McGeoch* et al. 1980; *Keene* et al. 1981a). These data therefore also indirectly support a critical role for terminal sequences in the phenomenon of VSV DI interference.

Perhaps the most important instance of factors modulating interference by VSV DI, at least from an evolutionary point of view, is the situation documented by *Horodyski* and *Holland* (1980) and referred to briefly in Section 2.3. The standard VSV genome under- goes rapid and extensive mutational drift during persistence in cell culture or during re- peated high multiplicity lytic passage in the presence of DI (*Holland* et al. 1979; *Rowlands* et al. 1980). As little as 34 days after initiation of virus persistence, the standard virus re- covered in some cases is no longer subject to interference by the VSV DI originally em- ployed to establish the persistent culture, and cannot act as a helper for their replication.

Clones from these standard virus mutants, however, can still generate "interfering type" DI de novo when passaged serially (*Horodyski* and *Holland* 1980). The basis of this phenomenon is undoubtedly related to the selection of standard virus mutations which specifically affect interference by VSV DI. *Semler* and *Holland* (1979), for example, demonstrated the occurrence of seven base substitutions in the first 46 nucleotides at the 5'-end of the standard genome after 5 years of persistence. These results once again emphasize the importance of the minus-strand genome replication origin in controlling interference by VSV DI since the genome 3'-end sequence mutates much less rapidly during persistence (*Rowlands* et al. 1980). Mutations affecting viral polymerase protein activity are also likely to occur under these conditions, and the coevolution of replicase and template RNA structures during persistence provides a novel and fascinating approach for the study of virus attenuation.

Lastly, a recent report demonstrates an additional unusual aspect of VSV DI interference in that one particular VSV DI (*DI 0.52*) invariably and efficiently outcompetes the replication of a smaller VSV DI (*DI 0.33* = DI-T) in a single cycle of replication (*Huang* et al. 1981). This observation, which is reminiscent of the situation with the unique transcribing VSV DI which is outcompeted by other VSV DI, is interesting because both DI RNAs in this case were generated independently from the same virus and correspond to type I structures (see Fig. 1). The stem sizes are 55 and 45 bp long for the larger and smaller RNAs respectively (*D. Rao* and *A.S. Huang*, personal communication). The basis for the replicative advantage of the larger DI is unknown but it is unlikely to be directly related to stem sizes since this parameter does not affect relative interfering ability in other VSV DI (see previous Section). The presence of different point mutations in each of these two DI RNAs which are not present in standard virus was also reported and is perhaps responsible for this odd behaviour (*Hagen* and *Huang*, 1981). The accumulation of point mutations in DI RNAs may be more widespread than hitherto suspected and may also be related to the phenomenon of mutational drift observed in standard virus RNA during DI-mediated virus persistence.

5.5 Interference Mechanisms of Other RNA Virus DI

The complexities relating to DI interference in VSV are certainly not unique to this virus. The absence of similar documentation in other RNA virus DI systems reflect the paucity of relevant studies. Except for togaviruses and picornaviruses virtually nothing is known regarding mechanisms of interference, other than the general concept of replicase competition. In some cases, such as host cell effects on interference (Sections 4.1 and 5.1), the results obtained are analogous to the VSV system. However, it is reasonable to suspect that interference mechanisms might reflect the differing replication strategies of each virus group. Moreover, in contrast to VSV and paramyxoviruses, the majority of DI RNAs in other viruses are internal deletions. The segmented influenza and reoviruses also present an intriguing problem since DI RNAs derived from specific gene segments may interfere with the "coordinate" replication of all segments.

Schlesinger et al. (1975) proposed a simple model for alphavirus DI interference based on straightforward competition for a limited amount of viral replicase synthesized by standard virus. *Bruton* et al. (1976), however, proposed a mechanism for DI interference in this virus group based on a more rapid synthesis of DI RNAs because of their small size. Assuming that elongation rate might be limiting during RNA synthesis in vivo, the shorter DI RNAs, which contain the original genome replication origins at their ends, might be expected to accumulate faster as a result of two competition processes operating sequentially, one for the synthesis of minus strands and one for synthesis of plus strands. Some support for this hypothesis comes from the aforementioned sequential deletion phenomenon observed when togavirus DI are passaged repeatedly (see Sections 3.4.1 and 4.1). It is not clear, however, whether this evolution towards smaller size DI molecules involves the same mechanism as the one responsible for interference in a single replication cycle. It also seems unlikely that elongation rates rather than initiation rates would govern overall accumulation of viral RNAs in infected cells. More detailed studies of interference parameters in togavirus infections are needed to clarify these points. The different rates of selection of smaller DI RNAs upon passage in different cells (*Stark* and *Kennedy* 1978) do argue strongly that other factors besides size (host cell factors, encapsidation constraints, etc.) play an important role in interference by togavirus DI.

The UV target size for interfering activity by togavirus DI is smaller than that of virus infectivity (*Dimmock* and *Kennedy* 1978; *Kowal* and *Stollar* 1980) as found for VSV (Section 5.4.1) and influenza DI (Section 3.3.2). In the case of SV DI produced in BHK cells, the target size was shown to correspond to the physical size of the DI molecule but, oddly enough, that of SV DI produced in *A. albopictus* cells was about 25–30% smaller than expected (*Kowal* and *Stollar* 1980). It is not clear whether the latter case is due to complications resulting from the use of a different host cell in the assay or whether it suggests a different mechanism of interference as in the case of the VSV *DI 0.46* (Section 5.4.1).

Interference by poliovirus DI is thought to result from two independent effects acting in concert (*Cole* 1975). In contrast to other RNA viruses, the total level of viral RNA synthesis in cells coinfected with standard and DI remains essentially the same (this may reflect the relatively lower levels of interference seen in this system). The replication of standard virus RNA is thus decreased by a percentage close to the percentage of DI in the inoculum (as mentioned previously in Section 5.2, poliovirus DI synthesize RNA as efficiently as standard virus). Synthesis of capsid precursors coded for by the standard genome only is therefore reduced by a similar amount. A prediction borne out by the results obtained is that the percentage of standard virus produced in coinfected cells is the square of the percentage of standard virus in the inoculum. This mechanism, however, does not account for the enrichment or preferential replication of poliovirus DI (about 5–8% per passage in the studies of *Cole* and colleagues). This crucial phenomenon remains unexplained but can be affected by temperature and transient treatment with cycloheximide (*Cole* and *Baltimore* 1973c). Some possible explanations involving preferential encapsidation or replication of DI RNAs, or more rapid completion of the first round of protein synthesis in the earliest events of infection were suggested (*Cole* 1975). As in other virus DI systems, however, the interference phenomenon is likely to be complex since the interference level of another picornavirus (mengovirus), is affected by the host cell (Section 5.1).

Overall, it seems clear that a detailed understanding of interference by RNA virus DI is limited by our current knowledge of standard virus replication. Progress in one area is often spurred by advances in the other. The elucidation of the exact segment composition of infectious influenza virions, for example, provided the basis for the characterization of DI RNAs. On the other hand, the discovery of stem structures in VSV DI

RNAs is paving the way for understanding initiation of RNA replication in standard virus.

6 DI of DNA Viruses – Brief Overview

For reasons outlined in the introduction to this review, DI of DNA viruses may be thought of as playing a less important role in nature than DI of RNA viruses. It is intriguing, however, to note the many parallels between these two different worlds of defective viruses. All DNA viruses, with the possible exception of adenoviruses and poxviruses, have been shown to generate DI. The best studied are the so-called evolutionary variants in the papovaviruses (reviewed in *Fareed* and *Davoli* 1977; *Kelly* and *Nathans* 1977; *Brockman* 1977; *Fried* and *Griffin* 1977). These clearly interfere with standard virus replication by virtue of reiterated origins of replication (*Lee* and *Nathans* 1979). They contain extensive rearrangements of the viral genome which are often linked to host cell DNA sequences. Some specificity in the type of host DNA selected may exist perhaps in view of substituting for viral functions (*Papamatheakis* et al. 1981; *Carroll* et al. 1981).

Parvovirus DI often contain internal genome deletions and snap-back DNAs (*Faust* and *Ward* 1979; *de la Maza* and *Carter* 1980) similar in structure to some VSV DI RNAs (Section 3.2.3). The origin of these snap-back DI DNAs probably differs from their VSV counterparts, however, since parvovirus standard DNA replicates via self-complementary or snap-back intermediates. Herpesviruses also generate DI which contain extensive genome rearrangements (*Murray* et al. 1975; *Kaplan* et al. 1976; *Henry* et al. 1979; *Stinski* et al. 1979; *Frenkel* et al. 1980). Even the filamentatous DNA bacteriophages were shown to produce DI (*Griffith* and *Kornberg* 1974; *Enea* and *Zinder* 1975; *Chen* and *Ray* 1978; *Ravetch* et al. 1979).

Recombinational mechanisms leading to generation of DI genomes of DNA viruses may well have features in common with general recombination in eucaryotic cells. Replication of small DNA viruses in particular is very much dependent on the host cell DNA replication enzymes. Nevertheless, there may be unknown recombinational features unique to the virus replication complex which govern DI generation. The recurring and independent emergence of very closely related evolutionary variants of SV40 (with identical host-viral DNA sequence junctions) suggests that some unknown mechanism leading to nonhomologous recombination between viral and host genomes is at play (*Singer* et al. 1978; *Papamatheakis* et al. 1981).

A host effect on the generation and/or amplification of papovavirus DI (*Norkin* et al. 1981; *O'Neill* and *Carroll* 1981), reminescent of that observed in RNA viruses, was also reported. The most intriguing parallel between the two virus systems, however, is the accumulating evidence that DI of DNA viruses also play a role in the establishment and/or maintenance of persistent infections. This has now been reported for SV40 and BKV (*Norkin* 1979; *O'Neill* and *Carroll* 1981), human cytomegalovirus (*Stinski* et al. 1979), and equine herpesvirus type 1 (*Robinson* et al. 1980). Of course, DNA viruses can also persist in host cells by means of integration. Perhaps DI confer evolutionary advantages in certain types of host virus associations. Whatever the case may be, the potential biological role of DI in DNA viruses is worthy of further exploration.

7 Concluding Remarks

The last decade has witnessed a major expansion of studies focused on DI biology. The diversity of genomic sequence rearrangements in these particles reflects the increased plasticity and evolutionary adaptability of viral genomes when they are no longer required to code for an infectious unit. DI genomes most likely accumulate by selective amplification of some defective molecules generated at low frequency during standard virus replication. The genomic rearrangements in DI of RNA viruses can best be explained by strand-switching of the viral replicase complex during synthesis. Some DI RNA structures strongly suggest that this strand-switching can occur between different genome templates. The parallels between this mechanism and homologous genetic recombination (see general model, Section 4.3.3) are intriguing and imply strongly that such recombination is universal among RNA viruses.

DI effectively outcompete their parent helper virus for multiplication without suppressing their growth entirely. The various DI template structures therefore teach us the minimal sequence requirements useful in controlling virus multiplication, a lesson which suggests strategies for preventing virus disease in the future.

The host cell often affects the replication and properties of DI independently of its influence on standard virus and more importantly, the interplay between infectious virus, DI, and host cell often leads to virus persistence in culture without cell killing. It would be surprising if DI were not involved in at least some aspects of virus multiplication in animal and human infections. Measles virus can certainly persist in humans for several years before it triggers subacute sclerosing panencephalitis. Other chronic or degenerative human diseases are also suspected to involve slow growing or latent viruses. DI could play a role in such infections but this may be difficult to establish if they exert their effects locally or during a restricted phase of virus spread.

Perhaps more important than the disease aspect, DI represent an important evolutionary element in nature. These subgenomes represent ideal vehicles for rapid evolution since they are much freer to mutate than infectious virus. Moreover, they appear to exert a mutational pressure on the standard virus itself by virtue of their interfering properties. It is conceivable that DI are only a subclass of virus-related sequences which interact with both host cells and infectious viruses. In analogy to the intimate relationship of DNA virus genomes and transposons with host cells, one can also imagine RNA virus sequences (DI?) remaining in association with their host in an episomal form, after losing the ability to be packaged and transmitted to other cells. The virus-like particles of fungi may in fact represent such an association.

The next decade of research on DI is likely to reveal fascinating aspects of virus growth control. A great deal of sequence analysis, now a favorite tool of nouveau molecular biologists, is likely to shed some light on mechanisms of origin and replication of DI. The basic conclusion that replication origin sequences are a major determinant of interference by these particles will undoubtedly be refined by the advent of in vitro systems of replication. Lastly, continued study of the role of DI in mutational drift during persistence is setting the stage for a much more dynamic understanding of virus evolution.

Acknowledgments. Work described in this review from the author's laboratory was supported by Research Grant No. AI 14365 from the National Institute of Allergy and Infectious Diseases and

Grant No. 1-734 from the March of Dimes Birth Defects Foundation. The author is recipient of a Research Career Development Award from the National Institutes of Health. I wish to especially thank Drs. *Sondra Schlesinger, Marcella McClure,* and *Stuart Nichol* for critical reading of the manuscript and many helpful suggestions. I also thank the many colleagues who have kindly supplied publication preprints and unpublished material, as well as *Laverne Wodraska* for typing the manuscript.

References

Adachi I, Lazzarini RA (1978) Elementary aspects of autointerference and the replication of defective virus particles. Virology 87:152-163

Adler R, Banerjee AK (1976) Analysis of the RNA species isolated from defective particles of vesicular stomatitis virus. J Gen Virol 33:51-60

Agol VI (1980) Structure, translation, and replication of picornaviral genomes. Prog Med Virol 26: 119-157

Ahmed R, Fields BN (1981) Reassortment of genome segments between reovirus defective interfering particles and infectious virus: Construction of temperature-sensitive and attenuated viruses by rescue of mutations from DI particles. Virology, (in press)

Ahmed R, Graham AF (1977) Persistent infections in L cells with temperature-sensitive mutants of reovirus. J Virol 23:250-262

Atabekov JG (1977) Defective and satellite plant viruses. In: Fraenkel-Conrat H, Wagner RR (eds) Comprehensive virology, vol 11, Plenum Press, New York, pp 143-193

Baltimore D (1971) Expression of animal virus genomes. Bacteriol Rev 35:235-241

Banerjee A (1980) The in vitro mRNA transcription process. In: Bishop DHL (ed) Rhabdoviruses, vol II, CRC Press, Florida, pp 35-50

Banerjee AK, Abraham G, Colonno RJ (1977) Vesicular stomatitis virus: Mode of transcription. J Gen Virol 34:1-8

Bay PHS, Reichmann ME (1979) UV inactivation of the biological activity of defective interfering particles generated by vesicular stomatitis virus. J Virol 32:876-884

Bay PHS, Reichmann ME (1981) In vivo inhibition of primary transcription of vesicular stomatitis virus by a defective interfering particle. In: Bishop DHL, Compans RW (eds) Replication of negative strand viruses. Elsevier North Holland, New York

Bean WJ, Simpson RW (1976) Transcription activity and genome composition of defective influenza virus. J Virol 18:365-369

Bellett AJD, Cooper PD (1959) Some properties of the transmissible interfering component of VSV preparations. J Gen Microb 21:498-509

Bishop DHL, Shope RE (1979) Bunyaviridae. In: Fraenkel-Conrat H, Wagner RR (eds) Comprehensive virology, vol 14. Plenum Press, New York, pp 1-132

Blumberg BM, Leppert M, Kolakofsky D (1981) Interaction of VSV leader RNA and nucleocapsid protein may control VSV genome replication. Cell 23:831-845

Blumenthal T, Carmichael GG (1979) RNA replication: Function and structure of $Q\beta$-replicase. Annu Rev Biochem 48:525-548

Bostian KA, Hopper JE, Rogers DT, Tipper DJ (1980) Translational analysis of the killer-associated virus-like particle ds RNA genome of S. cerevisiae: M ds RNA encodes toxin. Cell 19:403-414

Brockman WW (1977) Evolutionary variants of simian virus 40. Prog Med Virol 23:69-95

Bruenn JA (1980) Virus-like particles of yeast. Ann Rev Microbiol 34:49-68

Bruenn JA, Brennan VE (1980) Yeast viral double-stranded RNAs have heterogenous 3' termini. Cell 19:923-933

Bruenn J, Kane W (1978) Relatedness of the double-stranded RNAs present in yeast virus-like particles. J Virol 26:762-772

Bruton CJ, Kennedy SIT (1976) Defective-interfering particles of Semliki Forest virus: Structural differences between standard virus and defective-interfering particles. J Gen Virol 31:383-395

Bruton CJ, Porter A, Kennedy SIT (1976) Defective-interfering particles of Semliki Forest virus: Intracellular events during interference. J Gen Virol 31:397-416

Canaani E, Aaronson SA (1980) Isolation and characterization of naturally occurring deletion mutants of Moloney murine sarcoma virus. Virology 105:456–466

Carroll D, Hansen JL, Maryon EB, O'Neill F (1981) SV40 defectives selected during low multiplicity passage on A172 human glioblastoma cells. Virology, (in press)

Celma ML, Ehrenfeld E (1975) Translation of poliovirus RNA in vitro: Detection of two initiation sites. J Mol Biol 98:761–780

Chanda PK, Kang CY, Banerjee AK (1980) Synthesis in vitro of the full length complement of defective-interfering particle RNA of vesicular stomatitis virus. Proc Natl Acad Sci USA 77: 3927–3931

Chen T-C, Ray DS (1978) Replication of bacteriophage M13. XIII. Structure and replication of cloned M13 miniphage. J Mol Biol 125:107–121

Choppin PW (1969) Replication of influenza virus in a continuous cell line: High yield of infectious virus from cells inoculated at high multiplicity. Virology 39:130–134

Choppin PW, Compans RW (1975) Reproduction of paramyxoviruses. In: Fraenkel-Conrat H, Wagner RR (eds) Comprehensive virology, vol 4. Plenum Press, New York, pp 95–178

Choppin PW, Pons MW (1970) The RNAs of infective and incomplete influenza virions grown in MDBK and HeLa cells. Virology 42:603

Chow JM, Schnitzlein WM, Reichmann ME (1977) Expression of genetic information contained in the RNA of a defective interfering particle of vesicular stomatitis virus. Virology 77:579–588

Clerx-Van Haaster CM, Clewly JP, Bishop DHL (1980) Oligonucleotide sequence analyses indicate that VSV LT defective interfering virus particle RNA is made by internal deletion, and evidence for similar transcription polyadenylation signals for the synthesis of all VSV mRNA species. J Virol 33:807–817

Clewley JP, Bishop DHL (1978) Evolution of rhabdovirus genomes. In: Mahy BWJ, Barry RD (eds) Negative strand viruses and the host cell. Academic Press, London, pp 599–606

Clewley JP, Bishop DHL, Kang C-Y, Coffin J, Schnitzlein WM, Reichmann ME, Shope RE (1977) Oligonucleotide fingerprints of RNA species obtained from rhabdoviruses belonging to the vesicular stomatitis virus subgroup. J Virol 23:152–166

Cole CN (1975) Defective interfering (DI) particles of poliovirus. Prog Med Virol 20:180–207

Cole CN, Baltimore D (1973a) Defective interfering particles of poliovirus. II. Nature of the defect. J Mol Biol 76:325–343

Cole CN, Baltimore D (1973b) Defective interfering particles of poliovirus. III. Interference and enrichment. J Mol Biol 76:345–361

Cole CN, Baltimore D (1973c) Defective interfering particles of poliovirus. IV. Mechanisms of enrichment. J Virol 12:1414–1426

Cole CN, Smoler D, Wimmer E, Baltimore D (1971) Defective interfering particles of poliovirus. I. Isolation and physical properties. J Virol 7:478–485

Colonno RJ, Banerjee AK (1978) Complete nucleotide sequence of the leader RNA synthesized in vitro by vesicular stomatitis virus. Cell 15:93–101

Colonno RJ, Banerjee AK (1978b) Nucleotide sequence of the leader RNA of the New Jersey serotype of vesicular stomatitis virus. Nucleic Acids Res 5:4165–4176

Colonno RJ, Lazzarini RA, Keene JD, Banerjee AK (1977) In vitro synthesis of messenger RNA by a defective interfering particle of vesicular stomatitis virus. Proc Natl Acad Sci USA 74: 1884–1888

Cooper PD (1977) Genetics of picornaviruses. In: Fraenkel-Conrat H, Wagner RR (eds) Comprehensive virology, vol 9. Plenum Press, New York, pp 133–207

Cords CE, Holland JJ (1964) Replication of poliovirus RNA induced by heterologous virus. Proc Natl Acad Sci USA 51:1080–1082

Coward JE, Harter DH, Hsu KC, Morgan C (1971) Electron microscopic study of development of vesicular stomatitis virus using ferritin-labeled antibodies. J Gen Virol 13:27–34

Crumpton WM, Dimmock NJ, Minor PD, Avery RJ (1978) The RNAs of defective-interfering influenza virus. Virology 90:370–373

Crumpton WM, Clewley JP, Dimmock NJ, Avery RJ (1979) Origin of subgenomic RNAs in defective-interfering influenza virus. FEMS Microbiol Lett 6:431–434

Crumpton WM, Avery RJ, Dimmock NJ (1981) Influence of the host cell on the genomic and subgenomic RNA content of defective-interfering influenza virus. J Gen Virol 53:173–177

Darnell MB, Koprowski H (1974) Genetically determined resistance to infection with group B arboviruses. II. Increased production of interfering particles in cell cultures from resistant mice. J Infect Dis 129:248–256

Davis AR, Nayak DP (1979) Sequence relationships among defective interfering influenza viral RNAs. Proc Natl Acad Sci USA 76:3092–3096

Davis AR, Hiti AL, Nayak DP (1980) Influenza defective interfering viral RNA is formed by internal deletion of genomic RNA. Proc Natl Acad Sci USA 77:215–219

De BK, Nayak DP (1980) Defective interfering influenza viruses and host cells: Establishment and maintenance of persistent influenza virus infection in MDBK and HeLa cells. J Virol 36:847–859

de la Maza LM, Carter BJ (1980) Molecular structure of adeno-associated virus variant DNA. J Biol Chem 255:3194–3203

Dimmock NJ, Kennedy SIT (1978) Prevention of death in Semliki Forest virus infected mice by administration of defective interfering Semliki Forest Virus. J Gen Virol 39:231–242

Dohner D, Monroe S, Weiss B, Schlesinger S (1979) Oligonucleotide mapping studies of standard and defective Sindbis virus RNA. J Virol 29:794–798

Domingo E, Sabo D, Taniguchi T, Weissman C (1978) Nucleotide sequence heterogeneity of an RNA phage population. Cell 13:735–744

Dubin DT, Timko K, Gillies S, Stollar V (1979) The extreme 5′ terminal sequences of Sindbis virus 26 and 42s RNA. Virology 98:131–141

Duesberg PH (1968) The RNA's of influenza virus. Proc Natl Acad Sci USA 59:930–937

Dutko FJ, Pfau CJ (1978) Arenavirus defective interfering particles mask the cell-killing potential of standard virus. J Gen Virol 38:195–208

Eaton BT (1975) Defective-interfering particles of Semliki Forest virus generated in BHK cells do not interfere with viral RNA synthesis in Aedes albopictus cells. Virology 68:534–538

Eaton BT (1977) Evidence for the synthesis of defective particles by Aedes albopictus cells persistently infected with Sindbis virus. Virology 77:843–848

Eaton BT, Faulkner P (1973) Altered pattern of viral RNA synthesis in cells infected with standard and defective Sindbis virus. Virology 51:85–93

Emerson SU, Wagner RR (1972) Dissociation and reconstitution of the transcriptase and template activities of vesicular stomatitis B and T virions. J Virol 10:297–309

Emerson SU, Dierks PM, Parsons JT (1977) In vitro synthesis of a unique RNA species by a T particle of vesicular stomatitis virus. J Virol 23:708–716

Enea V, Zinder ND (1975) A deletion mutant of bacteriophage fl containing no intact cistrons. Virology 68:105–114

Epstein DA, Herman RC, Chien I, Lazzarini RA (1980) Defective interfering particle generated by internal deletion of the vesicular stomatitis virus genome. J Virol 33:818–829

Estis LF, Temin HM (1979) Suppression of multiplication of avian sarcoma virus by rapid spread of transformation-defective virus of the same subgroup. J Virol 31:389–397

Fareed GC, Davoli D (1977) Molecular biology of papovaviruses. Annu Rev Biochem 46:471–522

Faulkner GP, Lazzarini RA (1980) Homologous interference by defective virus particles. In: Bishop DHL (ed) Rhabdoviruses, vol II, CRC Press, Florida, pp 163–176

Faust EA, Ward DC (1979) Incomplete genomes of the parvovirus minute virus of mice: Selective conservation of genome termini, including the origin for DNA replication. J Virol 32:276–292

Flamand A (1980) Rhabdovirus genetics. In: Bishop DHL (ed) Rhabdoviruses, vol II, CRC Press, Florida, pp 115–140

Freeman GJ, Rao DD, Huang AS (1978) Genome organization of vesicular stomatitis virus: Mapping ts G 41 and the defective interfering T particle. In: Mahy BWJ, Barry RD (eds) Negative strand viruses and the host cell. Academic Press, London, pp 261–270

Frenkel N, Locker H, Vlazny DA (1980) Studies of defective herpes simplex viruses. Ann NY Acad Sci 354:347–370

Frey TK, Jones EV, Cardamone Jr JJ, Youngner JS (1979) Induction of interferon in L cells by defective interfering (DI) particles of vesicular stomatitis virus: lack of correlation with content of [±] snapback RNA. Virology 99:95–102

Frey TK, Frielle DW, Youngner JS (1981) Standard vesicular stomatitis virus is required for interferon induction in L cells by defective interfering particles. In: Bishop DHL, Compans RW (eds) Replication of negative strand viruses. Elsevier North Holland, New York

Fried HM, Fink GR (1978) Electron microscopic heteroduplex analysis of "killer" double-stranded RNA species from yeast. Proc Natl Acad Sci USA 75:4224–4228

Fried M, Griffin BE (1977) Organization of the genomes of polyoma virus and SV40. Adv Cancer Res 24:67–113

Friedman RM, Costa JR (1976) Fate of interferon treated cells. Infect Immun 13:487–493

Furman PA, Hallum JV (1973) RNA-dependent DNA polymerase activity in preparations of a mutant of Newcastle disease virus arising from persistently infected L cells. J Virol 12:548–555

Gaidamovich SY, Cherednichenko YN, Zhdanov VM (1978) On the mechanism of the persistence of lymphocytic choriomeningitis virus in the continuous cell line Detroit-6. Intervirology 9:156–161

Garoff H, Frischauf A-M, Simons K, Lehrach H, Delius H (1980a) Nucleotide sequence of cDNA coding for Semliki Forest virus membrane glycoproteins. Nature 288:236–241

Garoff H, Frischauf A-M, Simons K, Lehrach H, Delius H (1980b) The capsid protein of Semliki Forest virus has clusters of basis amino acids and prolines in its amino-terminal region. Proc Natl Acad Sci USA 77:6376–6380

Gillies S, Stollar V (1980a) The production of high yields of infectious vesicular stomatitis virus in *A. albopictus* cells and comparisons with replication in BHK-21 cells. Virology 107:509–513

Gillies S, Stollar V (1980b) Generation of defective interfering particles of vesicular stomatitis virus in Aedes albopictus cells. Virology 107:497–508

Gimenez HB, Compans RW (1980) Defective interfering Tacaribe virus and persistently infected cells. Virology 107:229–239

Griffith J, Kornberg A (1974) Mini M13 bacteriophage: Circular fragments of M13 DNA are replicated and packaged during normal infections. Virology 59:139–152

Guild GM, Stollar V (1975) Defective interfering particles of Sindbis virus. III. Intracellular viral RNA species in chick embryo cell cultures. Virology 67:24–41

Guild GM, Stollar V (1977) Defective interfering particles of Sindbis virus. V. Sequence relationships between SV$_{STD}$ 42S RNA and intracellular defective viral RNAs. Virology 77:175–188

Guild GM, Flores L, Stollar V (1977) Defective interfering particles of Sindbis virus. IV. Virion RNA species and molecular weight determination of defective double-stranded RNA. Virology 77:158–174

Haase AT, Stowring L, Ventura P, Traynor B, Johnson K, Swoaveland P, Smith M, Britten-Darnall MB, Faras A, Narayan O (1977) Role of DNA intermediates in persistent infections caused by RNA viruses. In: Schlessinger D (ed) Microbiology–1977. American Society for Microbiology, Washington DC, pp 478–483

Hagen FS, Huang AS (1981) Comparison of ribonucleotide sequences from the genome of vesicular stomatitis virus and two of its defective-interfering particles. J Virol 37:363–371

Hastie ND, Brennan V, Bruenn JA (1978) No homology between double stranded RNA and nuclear DNA of yeast. J Virol 28:1002–1005

Henry BE, Newcomb WW, O'Callaghan DJ (1979) Biological and biochemical properties of defective interfering particles of equine herpesvirus type 1. Virology 92:495–506

Herman RC, Adler S, Lazzarini RA, Colonno RJ, Banerjee AK, Westphal H (1978) Intervening polyadenylate sequences in RNA transcripts of vesicular stomatitis virus. Cell 15:587–596

Hill VM, Simonsen CC, Summers DF (1979) Characterization of vesicular stomatitis virus replicating complexes isolated in renografin gradients. Virology 99:75–83

Holland JJ, Villarreal LP (1974) Persistent non-cytocidal vesicular stomatitis virus infections mediated by defective T particles that suppress virion transcriptase. Proc Natl Acad Sci USA 71:2956–2960

Holland JJ, Villarreal LP (1975) Purification of defective interfering T particles of vesicular stomatitis and rabies viruses generated in vivo in brains of newborn mice. Virology 67:438–449

Holland JJ, Villarreal LP, Breindl M (1976a) Factors involved in the generation and replication of rhabdovirus defective T particles. J Virol 17:805–815

Holland JJ, Villarreal LP, Breindl M, Semler BL, Kohne D (1976b) Defective interfering virus particles attenuate virus lethality in vivo and in vitro. In: Baltimore D, Huang AS, Fox CF (eds) Animal virology. ICN-UCLA Symposia on molecular and cellular biology, vol IV. Academic Press, New York, pp 773–786

Holland JJ, Villarreal LP, Welsh RM, Oldstone MBA, Kohne D, Lazzarini R, Scolnick E (1976c) Long-term persistent vesicular stomatitis virus and rabies virus infection of cells in vitro. J Gen Virol 33:193–211

Holland JJ, Semler BL, Jones C, Perrault J, Reid L, Roux L (1978) Role of DI, virus mutation, and host response in persistent infections by envelope RNA viruses. In: Stevens JG, Todaro GJ, Fox CP (eds) Persistent viruses. ICN-UCLA Symposia on molecular and cellular biology, vol XI. Academic Press, New York, pp 57–73

Holland JJ, Grabau EA, Jones CL, Semler BL (1979) Evolution of multiple genome mutations during long-term persistent infection by vesicular stomatitis virus. Cell 16:495–504

Holland JJ, Kennedy SIT, Semler BL, Jones CL, Roux L, Grabau EA (1980) Defective interfering RNA viruses and the host cell response. In: Fraenkel-Conrat H, Wagner RR (eds) Comprehensive virology, vol. 16. Plenum Press, New York, pp 137–192

Horodyski FM, Holland JJ (1980) Viruses isolated from cells persistently infected with vesicular stomatitis virus show altered interactions with defective interfering particles. J Virol 36:627–631

Huang AS (1973) Defective interfering viruses. Ann Rev Microbiol 27:101–117

Huang AS (1977) Viral pathogenesis and molecular biology. Bacteriol Rev 41:811–821

Huang AS, Baltimore D (1970) Defective viral particles and viral disease processes. Nature 226: 325–327

Huang AS, Baltimore D (1977) Defective interfering animal viruses. In: Fraenkel-Conrat H, Wagner RR (eds) Comprehensive virology, vol 10. Plenum Press, New York, pp 73–106

Huang AS, Manders EK (1972) Ribonucleic acid synthesis of vesicular stomatitis virus. IV. Transcription by standard virus in the presence of defective interfering particles. J Virol 9:909–916

Huang AS, Little SP, Oldstone MBA, Rao D (1978) Defective interfering particles: Their effect on gene expression and replication of vesicular stomatitis virus. In: Stevens JG, Todaro GH, Fox CF (eds) Persistent viruses. ICN-UCLA Symposia on molecular and cellular biology, vol VI. Academic Press, New York, pp 399–408

Huang AS, Rao DD, Lanman G (1981) Defective interfering particles of vesicular stomatitis virus: structure-function relationships. Ann NY Acad Sci 354:238–250

Humphries S, Knauert F, Ehrenfeld E (1979) Capsid protein precursor is one of two initiated products of translation of poliovirus RNA in vitro. J Virol 30:481–488

Igarashi A, Stollar V (1976) Failure of defective-interfering particles of Sindbis virus produced in BHK or chicken cells to affect viral replication in Aedes albopictus cells. J Virol 19:398–408

Igarashi A, Koo R, Stollar V (1977) Evolution and properties of Aedes albopictus cell cultures persistently infected with Sindbis virus. Virology 82:69–83

Jacobson S, Dutko FJ, Pfau CJ (1979) Determinants of spontaneous recovery and persistence in MDCK cells infected with lymphocytic choriomeningitis virus. J Gen Virol 44:113–121

Janda JM, Nayak DP (1979) Defective influenza viral ribonucleoproteins cause interference. J Virol 32:697–702

Janda JM, Davis AR, Nayak DP, De BK (1979) Diversity and generation of defective interfering influenza virus particles. Virology 95:45–48

Johnson LD, Lazzarini RA (1977a) The 5' terminal nucleotide of RNA from vesicular stomatitis virus defective interfering particles. Virology 77:836–866

Johnson LD, Lazzarini RA (1977b) Replication of viral RNA by a defective interfering vesicular stomatitis virus particles in the absence of helper virus. Proc Natl Acad Sci USA 74:4387–4391

Johnson LD, Lazzarini RA (1978) Gene expression by a defective interfering particle of vesicular stomatitis virus. In: Stevens JG, Todaro GJ, Fox CF (eds) Persistent virus. ICN-UCLA Symposia on molecular and cellular biology, vol XI. Academic Press, New York, pp 409–416

Johnson LD, Lazzarini RA (1980) RNA synthesis by defective interfering vesicular stomatitis virus particles. In: Bishop DHL (ed) Rhabdoviruses, vol II. CRC Press, Florida, pp 177–188

Johnston RE, Tovell DR, Brown DT, Faulkner P (1975) Interfering passages of Sindbis virus: concomitant appearance of interference, morphological variants and truncated viral RNA. J Virol 16:951–958

Joklik WK (1980) The structure and function of the reovirus genome. Ann NY Acad Sci 354:107–124

Kääriäinen L, Soderlund H (1978) Structure and replication of α-viruses. Curr Top Microb Immunol 82:15–69

Kane WP, Pietras DF, Bruenn JA (1979) Evolution of defective-interfering double-stranded RNAs of the yeast killer virus. J Virol 32:692–696

Kang CY (1980) Interference induced by defective interfering particles. In: Bishop DHL (ed) Rhabdoviruses, vol II. CRC Press, Florida, pp 201–220

Kang CY, Allen R (1978) Host function-dependent induction of defective-interfering particles of vesicular stomatitis virus. J Virol 25:202–206

Kang CY, Tischfield JA (1978) Host-gene control in generation of vesicular stomatitis defective interfering virus particles. In: International virology IV. Centre for Agricultural Publishing and Documentation, Wageningen, p 240

Kang CY, Glimp T, Clewley JP, Bishop DHL (1978a) Studies on the generation of vesicular stomatitis virus (Indiana serotype) defective interfering particles. Virology 84:142–152

Kang CY, Glimp T, Allen R (1978b) Host cell function dependent induction of defective interfering particles of vesicular stomatitis virus. In: Mahy BWJ, Barry RD (eds) Negative strand viruses and the host cell. Academic Press, London, pp 501–513

Kaplan AS, Ben-Porat T, Rubenstein AS (1976) On the mechanism of herpesvirus DNA replication and the genesis of defective particles. In: Borek C, King DW (eds) Cancer biology, vol III: Epidemiology, molecular events, oncogenicity and therapy. Stratton Intercontinental Medical Book, New York, pp 61–86

Kascsak RJ, Lyons MJ (1978) Bunyamvera Virus. II. The generation and nature of defective interfering particles. Virology 89:539–546

Kawai A, Matsumoto S (1977) Interfering and noninterfering defective particles generated by a rabies small plaque variant virus. Virology 76:60–71

Keene JD, Rosenberg M, Lazzarini RA (1977) Characterization of the 3′ terminus of RNA isolated from vesicular stomatitis virus and from its defective interfering particles. Proc Natl Acad Sci USA 74:1353–1357

Keene JD, Schubert M, Lazzarini RA, Rosenberg M (1978) Nucleotide sequence homology at the 3′ termini of RNA from vesicular stomatitis virus and its defective interfering particles. Proc Natl Acad Sci USA 75:3225–3229

Keene JD, Schubert M, Lazzarini RA (1979) Terminal sequences of vesicular stomatitis virus RNA are both complementary and conserved. J Virol 32:167–174

Keene JD, Schubert M, Lazzarini RA (1980) Intervening sequence between the leader region and the nucleocapsid gene of vesicular stomatitis virus RNA. J Virol 33:789–794

Keene JD, Pironica-Worms H, Isaac CL (1981a) Structure and origin of terminal complementarity in the RNA of DI-LT(HR) and sequence arrangements at the 5′ ends of VSV RNA. In: Bishop BHL, Compans RW (eds) Replication of negative strand viruses. Elsevier North Holland, New York

Keene JD, Chien IM, Lazzarini RA (1981b) Vesicular stomatitis defective interfering particle containing a muted, internal leader RNA gene. Proc Natl Acad Sci USA 18:2090–2094

Kelly TJ, Nathans D (1977) The genome of simian virus 40. Adv Virus Res 21:85–173

Kennedy SIT (1976) Sequence relationships between the genome and the intracellular RNA species of standard and defective-interfering Semliki Forest virus. J Mol Biol 108:491–511

Kennedy SIT (1980) Synthesis of alphavirus RNA. In: Schlesinger RW (ed) The togaviruses, biology, structure, replication. Academic Press, New York, pp 351–368

Kennedy SIT, Bruton CJ, Weiss B, Schlesinger S (1976) Defective interfering passages of Sindbis virus: Nature of the defective virion RNA. J Virol 19:1034–1043

Khan SR, Lazzarini RA (1977) The relationship between autointerference and the replication of a defective interfering particle. Virology 77:189–201

King CC, King MW, Garry RF, Wan KM, Ulug ET, Waite MRF (1979) Effect of incubation time on the generation of defective-interfering particles during undiluted serial passage of Sindbis virus in Aedes albopictus and chick cells. Virology 96:229–238

Kingsbury DW (1977) Paramyxoviruses. In: Nayak DP (ed) The molecular biology of animal viruses, vol 1. Marcel Dekker, New York, pp 349–382

Kingsbury DW, Portner A (1970) On the genesis of incomplete Sendai virions. Virology 42:872–879

Kingsbury DW, Portner A, Darlington RW (1970) Properties of incomplete Sendai virions and subgenomic viral RNA's. Virology 42:857–871

Kitamura N, Adler C, Wimmer E (1980) Structure and expression of the picornavirus genome. Ann NY Acad Sci 354:183–201

Kolakofsky D (1976) Isolation and characterization of Sendai virus DI-RNAs. Cell 8:547–555

Kolakofsky D (1979) Studies on the generation and amplification of Sendai virus defective-interfering genomes. Virology 93:589–593

Kowal KJ, Stollar V (1980) Differential sensitivity of infectious and defective-interfering particles of Sindbis virus to ultraviolet irradiation. Virology 103:149–157

Kowal K, Stollar V, Dubin DT (1980) The 5′-terminal sequences of Sindbis virus defective RNA [Abstr] Am Soc Microb 1980, p 240

Krug RM, Bouloy M, Plotch SJ (1981) The 5' ends of influenza viral messenger RNAs are donated by capped cellular RNAs. Trends in Biochem Sci 6:7–10

Lamb RA, Lai C-J (1980) Sequence of interrupted and uninterrupted mRNAs and cloned DNA coding for the two overlapping nonstructural proteins of influenza virus. Cell 21:475–485

Lazzarini RA, Weber GH, Johnson LD, Stamminger GM (1975) Covalently linked message and anti-message (genomic) RNA from a defective vesicular stomatitis virus particle. J Mol Biol 97:289–308

Leamnson RN, Reichmann ME (1974) The RNA of defective vesicular stomatitis virus particles in relation to viral cistrons. J Mol Biol 85:551–568

Lee TNH, Nathans D (1979) Evolutionary variants of simian virus 40: replication and encapsidation of variant DNA. Virology 92:291–298

Lenard J, Compans RW (1975) Polypeptide composition of incomplete influenza virus grown in MDBK cells. Virology 65:418–426

Leppert M, Kolakofsky D (1980) Effect of defective interfering particles on plus and minus strand leader RNAs in vesicular stomatitis virus-infected cells. J Virol 35:704–709

Leppert M, Kort L, Kolakofsky D (1977) Further characterization of Sendai virus DI-RNAs: A model for their generation. Cell 12:539–552

Leppert M, Rittenhouse L, Perrault J, Summers DF, Kolakofsky D (1979) Plus and minus strand leader RNAs in negative-strand virus-infected cells. Cell 18:735–748

Levin JG, Ramseur JM, Grimley PM (1973) Host effect on arbovirus replication: Appearance of defective-interfering particles in murine cells. J Virol 12:1401–1406

Logan KB (1979) Generation of defective interfering particles of Semliki Forest virus in a clone of Aedes albopictus (mosquito) cells. J Virol 30:38–44

Lundquist RE, Sullivan M, Maizel JV (1979) Characterization of a new isolate of poliovirus defective interfering particles. Cell 18:759–769

Lunger PD, Clark HF (1977) Host effect on vesicular stomatitis virus morphogenesis and "T" particle formation in reptilian, avian, and mammalian cell lines. In Vitro 11:239–246

Lynch S, Kolakofsky D (1978) Ends of the RNA within Sendai virus defective interfering nucleocapsids are not free. J Virol 28:584–589

MacDonald RD, Yamamoto T (1978) Quantitative analysis of defective interfering particles in infectious pancreatic necrosis virus preparations. Arch of Virol 57:77–89

MacDonald RD, Kennedy JC (1979) Infectious pancreatic necrosis virus persistently infects Chinook Salmon embryo cells independent of interferon. Virology 95:260–264

Marcus PI, Sekellick MJ (1977) Defective interfering particles with covalently linked (±) RNA induce interferon. Nature 266:815–819

Marcus PI, Sekellick MJ, Johnson LD, Lazzarini RA (1977) Cell killing by viruses. V. Transcribing defective interfering particles of vesicular stomatitis virus function as cell-killing particles. Virology 82:242–246

McClaren LC, Holland JJ (1974) Defective interfering particles from poliovirus vaccine and vaccine reference strains. Virology 60:549–583

McClure MA, Holland JJ, Perrault J (1980) Generation of defective interfering particles in picornaviruses. Virology 100:408–418

McGeoch DJ (1979) Structure of the gene N: gene NS intercistronic junction in the genome of vesicular stomatitis virus. Cell 17:673–681

McGeoch DJ, Dolan A (1979) Sequences of 200 nucleotides at the 3' terminus of the genome RNA of vesicular stomatitis virus. Nucleic Acids Res 6:3199–3211

McGeoch DJ, Turnbull NU (1978) Analysis of the 3' terminal nucleotide sequence of vesicular stomatitis virus N protein mRNA. Nucleic Acids Res 5:4007–4024

McGeoch DJ, Dolan A, Pringle CR (1980) Comparison of nucleotide sequences in the genomes of the New Jersey and Indiana serotypes of vesicular stomatitis virus. J Virol 33:69–77

Metzel PS, Schnitzlein WM, Reichmann ME (1978) Characterization of distinct vesicular stomatitis virus, New Jersey serotype, isolates with respect to nucleic acid homologies, interference by DI particles and protein structure. In: Mahy BWJ, Barry RD (eds) Negative strand viruses and the host cell. Academic Press, London, pp 515–526

Mills DR, Peterson RL, Spiegelman S (1967) An extracellular Darwinian experiment with a self-duplicating nucleic acid molecule. Proc Natl Acad Sci USA 58:217–224

Moyer SA, Gatchell SH (1979) Intracellular events in the replication and defective interfering particles of vesicular stomatitis virus. Virology 92:168–179

Moyer SA, Holmes KS (1981) The formation of defective interfering particles of vesicular stomatitis virus is limited by the synthesis of the G and M proteins. (personal communication)

Murphy BR, Tolpin MD, Massicot JG, Kim HY, Parrott RH, Chanock RM (1980) Escape of a highly defective influenza A virus mutant from its temperature sensitive phenotype by extragenic suppression and other types of mutation. Ann NY Acad Sci 354:172–182

Murray BK, Biswal N, Bookout JB, Lanford RE, Courtney RJ, Melnick JL (1975) Cyclic appearance of defective interfering particles of herpes simplex virus and the concomitant accumulation of early polypeptide VP 175. Intervirology 5:173–184

Nakajima K, Ueda M, Sugiura A (1979) Origin of small RNA in von Magnus particles of influenza virus. J Virol 29:1142–1148

Nayak DP (1972) Defective virus RNA synthesis and induction of incomplete influenza virus in chick embryo cells. J Gen Virol 14:63–67

Nayak DP (1980) Defective interfering influenza viruses. Ann Rev Microbiol 34:619–644

Nayak DP, Tobita K, Janda JM, David AR, De BK (1978) Homologous interference mediated by defective interfering influenza virus derived from a temperature-sensitive mutant of influenza virus. J Virol 28:375–386

Nomoto A, Jacobson A, Lee YF, Dunn J, Wimmer E (1979) Defective interfering particles of poliovirus: Mapping of the deletion and evidence that the deletions in the genomes of DI (1), (2), and (3) are located in the same region. J Mol Biol 128:179–196

Nonoyama M, Graham AF (1970) Appearance of defective virions in clones of reovirus. J Virol 6:693–694

Nonoyama M, Watanabe Y, Graham AF (1970) Defective virions of reovirus. J Virol 6:226–236

Norkin LC (1979) The emergence of simian virus 40 variants in a persistent infection of Rhesus monkey kidney cells, and their interactions with standard simian virus 40. Virology 95:598–603

Norkin LC, Wojcik JB, Groguen CA (1981) Effect of the host cell on the generation of defective simian virus 40 during undiluted serial passages and persistent infection. Virology 108:525–530

Norval M (1979) Mechanism of persistence of rubella virus in LLC-MK$_2$ cells. J Gen Virol 43:289–298

Nottay BK, Kew OM, Hatch MH, Heyward JT, Objeski JF (1981) Molecular variation of type 1 vaccine-related and wild polioviruses during replication in humans. Virology 108:405–423

O'Neill FJ, Carroll D (1981) Amplification of papovavirus defectives during serial low multiplicity infection of neural and non-neural cells. Virology, (in press)

Otsuki Y, Takebe I, Ohno T, Fukuda M, Okada Y (1977) Reconstitution of tobacco mosaic virus rods occurs bidirectionally from an internal initiation region: Demonstration by electron microscopic serology. Proc Natl Acad Sci USA 74:1913–1917

Ou J-H, Strauss EG, Strauss JH (1981) Comparative studies of the 3' terminal sequences of several alphavirus RNAs. Virology 109:281–289

Palese P (1977) The genes of influenza virus. Cell 10:1–10

Palma EL, Huang AS (1974) Cyclic production of vesicular stomatitis virus caused by defective interfering particles. J Infect Dis 129:402–410

Palma EL, Perlman SM, Huang AS (1974) Ribonucleic acid synthesis of vesicular stomatitis virus. VI. Correlation of defective particle RNA synthesis with standard RNA replication. J Mol Biol 85:127–136

Papamatheakis J, Lee TH, Thayer RE, Singer MF (1981) Recurring defective variants of simian virus 40 containing monkey DNA segments. J Virol 37:295–306

Pedersen IR (1979) Structural components and replication of arenaviruses. Adv Virus Res 24:277–330

Perrault J (1976) Cross-linked double stranded RNA from a defective vesicular stomatitis virus particle. Virology 70:360–371

Perrault J, Holland JJ (1972a) Variability of vesicular stomatitis virus autointerference with different host cells and virus serotypes. Virology 50:148–158

Perrault J, Holland JJ (1972b) Absence of transcriptase activity and transcription-inhibiting ability in defective interfering particules of vesicular stomatitis virus. Virology 50:159–170

Perrault J, Leavitt RW (1977a) Characterization of snap-back RNAs in vesicular stomatitis defective interfering virus particles. J Gen Virol 38:21–34

Perrault J, Leavitt RW (1977b) Inverted complementary terminal sequences in single-stranded RNAs and snap-back RNAs from vesicular stomatitis defective interfering virus particles. J Gen Virol 38:35–50

Perrault J, Semler BL (1979) Internal genome deletions in two distinct classes of defective inter-fering particles of vesicular stomatitis virus. Proc Natl Acad Sci USA 76:6191–6195

Perrault J, Semler BL, Leavitt RW, Holland JJ (1978) Inverted complementary terminal sequences in defective interfering particle RNAs of vesicular stomatitis virus and their possible role in autointerference. In: Mahy BWJ, Barry RD (eds) Negative strand viruses and the host cell. Academic Press, New York, pp 527–538

Petric M, Prevec L (1970) Vesicular stomatitis virus – A new interfering particle, intracellular structures, and virus-specific RNA. Virology 41:615–630

Pettersson RF (1981) 5′ Terminal nucleotide sequence of Semliki Forest virus 18S defective inter-fering RNA is heterogeneous and different from the genomic 42S RNA. Proc Nat Acid Sci USA 78:115–119

Pettersson RF, Soderlund H, Kääriäinen L (1980) The nucleotide sequence of the 5′ terminal T1 oligonucleotides of Semliki Forest virus 42S and 26S RNAs are different. Eur J Biochem 105: 435–443

Phillips BA, Lundquist RE, Maizel Jr JV (1980) Absence of subviral particles and assembly activity in HeLa cells infected with defective-interfering (DI) particles of poliovirus. Virology 100:116–124

Pons MW (1980) The genome of incomplete influenza virus. Virology 100:43–52

Potter KN, Stewart RB (1976) Comparison of vesicular stomatitis virus defective interfering particle synthesis in chick embryo and L cells. Can J Microbiol 22:1458–1463

Prevec L, Kang CY (1970) Homotypic and heterotypic interference by defective particles of vesi-cular stomatitis virus. Nature 228:25–27

Pringle CR (1977) Genetics of rhabdoviruses. Fraenkel-Conrat H, Wagner RR (eds) Comprehen-sive virology, vol 9. Plenum Press, New York, pp 239–289

Pringle CP, Cash P, Gimeney HB, Shirodaria PV (1978) Cytocidal and persistent infection of BSC-1 cells by respiratory syncytial virus. In: Mahy BWJ, Barry RD (eds) Negative strand viruses and the host cell. Academic Press, New York, pp 645–652

Ramig RF, Fields BN (1979) Revertants of ts mutants of reovirus: evidence for frequent extragenic suppression. Virology 92:155–167

Rao DD, Huang AS (1979) Synthesis of a small RNA in cells coinfected by standard and defective interfering particles of vesicular stomatitis virus. Proc Natl Acad Sci USA 76:3742–3745

Rao DD, Huang AS (1980) RNA synthesis of vesicular stomatitis virus. X. Transcription and rep-lication by defective interfering particles. J Virol 36:756–765

Ravetch JV, Horiuchi K, Zinder ND (1979) DNA sequence analysis of the defective interfering particles of bacteriophage fl. J Mol Biol 128:305–318

Reichmann ME, Schnitzlein WM (1977) Defective interfering particles of vesicular stomatitis virus. In: Schlessinger D (ed) Microbiology–1977. Am Soc Microbiol, Washington DC, pp 439–444

Reichmann ME, Schnitzlein WM (1979) Defective interfering particles of rhabdoviruses. Curr Top Microbiol Immunol 86:123–168

Reichmann ME, Schnitzlein WM (1980) Rhabdovirus defective particles: Origin and genome as-signments. In: Bishop DHL (ed) Rhabdoviruses, vol II. CRC Press, Florida, pp 189–200

Reichmann ME, Pringle CR, Follett EAC (1971) Defective particles in BHK cells infected with temperature-sensitive mutants of vesicular stomatitis virus. J Virol 8:154–160

Reichmann ME, Villarreal LP, Kohne D, Lesnaw JA, Holland JJ (1974) RNA polymerase activity and poly(A) synthesizing activity in defective T particles of vesicular stomatitis virus. Viro-logy 58:240–249

Reichmann ME, Schnitzlein WM, Bishop DHL, Lazzarini RA, Beatrice ST, Wagner RR (1978) Classification of the New Jersey serotype of vesicular stomatitis virus into two subtypes. J Virol 25:446–449

Reichmann ME, Bishop DHL, Brown F, Crick J, Holland JJ, Kang C-Y, Lazzarini R, Moyer S, Perrault J, Prevec L, Pringle CR, Wagner RR, Youngner JS, Huang AS (1980) Proposal for a uniform nomenclature for defective interfering viruses of vesicular stomatitis virus. J Virol 34:792–794

Rice CM, Strauss JH (1981) Nucleotide sequence of the 26S mRNA of Sindbis virus and deduced sequence of the encoded virus structural proteins. Proc Natl Acad Sci USA 18:2062–2066

Rima BK, Davidson WB, Martin SJ (1977) The role of defective interfering particles in persistent infection of Vero cells by measles virus. J Gen Virol 35:89–97

Robb JA, Bond CW (1979) Coronaviridae. In: Fraenkel-Conrat H, Wagner RR (eds) Comprehensive virology, vol 14. Plenum Press, New York, pp 19–237

Robinson RA, Vance RB, O'Callaghan DJ (1980) Oncogenic transformation by equine herpesviruses. II. Establishment of persistent infection and oncogenic transformation of hamster embryo cells by equine herpesvirus type 1 preparations enriched for defective interfering particles. J Virol 36:204–219

Roman JM, Simon EH (1976) Defective interfering particles in monolayer-propagated Newcastle Disease virus. Virology 69:298–303

Romanova LI, Talskaya EA, Kolesnikova MS, Agol VI (1980) Biochemical evidence for intertypic genetic recombination of polioviruses. FEBS Lett 118:109–112

Rose JK (1980) Complete intergenic and flanking gene sequences from the genome of vesicular stomatitis virus. Cell 19:415–421

Rose JK, Iverson L (1979) Nucleotide sequences from the 3′ ends of vesicular stomatitis virus mRNAs as determined from cloned DNA. J Virol 32:404–411

Rose JK, Welch WJ, Sefton BM, Esch FS, Ling NL (1980a) Vesicular stomatitis virus glycoprotein is anchored in the viral membrane by a hydrophobic domain near the COOH terminus. Proc Natl Acad Sci USA 77:3884–3888

Rose JK, Welch WJ, Sefton BM, Iverson LE (1980b) Analysis of VSV glycoprotein structure and genome structure using cloned DNA. In: Fields BN, Jaenisch R, Fox CF (eds) Animal virus genetics. ICN-UCLA Symposia on molecular and cellular biology, vol XVIII. Academic Press, New York, pp 81–93

Rosenberg M, Court D (1979) Regulatory sequences involved in the promotion and termination of RNA transcription. Ann Rev Genet 13:319–353

Rowlands DJ (1979) Sequences of vesicular stomatitis virus RNA in the region coding for the leader RNA, N protein mRNA, and their junction. Proc Natl Acad Sci USA 76:4793–4797

Rowlands D, Grabau E, Spindler K, Jones C, Semler B, Holland J (1980) Virus protein changes and RNA termini alterations evolving during persistent infection. Cell 19:871–880

Roy P, Pepik P, Hefti E, Bishop DHL (1973) Complementary RNA species isolated from vesicular stomatitis (HR strain) defective virions. J Virol 11:915–925

Schaffer FL (1979) Caliciviruses. In: Fraenkel-Conrat H, Wagner RR (eds) Comprehensive Virology, vol 13. Plenum Press, New York, pp 249–278

Schlesinger S, Weiss, B, Dohner D (1975) Defective particles in alphavirus infections. Med Biol 53:372–379

Schmaljohn C, Blair CD (1977) Persistent infection of cultured mammalian cells by Japanese encephalitis virus. J Virol 24:580–589

Schnitzlein WM, Reichmann ME (1976) The size and the cistronic origin of defective vesicular stomatitis virus particle RNAs in relation to homotypic and heterotypic interference. J Mol Biol 101:307–325

Schnitzlein WM, Reichmann ME (1977a) Interference and RNA homologies of New Jersey serotype isolates of vesicular stomatitis virus and their defective particles. Virology 77:490–500

Schnitzlein WM, Reichmann ME (1977b) A possible effect of viral proteins on the specificity of interference by defective vesicular stomatitis virus particles. Virology 80:275–288

Schnurr DS, Hardy JL (1980) Autointerference of Turlock virus in duck embryonic and Culex tarsaris cell cultures by defective interfering particles. Abstracts, Amer Soc Microb 1980, p 262

Scholtissek C (1978) The genome of the influenza virus. Curr Top Microbiol Immunol 80:139–169

Schubert M, Lazzarini RA (1981) Studies on the structure and origin of a snap back DI particle of vesicular stomatitis virus. J Virol 37:661–672

Schubert M, Keene JD, Lazzarini RA, Emerson SU (1978) The complete sequence of a unique RNA species synthesized by a DI particle of VSV. Cell 15:103–112

Schubert M, Keene JD, Lazzarini RA (1979) A specific internal RNA polymerase recognition site of VSV RNA is involved in the generation of DI particles. Cell 18:749–757

Schubert M, Keene JD, Herman RC, Lazzarini RA (1980) Site on the vesicular stomatitis virus genome specifying polyadenylation and the end of the L gene mRNA. J Virol 34:550–559

Schuerch AR, Matsuhisa T, Joklik WK (1974) Temperature-sensitive mutants of reovirus. VI. Mutant ts447 and ts556 particles that lack either one or two genome segments. Intervirology 3:36–46

Sekellick MJ, Marcus PI (1978) Persistent infection I. Interferon-inducing defective-interfering particles as mediators of cell sparing: possible role in persistent infection by vesicular stomatitis virus. Virology 85:175–186

Sekellick MJ, Marcus PI (1980) Viral interference by defective particles of vesicular stomatitis virus measured in individual cells. Virology 104:247–252

Semler BL, Holland JJ (1979) Persistent vesicular stomatitis virus infection mediates base substitutions in viral RNA termini. J Virol 32:420–428

Semler BL, Perrault J, Abelson J, Holland JJ (1978) Sequence of a RNA templated by the 3'-OH RNA terminus of defective interfering particles of vesicular stomatitis virus. Proc Natl Acad Sci USA 75:4704–4708

Semler BL, Perrault J, Holland JJ (1979) The nucleotide sequence of the 5' terminus of vesicular stomatitis virus RNA. Nucleic Acids Res 6:3923–3931

Shalitin C, Fischer I (1975) Abundant species of poly(A)-containing RNA from Saccharomyces cerevisiae. Biochim Biophys Acta 414:263–272

Shatkin AJ, Sipe JD (1968) RNA polymerase activity in purified reoviruses. Proc Natl Acad Sci 61:1462–1469

Shenk TE, Stollar V (1972) Viral RNA species in BHK-21 cells infected with Sindbis virus serially passaged at high multiplicity of infection. Biochem Biophys Res Commun 49:60–67

Simpson RW, Inuma M (1975) Recovery of infectious proviral DNA from mammalian cells infected with respiratory syncytial virus. Proc Natl Acad Sci USA 72:3233–3234

Singer MF, Rosenberg M, Rosenberg H, McCutchan T, Wakamiya T, Segal S (1978) Monkey DNA sequences in defective simian virus 40 variants. In: Stevens JG, Todaro GJ, Fox CF (eds) Persistent viruses. ICN-UCLA Symposia on molecular and cellular biology, vol XI. Academic Press, New York, pp 445–460

Soria M, Little SP, Huang AS (1974) Characterization of vesicular stomatitis virus nucleocapsids. I. Complementary 40S RNA molecules in nucleocapsids. Virology 61:270–280

Spandidos DA, Graham AF (1975) Complementation between temperature-sensitive and deletion mutants of reovirus. J Virol 16:1444–1452

Spandidos DA, Graham AF (1976) Generation of defective virus after infection of newborn rats with reovirus. J Virol 20:234–247

Spandidos DA, Krystal G, Graham AF (1976) Regulated transcription of the genomes of defective virions and temperature-sensitive mutants of reovirus. J Virol 18:7–19

Stamminger G, Lazzarini RA (1974) Analysis of the RNA of defective VSV particles. Cell 3:85–93

Stamminger GM, Lazzarini RA (1977) RNA synthesis in standard and autointerfered vesicular stomatitis virus infections. Virology 77:202–211

Stampfer M, Baltimore D, Huang AS (1969) Ribonucleic acid synthesis of vesicular stomatitis virus. I. Species of ribonucleic acid found in Chinese hamster ovary cells infected with plaque-forming and defective particles. J Virol 4:154–151

Stark C, Kennedy SIT (1978) The generation and propagation of defective-interfering particles of Semliki Forest virus in different cell types. Virology 89:285–299

Stinski MF, Mocarski ES, Thomsen DR (1979) DNA of human cytomegalovirus: size heterogeneity and defectiveness resulting from serial undiluted passage. J Virol 31:231–239

Stollar V (1979) Defective interfering particles of togaviruses. Curr Top Microbiol Immunol, vol 86: 35–66

Stollar V (1980) Defective interfering alphaviruses. In: Schlesinger RW (ed) The togaviruses, biology, structure, replication. Academic Press, New York, pp 427–455

Stollar V, Shenk TE, Koo R, Igarashi A, Schlesinger RW (1975) Observations on Aedes albopictus cell cultures persistently infected with Sindbis virus. Ann NY Acad Sci 266:214–231

Testa D, Chanda PK, Banerjee AK (1980) Unique mode of transcription in vitro by vesicular stomatitis virus. Cell 21:267–275

Tooker P, Kennedy SIT (1981) Semliki Forest virus multiplication in clones of Aedes albopictus cells. J Virol 37:589–600

Tzen JC, Somers JM, Mitchell DJ (1974) A ds-RNA analysis of suppressive sensitive mutants of "killer" Saccharomyces cerevisiae Heredity 33:132

Ueda M, Nakajima K, Sugiura A (1980) Extra RNAs of von Magnus particles of influenza virus cause reduction of particular polymerase genes. J Virol 34:1–8

Verwoerd DW, Huismans H, Erasmus BJ (1979) Orbiviruses. In: Fraenkel-Conrat H, Wagner RR (eds) Comprehensive virology, vol 14. Plenum Press, New York, pp 285–332

Villa-Komaroff L, Guttman N, Baltimore D, Lodish HF (1975) Complete translation of poliovirus RNA in a eukaryotic cell-free system. Proc Natl Acad Sci USA 72:4157–4161

Vodkin M (1977) Homology between double-stranded RNA and nuclear DNA of yeast. J Virol 21: 516–521

Vodkin M, Katterman F, Fink GR (1974) Yeast killer mutants with altered double-stranded ribonucleic acid. J Bacteriol 117:681–686

von Magnus P (1954) Incomplete forms of influenza virus. Adv Virus Res 2:59–79

Wagner RR (1975) Reproduction of rhabdoviruses. In: Fraenkel-Conrat H, Wagner RR (eds) Comprehensive virology, vol 4, Plenum Press, New York, pp 1–93

Wechsler SL, Rustigian R, Stallcup KC, Byers KB, Winston SH, Fields BN (1979) Measles virus-specified polypeptide synthesis in two persistently infected HeLa cell lines J Virol 31:677–684

Weiss B, Schlesinger S (1973) Defective interfering passages of Sindbis virus: chemical composition, biological activity, and mode of interference. J Virol 12:862–871

Weiss B, Schlesinger S (1981) Defective interfering particles of Sindbis virus do not interfere with the homologous virus obtained from persistently infected BHK cells but do interfere with Semliki Forest virus. J Virol 37:840–844

Weiss B, Goran D, Cancedda R, Schlesinger S (1974) Defective-interfering passages of Sindbis virus: Nature of the intracellular defective viral RNA. J Virol 14:1189–1198

Weiss B, Rosenthal R, Schlesinger S (1980) Establishment and maintenance of persistent infection by Sindbis virus in BHK cells. J Virol 33:463–474

Wengler G, Wengler G, Gross HJ (1979) Replicative form of Semliki Forest virus RNA contains an unpaired guanosine. Nature 282:754–756

Wickner RB, Leibowitz MJ (1977) Dominant chromosomal mutation bypassing chromosomal genes needed for killer RNA plasmid replication in yeast. Genetics 87:453–469

Wimmer E (1979) The genome-linked protein of picornaviruses: Discovery, properties and possible functions. In: Perez-Bercoff R (ed) The molecular biology of picornaviruses, Plenum Press, New York, pp 175–188

Winship TR, Thacore HR (1979) Inhibition of vesicular stomatitis virus-defective interfering particle synthesis by Shope fibroma virus. Virology 93:515–526

Youngner JS, Jones EV, Kelly M, Frielle DW (1981) Generation and amplification of temperature-sensitive mutants during serial undiluted passages of vesicular stomatitis virus. Virology 108: 87–97

Zhdanov VM (1975) Integration of viral genomes. Nature 256:471–473

Zhdanov VM, Parfanovich MI (1974) Integration of measles virus nucleic acid into the cell genome. Arch of Virol 45:225–234

Zhdanov VM, Bogomolova NN, Gavrilov VI, Andyhaparidize DG, Deryabin PG, Astakhova AN (1974) Infectious DNA of tickborne encephalitis virus. Arch of Virol 45:215–224

Zimmern D (1977) The nucleotide sequence at the origin for assembly on tobacco mosaic virus RNA. Cell 11:463–482

Subject Index

Adenoviral late mRNA   57
  polyadenylation at five sites   59
  5′-tripartite leader   57
adenovirus   51, 93, 94, 105, 107–109
  acceptor sites   53
  early regions   52
  mRNA polyadenylation   56
  splice donor sites   53
  SV 40 hybrid   8
  type 2 late genes   56
  VA RNA genes   28
alphaviruses DI RNAs   167
ATPase   18
autointerference   152

Brome mosaic virus   95, 100, 107

Cap (see translation)
cap-binding protein   106, 108
capstructure   1
capped cellular RNAs   142
  5′-end heterogeneity   142
capped fragments   138
  A cleavage   138
cellular DNA replication   18
chromatin structure   30
cloned SV 40 origin   17
  hybrid plasmid vectors   18
  pseudorevertants   17
conserved replication and encapsidation
  origins   185
  minimum sequence   186
  packaging constraints   187
  mutational drift   191
cooperative binding   12
  three sites   11
copy-back model   174, 175
  viral replicase   174
  fall-off and resumption   175
coterminal mRNA species   49

DI RNA transcriptional and translational
  activities   182

plus-strand leader RNA   182, 189
minus-strand leader RNA   183, 189
  interferon-inducing   183
  primary transcription   188
  secondary transcription   188
D2 protein   8
  electron micrographs   12
defective interfering particles   151
  occurrence in RNA viruses   153
definition of DI   154
DNA binding protein   9
  filter binding assay   11
  DNase footprinting   11
  DMS protection   11
DNA virus DI particles   194
  snap-back   194
double-strand viruses   169
  reovirus   169
  S cerevisiae   170
drosophila heat shock mRNAs   88

E1A adenoviral polypeptides   53
E1B coding sequences   53
edeine   95
enzymatic properties of T   18
error-prone RNA polymerase   174
eukaryotic genetic expression   1

Flavivirus   101
foot-and-mouth disease virus   94, 99, 105,
  109

Generation of DI RNAs   170, 171
genome rearrangements   152, 155, 177
  negative-strand viruses   156
  rhabdovirus   156
  paramyxoviruses   156
  positive-strand RNA virus   156
  double-strand RNA viruses   156
globin mRNA   92, 93, 99, 107–108

Helper virus   154

Influenza   163
    DI RNAs   164
    m RNA synthesis   126
    mRNAs   54
        NS1   54
        NS2   54
        Segment 8 RNA   55
    virus   125
inhibitors of influenza transcription   141
    secondary structures   141
    multistranded polyA. polyU   141
    polyS^{4}U   141
initiating SV 40 DNA replication   17
    deletion mapping   17
initiation codon   89
    failure to initiate at GUG   91
    redundant AUG codons   105
initiation factors (see translation)
initiator oligonucleotides   3
    RNA priming   3
    preformed 5′-ends   3
interference mechanisms   187
    replicase competition   187
    replicative advantage   187
    heterotypic interference   189
interfering properties of DI RNAs   181
    low vs. high interference cells   181
internal genome deletions   161, 162, 177
    splicing   177
    breakage and union   177
    transcriptive or replicative error   177

Large T antigen   7
    primary structure   7
    purification   7
    levels from different cells   9
    SV 80   7
    monoclonal antibodies   18
late SV 40 transcription control   16

m 7 G(5′)ppp(5′)N   1
mechanism for recombination   179, 180
mechanism of splicing   64
    signals   64
    consensus sequences   65
    components   67
    small nuclear RNAs   68
messenger RNA
    monocistronic character   96–98
    ribosome-protected fragments   85, 95,
        100, 102
    secondary structure   92, 93, 99, 107
    5′ cap (see translation)
    5′ terminal heterogeneity   84, 88, 104
    poly(A) tail, role in translation   108

differences between viral and cellular
    88, 108–109
    5′-linked protein   109
    denaturation   92, 92, 99, 103, 106–107
    fragmentation   92, 93, 94, 100
6-methyladenosine   144
methylated cap   126
    2′-O-methyl group   128
mRNA capping   2
    cap binding protein   2
    enzyme activities   2
    steps involved   2
mRNA structure   48
    translated sequences   48

Nucleus   145
    primary transcription site   146
    cellular transcription   146

Origin of DI RNAs   170
    host cell effects   170
origin of viral DNA replication   10
    BK   10
    papovaviruses   10
    polyoma   10
    T antigen binding sites   10

Papovavirus early mRNA   56
parvoviruses   63
    RNA species   63
    AAV genome   63
picornaviruses   168
    poliovirus   168
    mengovirus   168
poliovirus   97–98, 100, 105, 108, 109
poly(A) tail on mRNA
    role in translation   108
polyoma late mRNA   62
    3′-coterminal family   62
    heterogeneous 5′-terminal leader   62
polymerase II control region   33
    TATAA box   33
    5′-flanking regions   34
    conserved sequences   34
polymerase II in vivo   37
    initiation   37
    regulatory polypeptides   38
polymerase III control regions   26
polyoma   50
    early region   50
    small T antigen   50
    middle T antigen   50
    large T antigen   50
posttranscriptional processing   47
primer RNAs   127

priming, mechanism of   129
   hydrogen bonding   129
   capped ribopolymers   129
   dinucleotides   131
protein synthesis (see translation)
provirus hypothesis   173
psoralen   92

Regulation of early SV 40 transcription   13
   autoregulation   16
   in vitro system   14
   RNA polymerase II promoter   14
   run off products   14
   T antigen as repressor   13
   TATA box   14
reovirus   92–95, 100, 107–109
replication of DI RNAs   181
   host cell modulation   181
retrovirus proviral DNA   59
   mRNA species   60
   long terminal repeats   60
   5′-terminal leader   61
ribosomal RNA
   complementarity to messenger RNA
      81, 92–93
ribosome binding sites in mRNA   85
ribosomes   81
   protection of initiation sites in mRNA
      85, 95, 100, 102
RNA polymerase II   31, 126
   heterogeneous nuclear RNA   31
   initiation sites   31
   cap sites   31
   cell-free transcription   32
RNA polymerase III   26
   cell free transcription   26
RNA virus persistence   155
Rous sarcoma virus   94, 102, 104

7S ribonucleoprotein complex   30
scanning mechanism for translational
   initiation   91, 94–99
   messages in which initiation is not
      limited to first AUG   101–102
   relaxed scanning mechanism   103
semliki forest virus   101, 102
sendai   163
silkworm tRNA ala gene   30
simian virus 40   5, 92, 99, 102–104
   agnoprotein   103
   gene regulation   5
   lytic infection   5
   replication   5
   transcription   5, 36
snap-back hairpin molecules   159, 161

sparsomycin   95, 100
splice junctions   65, 67, 69, 70
spliced viral mRNA   47
   structure   47
   synthesis   47
   processing patterns   47
   leaders   47
SV 40 A gene   6
SV 40 early mRNA   48
   small T antigen   48
   large T antigen   48
SV 40 late mRNA   61
   multiple leaders   62
SV 40 transcription   36
   control regions   36
   deletion mutants   36

Terminal sequence complementarity   159
   stem molecules   159
tobacco mosaic virus   89, 95
togaviruses   165
   Sindbis   165
   Semliki Forest   165
transfer RNA, initiator species   91, 95, 107
transformation, virally induced   6
transcription in vitro   139
   cleavage   139
   initiation   139
   elongation   139
   GppppG   140
   viral cores   140
translation in eukaryotes   81–123
   initiation factors   106
   role of 5′-terminal cap   85, 92, 94, 106
   synthetic ribopolymers   91, 92, 94, 95
   efficiency   92, 99, 106–108
   differences between prokaryotes and
      eukaryotes   81, 89–91
   using prokaryotic mRNA   98
   shut-off of host protein synthesis   108–
      109

U1 RNA   68, 69
5′-untranslated leader sequences in mRNA
   82–91
   length   85, 88–89, 95, 101, 107
   composition   88–89
   (occurrence of) terminator codons   90,
      102, 103
   nucleotides flanking initiator codon   89,
      90, 92, 96, 107–108
   occurrence of introns   91
   absence of AUG codons   91, 96
   perturbations   96, 99

Vaccinia virus 109
VA-RNA 69, 70
vesicular stomatitis DI RNAs 157
    types of rearrangements 158
vesicular stomatitis virus 89, 100, 105,
    107–109
viral DNA replication 18
    mechanisms 18
    unwinding proteins 19
    cellular 53,000 dalton phosphoprotein
      19

virion-associated nuclease 131
    endonuclease 135
    cap-dependent 135
    cleavage products 135
    purines 137

Xenopus 5S RNA gene 27
    37K dalton polypeptide 27

Yeast cytochrome c mutants 93, 96, 99, 108

Of Further Interest from this Series

Volume 86
1979. 29 figures, 22 tables. III, 168 pages
ISBN 3-540-09432-6

Contents: H.L. Bishop: Genetic Potential of Bunyaviruses. – V. Stollar: Defective Interfering Particles of Togaviruses. – P. Jolicoeur: The Fv-1 Gene of the Mouse and its Control of Murine Leukemia Virus Replication. – M.E. Reichmann, W.M. Schnitzlein: Defective Interfering Particles of Rhabdoviruses.

Volume 87
1979. 24 figures, 13 tables. III, 172 pages
ISBN 3-540-09433-4

Contents: A. Graessmann, M. Graessmann, C. Müller: Simian Virus 40 and Polyoma Virus Gene Expression Explored by the Microinjection Technique. – J.M. Taylor: DNA Intermediates of Avian RNA Tumor Viruses. – P. Lebowitz, S.M. Weissmann: Organization and Transcription of the Simian Virus 40 Genome.

Volume 88
1979. 25 figures (one in color), 15 tables. III, 142 pages
ISBN 3-540-09415-6

Contents: W. Heumann: Rhizobium lupini Genetics. – R.G.Q. Leslie, M.D. Alexander: Cytophilic Antibodies. – M. Bustin: Immunological Approaches to Chromatin and Chromosome Structure and Function.

Volume 89
D. W. Weiss:
Tumor Antigenicity and Approaches to Tumor Immunotherapy
1980. IX, 83 pages
ISBN 3-540-09789-9

Contents: Tumor-Associated Antigenicity and Host Responsiveness: Basic Questions and Considerations. – Tumor Etiology and Antigenicity. – Approaches to Immunotherapy.

Volume 90
1980. 32 figures, 17 tables. III, 147 pages
ISBN 3-540-10181-0

Contents: J.H. Miller: Genetic Analysis of the lac Repressor. – H.-D. Klenk, R. Rott: Cotranslational and Posttranslational Processing of Viral Glycoproteins. – J. Rothman Scott: Immunity and Repression in Bacteriophages P1 and P7. – B. Norrild: Immunochemistry of Herpes Simplex Virus Glycoproteins. – H. Becht: Infectious Bursal Disease Virus. – D. Mergenhagen: Circadian Rhythms in Unicellular Organisms.

Volume 91
1981. Approx. 96 figures. Approx. 260 pages
ISBN 3-540-10722-3

Contents: B.N. Fields: Genetics of Reovirus. – R.L. Erikson: The Transforming Protein of Avian Sarcoma Viruses and Its Homologue in Normal Cells. – D.H. Spector: Gene-Specific Probes for Avian Retroviruses. – T. Ben-Porat: Replication of Herpes Virus DNA. – G. Wick, R. Boyd, L. de Carvalho, R.K. Cole, K. Hála, K. Kofler, P.U. Müller: The Obese Strain (OS) of Chicken with Spontaneous Autoimmune Thyroiditis: Review of the Recent Data. – H. Kleinkauf, H. von Döhren: Nucleic Acid-indepedent Synthesis of Peptides. – P.H. Krammer: The T-Cell Receptor Problem. – W.S. Hayward, B.G. Neel: Retroviral Gene Expression.

Volume 92
Natural Resistance to Tumors and Viruses
Editor: O. Haller
1981. 23 figures, approx. 28 tables. Approx. 150 pages
ISBN 3-540-10732-0

Contents: M.A. Brinton: Genetically Controlled Resistance to Flavivirus and Lactate-Dehydrogenase-Elevating Virus. – C. Lopez: Resistance to Herpes Simplex Virus-Type 1 (HSV-1). – O. Haller: Inborn Resistance of Mice to Orthomyxovirus. – J.-L. Virelizier: Role of Macrophages and Interferon in Natural Resistance to Mouse Hepatitis Virus Infection. – V. Kumar, M. Benett: Genetic Resistance to Friend Virus-Induced Erythroleukemia and Immunosuppression. – R.M. Welsh: Natural Cell-Mediated Immunity During Viral Infections. – R. Kiessling, H. Wigzell: Surveillance of Primitive Cells by Natural Killer Cells.

Springer-Verlag Berlin Heidelberg New York

Reviews of Physiology, Biochemistry and Pharmacology

Editors: R.H. Adrian, H. zur Hausen,
E. Helmreich, H. Holzer, R. Jung, O. Krayer,
R.J. Linden, P.A. Miescher, J. Piiper,
H. Rasmussen, A.E. Renold, U. Trendelenburg,
K. Ullrich, W. Vogt, A. Weber

Volume 83
1978. 45 figures, 15 tables. IV, 196 pages
ISBN 3-540-08907-1

Contents: E. M. Wright: Transport Processes in the Formation of the Cerebrospinal Fluid. – L. B. Cohen, B. M. Salzberg: Optical Measurement of Membrane Potential. – L. Glaser: Cell-Cell Adhesion Studies with Embryonal and Cultured Cells. – P. Propping: Pharmacogenetics.

Volume 84
1978. 23 figures, 2 tables. III, 240 pages
ISBN 3-540-08984-5

Contents: H. P. Godfrey, P. G. H. Gell: Cellular and Molecular Events in the Delayed-Onset Hypersensitivities. – E. Wintersberger: DNA Replication in Eukaryotes. – H. Z. Movat: The Kinin System: Its Relation to Blood Coagulation, Fibrinolysis and the Formed Elements of the Blood.

Volume 85
1979. 64 figures, 7 tables. III, 231 pages (58 pages in German).
ISBN 3-540-09225-0

Contents: M. Lindauer: Orientierung der Tiere in Raum und Zeit. – U. E. Nydegger: Biologic Properties and Detection of Immune Complexes in Animal and Human Pathology. –S. Matern, W. Gerok: Pathophysiology of the Enterohepatic Circulation of Bile Acids.

Volume 86
1979. 44 figures, 3 tables. III, 206 pages
ISBN 3-540-09488-1

Contents: P. Thorén: Role of Cardiac Vagal C-Fibers in Cardiovascular Control. – R. J. Hogg, J. P. Kokko: Renal Countercurrent Multiplication System. – P. Scheid: Mechanisms of Gas Exchange in Bird Lungs.

Volume 87
1980. 26 figures, 6 tables. V, 232 pages (8 pages in German).
ISBN 3-540-09944-1

Contents: G. Moruzzi: In Memoriam Lord Adrian. – D. E. W. Trincker: Wilhelm Steinhausen. – U. Trendelenburg: A Kinetic Analysis of the Extraneuronal Uptake and Metabolism of Catecholamines. – J. T. Fitzsimons: Angiotensin Stimulation of the Central Nervous System. – L. D. Strawser, O. Touster: The Cellular Processing of Lysosomal Enzymes and Related Proteins.

Volume 88
1981. 29 figures. V, 264 pages (23 pages in German)
ISBN 3-540-10408-9

Contents: R. Jung: Walter R. Hess 1881–1973. – K. M. Spyer: Neural Organisation and Control of the Baroreceptor Reflex. – M. Haider, E. Groll-Knapp, J. A. Ganglberger: Event-Related Slow (DC) Potentials in the Human Brain. – K. Starke: α-Adrenoceptor Subclassification.

Volume 89
1981. 39 figures. V, 254 pages
ISBN 3-540-10495-X

Contents: E. H. Heinz: Walter Wildbrandt.– P. D. Snashall, J. M. B. Hughes: Lung Water Balance. – D. D. Bikle, R. L. Morrissey, D. T. Zolock, H. H. Rasmussen: The Intestinal Response to Vitamin D. – P. E. di Prampero: Energetics of Muscular Exercise.

Volume 90
1981. 31 figures, approx. 32 tables.
Approx. 300 pages
ISBN 3-540-10657-X

Contents: K. Decker: Feodor Lynen (1911–1979) – A. B. Borle: Control, Modulation, and Regulation of Cell Calcium – Z. S. Agus, S. Goldfarb, A. Wasserstein: Calcium Transport in the Kidney – M. E. Schlaefke: Central Chemosensitivity: A Respiratory Drive

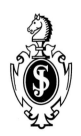

Springer-Verlag
Berlin
Heidelberg
NewYork